THE
SUNFOOD DIET
SUCCESS SYSTEM

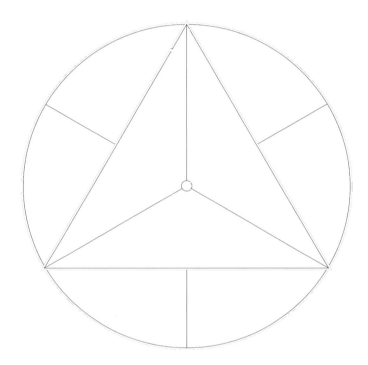

DAVID WOLFE

North Atlantic Books
Berkeley, California

This book contains little-known truths regarding the human body's amazing secrets.

A Note To The Reader: Each lesson in this book contains facts, concepts, and ideas that build upon the lessons before it. Therefore, on the first time through, we urge the reader to avoid skipping around. The reading will surely prove most fruitful if you begin at the Table of Contents and read straight through. It is our desire that a thousand years hence the contents of this book will be as up-to-date as at this moment. A lifestyle based on the cosmic laws is always in order and never becomes obsolete.

Unless otherwise noted, all poems are the author's work.

Published by North Atlantic Books, P.O. Box 12327, Berkeley, California 94712

North Atlantic Books' publications are available through most bookstores. For further information, call 800-733-3000 or visit our website at www.northatlanticbooks.com.

The Sunfood Diet Success System is sponsored by the Society for the Study of Native Arts and Sciences, a nonprofit educational corporation whose goals are to develop an educational and cross-cultural perspective linking various scientific, social, and artistic fields; to nurture a holistic view of arts, sciences, humanities, and healing; and to publish and distribute literature on the relationship of mind, body, and nature.

ISBN 978-1-55643-749-6

First Edition: April 1, 1999
Second Edition: January 1, 2000
Third Edition: October 1, 2000
Fourth Edition: October 1, 2001
Fifth Edition: October 1, 2002
Sixth Edition: April 1, 2006
Seventh Edition: March 1, 2008
Eighth Edition: December 1, 2009
10-Year Anniversary Edition: March 1, 2012

Outside Cover Art: JAVIER MICHALSKI AND AMY GAYHEART
Interior Color Art: JAVIER MICHALSKI, AMY GAYHEART, DAVID WOLFE
Total Book Design and Text Layout: DAVID WOLFE

Printed in the United States of America

Environmental Certificate
Printed on 70# Utopia II Recycled stock.
Compared to standard 70# coated white stock, Utopia II saves:

Trees: 24	Water: 11,081 gallons
Energy: 9.9 million BTUs	Solid Waste: 702 pounds
Greenhouse Gases: 17,921 pounds CO2 equivalent	

Environmental impact estimates were made using the Environmental Paper Network Paper Calculator: http://www.environmentalpaper.org

"The philosophy and teachings of **The Sunfood Diet Success System** are terrific. The foundational law is the key understanding of this book: 'one thing does lead to another.' David Wolfe, in a beautifully authentic way, plants the awareness of the power of a live-food diet and healthy thinking that is transforming to each individual and to the very planet itself. I will be highly recommending this book to all at the Tree Of Life Rejuvenation Center." – Gabriel Cousens M.D. (H) author of **Conscious Eating, Rainbow Green Live-Food Cuisine, Spiritual Nutrition**

"This breakthrough book not only demonstrates a profound understanding of Nature's physical laws of health-building, but also masterfully integrates the under-recognized motivational, mental, and emotional components needed to create overall success in life. A unique contribution to the field and I highly recommend it to all success seekers." – Viktoras Kulvinskas MS, author of **Survival Into The 21st Century**

"Just as a fragrant tropical mango, glistening in the Sun, is an open invitation to eat it, reading **The Sunfood Diet Success System** is an open invitation to live it. Written by one who clearly does, this book is an inspiring synthesis of life-proven success technologies and the author's understanding of Nature's unchanging laws." – Eliot Jay Rosen, author of Los Angeles Times bestselling book **Experiencing The Soul**

"David Wolfe has synergized a first class methodology for transitioning to and attaining limitless health and success on every level. With unyielding courage and compassion, David has removed the veils, pitfalls, and obstacles which keep us from achieving our full potential. He shares the simple, yet profound, truth of eating naturally. Put this book to work for you right now and start enjoying the results immediately. Sunfood is funfood!" – Jason Aberbach, Tucson, Arizona

"The only thing I can say is: what are we going to do with all the other books we've been selling?! This book is amazing. It encompasses the entire field of raw foods. It answers every question." – Barbara Rogers, herbalist, owner of **Simply Divine Botanicals**, Las Vegas, Nevada

"Reading your book was like eating a fresh, ripe durian for the first time. At first you don't know what it is, but you know in some profound way it is really good! It starts to strike some familiarity with you but you can't place a finger on it. Maybe you had it when you were a little kid? No, you definitely would have remembered it if you had. Then suddenly, it hits you! You start realizing that in some mysterious way it is awakening past life memories! You had the knowledge and experience of the durian in a past life and now this powerful, aromatic, sweet, rich fruit has brought that knowledge and experience to your consciousness once again! You knew it all along, it was just locked up inside of you, and that first bite was the key that opened the door. David, this is your book!" – Steve Adler, founder of www.sacredchocolate.com, Fairfax, California

Books, Programs, and Music by David Wolfe:

BOOKS

The Sunfood Diet Success System

Superfoods: The Food and Medicine of the Future

Eating For Beauty

Naked Chocolate
(with Shazzie)

Amazing Grace
(with Nick Good)

Chaga: King of the Medicinal Mushrooms

PROGRAMS

The LongevityNOW Program

MUSIC

The Healing Waters Band

David Wolfe is the drummer for The Healing Waters Band

This Cooked Planet
(10 songs, 60 minutes of music, released February 2004)

All Is One
(12 songs, 70 minutes of music, released February 2006)

DAVID WOLFE WEBSITES

www.davidwolfe.com

www.thebestdayever.com

www.ftpf.org

www.LongevityWarehouse.com

www.rawnutritioncertification.com

This book is dedicated to my Aunt Dee-Dee.

You knew. You always believed. Thank you.

ACKNOWLEDGMENTS

No one ever goes it alone. I thank every courageous person who helped to create this book and all those who have sought out this information, acted upon it, and informed others of the extraordinary possibilities that surround us always. Thank you. You deserve the highest praise.

A special thank you goes out to everyone who has engaged the world with a positive mental attitude and who has nourished love in their heart.

May freedom reign.

TABLE OF CONTENTS

A WORD FROM THE AUTHOR

The Age of Information is surrounding us, embracing us. Through the fantastic information available to all of us through the Internet, libraries and transformed individuals we now have the ability to create a whole new paradigm of health, wealth, happiness, success, prosperity and possibility!

It is my goal, in this book, to bring you up to speed on key transformational technologies, especially in the area of nutrition, now available to us all.

Throughout these pages we are going to participate together in an opening of opportunities that everywhere surround us.

The material contained here is designed for all people, whether you are healthy, sick, searching, curious, looking for the next level and/or seeking success physically and spiritually.

I cannot express how excited I am to present this information to all those interested in personal development and self-improvement. By availing yourself of this information you fulfill your destiny and simultaneously help fulfill my destiny of bringing **The Sunfood Diet Success System** to the world.

How I came to write this book is an interesting story. Both of my parents are medical doctors. My father had a general practice, then became an osteopath over his 35-year career. My mother was trained as an anesthesiologist. As a child, I spent a lot of time at my parents' office. I used to play with my brothers beneath the chairs in the waiting room. I even used to travel with my dad on house calls.

I have observed the inside of the medical profession with a unique perspective. What I noticed was that people, over the long term, did not get better taking medicine. Instead, they got worse. When I was about ten years old (probably younger), I decided I was not going to take medicine anymore for any reason. And though I fought with my mother over this for many years, I did not submit.

What I noticed was that when my two brothers and I would get sick, I would only be sick for one or two days, while their flus or colds would drag on for four or five days with the medicine. I learned then to just rest and drink only freshly-squeezed orange juice all day and soon I would feel better. That was a major revelation to me at that age and set me on a path that would markedly transform my destiny.

In my late teens I found that I was reacting to certain foods. I finally narrowed it down to dairy products. So, without really knowing anything about nutrition at that time, I cut out dairy products completely. I immediately lost 10 pounds (4.5 kilograms) and felt amazingly better! I soon reached a point where I would not eat any food that contained any dairy products whatsoever — even if it was the tenth ingredient.

It was the discipline of completely letting go of all dairy products which set up a "blueprint" for more dietary progress. Therein I learned a valuable lesson: all disciplines affect each other. A powerful discipline can transfer over from one area of your life to any other area.

Fortunately, I had been turned on to self-help, personal development and spiritual literature at the age of 14 and somehow was graced to have an insight that reading could help unveil the magic in the universe.

After letting go of all dairy products, I started to read every book and listen to every audio tape in the field of nutrition that we had in my house. I quickly found the book **Fit For Life** by Marilyn and Harvey Diamond that confirmed what I knew about the danger of pasteurized dairy products. I adopted the Fit For Life Diet and gradually moved over to a vegan diet by eliminating animal products from my life (the vegan lifestyle contains no animal foods or products which impact animal lives).

But I kept reading, I kept searching. All of my life I could not escape the feeling that I was missing something, overlooking something so obvious it had managed to escape me. Ever since the earliest days I could remember, I had a sense that I would one day stumble onto some great secret. Obviousness seemed to be the key, like the ancient allegory of the gods on Mount Olympus:

When the world was new, the gods on Mount Olympus enriched the Earth with the animals, the creatures of the sea, the plants, and all living things. After many eons of time, the gods at last looked upon those curious humans tampering with the forests and gardens of the world. They decided they would hide the Secret of Life until humans had grown and evolved in consciousness to the point where they would be ready for it.

The gods on Mount Olympus argued about where the Secret of Life should be hidden.

One said, "Let us hide it high upon the tallest mountain, they shall never find it there."

A goddess replied, "Humans have insatiable curiosity and ambition. They will eventually climb the tallest mountain."

Then another goddess suggested, "We should hide the Secret of Life at the bottom of the deepest ocean."

"You don't understand," said a god, "Humanity has a boundless imagination and a potent desire to explore the world. Sooner or later they will reach even the greatest ocean depths."

Finally, a goddess came up with a solution, "Let us hide the Secret of Life in the last place humans would ever look. A place they will only come to when they have exhausted all other possibilities and are finally ready."

"And where is the that?" asked the gods.

To which the goddess replied, "We will not hide it at all."

Through reading I found out about raw-food nutrition. When I first discovered that one could live primarily on raw plant food, it was a revelation to me. It resonated with my core — it sent chills throughout my body. Within three months of eating raw foods, I knew I had found a great key that could open and create many doors. I felt as if a great secret of the ages had been revealed. For me, it was an Earth-trembling discovery. I knew this was the way for me to achieve my maximum potential. I knew instantaneously that it was a major part of my mission in this life to bring this message to the world. I knew in that sparkling moment that I could and would revolutionize the personal-development world with this information. I saw massive potential. Within three words — raw plant food — is a major key to unlocking humanity's dormant powers.

I quickly found that this wonderful truth was not so evident to other people. And again I learned a great lesson. The greatest truths of the world, the ones which have shaken civilizations to their core, always appear insignificant to many other observers. But to the discoverer, the philosopher, that truth is priceless. To the one who has acted upon that truth and taken a new vantage, everything is clear and obvious. Through experience, a guess becomes knowledge, speculation becomes certainty. Part of the true world reveals itself and that in itself is a revelation.

I found out that just knowing to eat raw plant foods is not enough: variety is critical, peer pressure steps in, breaking addictions plays a role, the proper mindset is important, detoxification is a factor, as are emotions and balance. After many years of experimenting, reading and communicating with thousands of others on this path of eating raw plant foods, I finally perfected what I call **The Sunfood Diet Success System** and wrote the first edition of this book. That was in the summer and autumn of 1998.

The release of **The Sunfood Diet Success System** radically transformed my life. Book and lecture tours followed in early 1999 and continued unabated for years. The book attracted absolutely amazing people, events and circumstances. So many beautiful moments filled my days. Profound teachings found my ears and advanced my health education in exceptional ways. Extraordinary foods were laid before me. Adventures abounded in exotic locations all over the world. I feel so graced and fortunate for all these awesome gifts — all brought by this book!

As you read through these pages, my hope is that you find yourself discovering the tremendous importance of this message for the future of the world; this information allows the Earth to heal and prosper. You may find new wonder and hope. You may perceive that your life can be transformed in a most profound way.

At this moment I am overcome with the emotion of gratitude for having reached the level of health I have been blessed to experience and for having the opportunity to present this health information to you. Thank you for choosing this book. I invite you as a guest into a new realm of possibility. I wish you the greatest prosperity.

Have The Best Day Ever!

DAVID "Avocado" WOLFE
Hawaii
April 2011

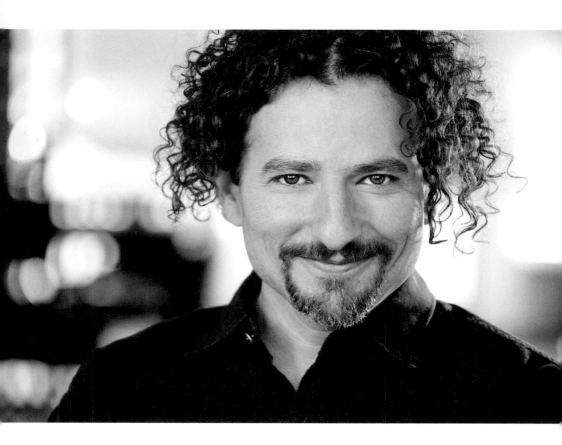

INTRODUCTION

The Sunfood Diet is the promise that we can become something more — that there is a better way to live. You can be totally rejuvenated. You can walk the Earth barefoot again as you did as a child, feeling the blades of grass beneath your feet, touching the flower petals, chasing the butterflies, watching the ants, thinking clearly and calmly.

Within you is a power which will astonish you. Within you are the seeds of greatness, of beauty, of discipline, of excellence, of destiny. This is the last moment of the way you used to be. It is time to give yourself permission to reach the absolutely highest possible state of health.

What good are all the possessions in the world if you do not have your health? What good are material experiences if you do not have the intense vibrancy to enjoy them?

The Sunfood Diet is the product of a new will-to-health, a new will-to-life, arising from ashen foods like a phoenix all over the world. The Sunfood Diet identifies those foods that allow the body to work to its maximum potential. The Sunfood lifestyle teaches that robust health is the natural state; inspired energy is our natural birthright. It demonstrates how to purify your physical body and unlock the key to your maximum potential.

Sunfoods beautify the body, mind and spirit. They carry with them the vitality of health and life — the vibrant Sun energy that nourishes all life on Earth. By taking in the energy of vibrant Sunfoods you can overcome any health challenge. The Sun is a transformer. By eating Sunfoods you can improve your life in every way. When your health improves, every other aspect of your life improves simultaneously.

To strive for health, wealth, happiness and success is as natural to your creative urges as it is natural for a tree to strive for its maximum fulfillment. In

Nature, there are no limits to what you can have, be or do. You deserve to reach the highest goal possible: vibrant happiness.

This book, **The Sunfood Diet Success System**, is first and foremost a philosophy. It is a study of secret fundamental things that are not part of everyday conversation. This message is about getting close to Nature and natural laws. It is the idea that people living close to Nature tend to be noble. Living close to Nature is the greatest wonder we can experience for our spiritual, emotional, mental and physical health. The more natural we are, the healthier and happier we are (and there is no limit as to how healthy and happy we can become!).

Many books are filled with words about words, they are filled with researched research; the authors themselves have not experienced what they are writing about. What I teach is based on real-life experience. I have discovered powerful distinctions we can use immediately to dramatically improve our health today.

If you are tired of the crumbs and ashes of life, if a mediocre existence has become a burden upon you, then take this book to heart and read it deeply. For within these pages is a distillation of many wonderful principles of life transformation. These pages invite you to open your spirit to the full abundance life offers the seeker.

This is an abundant universe. Grasp your birthright. Success is a massive abundance of physical, mental, emotional and spiritual health.

The divine power within you is the healing and creative power in your life. As long as you have a single spark of vitality within you, there is great hope. You are a physical, mental, emotional and spiritual being capable of achieving incredible prosperity at all levels. You are priceless. Treat your body better than a Rolls Royce. No technology will ever surpass the magnificence of your own biological design.

The real lesson here is that you are in control of your destiny. The apple never falls far from the tree. If you do not like the health you are experiencing, you can change it! If you do not like the video being played across your mind, you can change it! If you do not enjoy the food you are eating, you can change it! You feel positive about yourself to the degree you feel you are in control of your life. You feel negative about yourself to the degree you feel you are not in control of your life. When you feel out of control, you experience stress, fear and psycho-somatic illness. Overcome negativity by understanding that you are always in control. No one outside of you controls how you feel; you are responsible. I congratulate you, because by reading this book, you have made the decision to take control; you have already begun to achieve vibrant health.

All books are not created equal. Of what account is a book that does not carry us away beyond all books? We learn in order to acquire distinctions: little clues which improve the value of our lives. Each distinction becomes a fresh new opportunity. Tune into the information that contains the most distinctions. The best books contain a maximum amount of distinctions we can use immediately to produce incredible results now.

The most successful people in life have the best information. Through my businesses and organizations I have been privy to some of the best personal-development information available. In our company library, we have some of the best, rarest and most exclusive self-help information resources, gathered from around the world. Information drawn from these resources is contained herein. In fact, all the greatest transformative lessons I have ever encountered are planted here within these pages. The distinctions provided in this book have been proven by real-life testing. My own experience has made me a science project for these facts. Intense research has unlocked health secrets that can only be called "magical."

Nothing succeeds like success, and there is no better proof of something's worthiness than good results. The success, joy and exuberance for life I enjoy each moment is proof-positive of the incredible power of the concepts in this book.

Stop listening to anyone, in any field, who is not getting the results that you desire. Stop. Read that sentence three times in a row. Would you go to a beggar for financial advice? Only listen to those who are getting the results you desire in any given area of life. I have achieved an extraordinary aliveness, and I will show you how you can achieve it too by the lessons provided within these pages.

The information within this book is meant for you to not only read, but to study and act upon. Expect the maximum possible value from each page. As you read, see, listen and feel this message. Highlight your favorite passages. Take notes. Specifically: first read the book through entirely; second, read each chapter twice (before moving on to the next chapter) and highlight your favorite passages; third, immediately act upon the information by using the action steps provided at the end of each lesson; fourth, purchase and use a journal with which to record your progress.

The content of this book is revolutionary in scope. Any given person can begin to function at extraordinary levels once they have realized in which way lies their true line of progress. That line of progress is internal purification through the application of a success system — a methodology to achieving goals. Internal purification allows one to begin remembering how the mind and heart work together and how to use that knowledge to achieve superior health. A wise adage states, "All this struggling to learn, when all we have to do is remember." All the wisdom we require is already within us.

To direct this planet into a new era of massive prosperity, we are going to require a new level of physical health. A healthy body allows us to access the dormant areas of our nervous system. We access those areas through internal purification, positive thinking, spiritual connection and by activating the glands (including the "spiritual" pineal gland, located in the mid-brain). When our nervous system is clear of toxicity, we can receive clear information and then take action.

This is powerful information. The Sunfood Diet creates a whole new paradigm of possibility. Many, many people I have met have searched throughout the personal development, self-help genre of literature for a book on living foods and success. Many of the success philosophers of the newest age have missed this vital link. Only a few books hint of the connection, Anthony Robbins' **Unlimited Power** (Chapter X) is the foremost example, which comes to mind. In his book, Robbins describes that a successful individual must be fueled by a healthy diet. The connection between success and diet is absolutely crucial.

The time has come to bring this diet information to the personal-development audience. I have tapped a magic power and I will show you how you can too. And so, I present to you the dietary approach to self-mastery and massive abundance:

The Sunfood Diet Success System
or
Living Foods and Life Transformation
or
How To Unlock Your Magical Powers

This book can show you how to achieve perfect health and perfect digestion as I have done. In the following 36 lessons are many seeds that you may nourish to discover a new destiny. This book is not only about nutrition; it is about a complete health transformation that begins with the proper frame of mind. I invite you to grasp the distinctions provided in these pages. Swallow this elixir of knowledge and experience the true beauty of living!

All confusion fades once the facts are known...

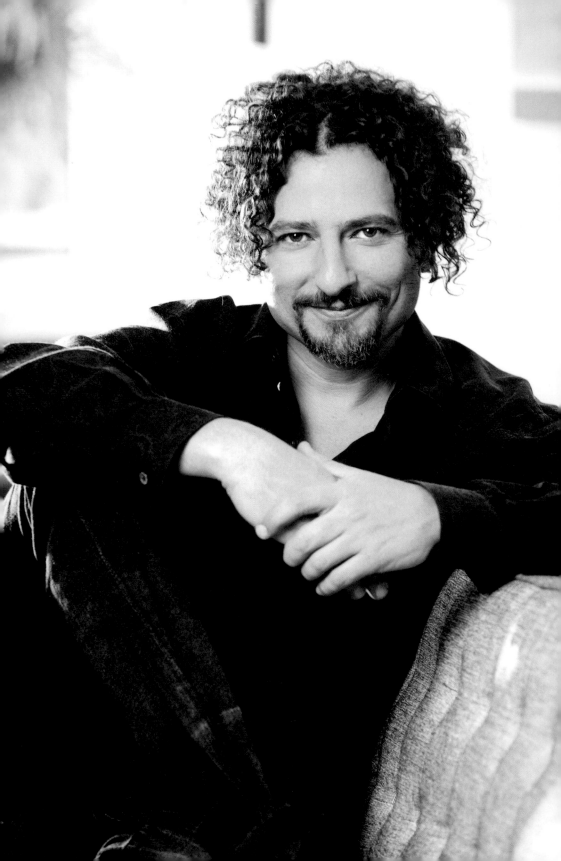

THE PRINCIPLE OF LIFE TRANSFORMATION

"In order to have something,
you must first be something." — Goethe

"The outer situation is always a reflection of
the collective inner situation." — Peace Pilgrim

You are not what you are, rather, what you are, is what you can be. The most interesting thing about life is that you can become more than you were before. You can become stronger, wiser, healthier than you ever dreamed possible. You can achieve your true potential. You can completely re-form your physical structure, your intelligence, your emotional poise, your spiritual power. This book is about how to biologically transmutate the lead of life into the white gold of glory.

The Principle of Life Transformation is that life change comes from the inside out. All transformation begins with one person — you. As above, so below. Everything happening around you is only a reflection of what is going on inside you. If you want the world to change, you have to change.

We are all personally responsible for the state of the entire world because the world only mirrors our inner selves. Pollution, famine, and disease are reflective of the inner crisis gripping us individually, and therefore collectively. These "realities" are fragments of our collective consciousness projected outward upon our environment.

Your idea of the world (what you believe the world is) manifests everything in your life. When you change your idea of the world, the world itself changes. Essentially, your mission is not to set the world right, but simply to set yourself right. Then, and only then, will the world begin to be set right. I tell my seminar listeners: "The world does not change — we change."

Life transformation is an inner journey. To succeed in life you have to work harder. But not on your family, or on your friends, or on your job, or on whatever comes your way. You have to work harder on yourself first.

Your own happiness is your number one priority. Many have the idea that they have to undergo a process of stress and pain in order to provide for themselves and their families. They do so with the idea that at some future date they will all be happy. If this is you, please understand that you cannot make anyone else happy by being unhappy yourself. Only happy people make others happy. Instead of achieving to be happy, happily achieve.

When we strive to become better ourselves, everything around us becomes better too. The environment we live in will become better or worse depending on whether we become better or worse. The people we associate with will become better or worse depending on whether we become better or worse. You automatically achieve improved results, when you become an improved person.

It seems the whole works of humankind are backwards. Most are trying to convince, instruct, and purify everyone else — without first purifying themselves. To enlighten others we have to enlighten ourselves.

The best way to make others healthy is to become incredibly healthy yourself!

Health is not something we can get; rather, it is something we attract by the person we become. If we chase after health, it will elude us like a butterfly. However, if we calmly attract health by becoming the type of person who can be radiantly healthy, it will land upon us with a most radiant flutter.

Once we understand that life change comes from the inside out, and that it is in becoming something new that we achieve something new, then we decide to take full responsibility for our lives. The success philosopher Earl Nightingale expressed this understanding when he said: "All of us are self-made, but only the successful will admit it."

You will make incredible progress in your life when you accept 100% responsibility for everything that happens to you. You are where you are and who you are because of one person — yourself.

Take full responsibility for everything that happens in your life. As the saying goes: "When you point your finger at someone, you have three fingers pointing back at you." People accuse others of what they themselves are guilty of.

Winners take full responsibility for everything that happens to them — even when those things seem remote and are not directly attributable to their actions. Taking 100% responsibility for everything in your life transforms you into a new type of person because it forces you to research all "effects" back to their "causes." Understanding "causes" is the science of life transformation.

Our focus here in this book is vibrant, superior health. If you are suffering from ill health, there is only one person responsible — yourself. Blaming others will not empower you. Concepts such as the germ/bad luck theory are the end products of efforts to put the blame of ill health on someone or something outside of oneself — to remove responsibility from the individual. To achieve our goal of superior health, we must take 100% responsibility.

THE PRINCIPLE OF LIFE TRANSFORMATION

1 Purchase and begin writing in a journal to record your progress through this book and beyond. Success philosopher Anthony Robbins says: "If your life is worth living, it is worth recording." Write down your wonderful thoughts. Begin now to descr be your health transformation. Release worries, doubts, and fears by writing them down. What an amazing gift your journals can be to your children and their children — they can learn from you and feel a connection with you even when you are gone!

2 The first day you begin this book, take a "before" picture.

3 Instead of trying to remedy everything "out there," decide now to turn your focus inward to beautify your physical, mental, emotional and spiritual potential. Write down the answer to the following questions in your journal: "What type of person do I have to become to experience radiant health?" "How do I become that type of person as quickly as possible while enjoying the process?"

4 Say to yourself daily: "I am fully responsible for my own great health. My daily habits create my great health." Write this affirmation on the first page of your journal and on your bathroom mirror.

"CORRECTING ONESELF IS CORRECTING THE WHOLE WORLD.
THE SUN IS SIMPLY BRIGHT. IT DOES NOT CORRECT ANYONE.
BECAUSE IT SHINES, THE WHOLE WORLD IS FULL OF LIGHT.
TRANSFORMING YOURSELF IS A MEANS OF GIVING LIGHT
TO THE WHOLE WORLD." — *Ramana Maharshi*

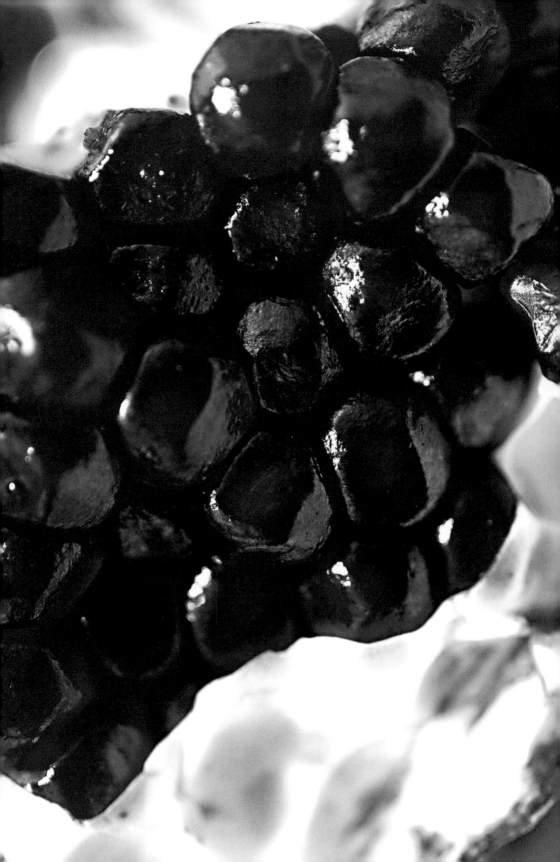

2

THE FOUNDATIONAL LAW

There is a law that was decreed during the foundation of the world. It is the law upon which all things are based. It is immortal and true, even for the few. The law is that things produce after their own kind. It is the primal law of cause and effect: the Law of Production. "As ye sow, so shall ye reap" (Galatians 6:7). Those seeds planted must return to us their kind — in abundance. This law knows no exception. The Law of Production does not bend for anyone.

The profound truth is: one thing does lead to another.

Excellent food choices lead to more excellent food choices. Excellent habits create a fertile ground for more excellent habits. Excellent decisions lead to more excellent decisions.

If you sow that which is beneficial to all, you will receive that which is beneficial to you. If you sow compassion for all animals, you will receive the compassion of all animals. If you sow beautiful living, you will receive a beautiful life. We have the choice as to what vibrations we send out into the cosmos.

Once the seeds are planted they sprout and grow into realities. They produce after their own kind and, with concentration and emotion, spread prolifically.

In **The Dispersion Of Seeds**, Henry David Thoreau wrote: "Though I do not believe that a plant will spring up where no seed has been, I have great faith in a seed. Convince me that you have a seed there, and I am prepared to expect wonders."

Seeds are karmic substances; they have a potential, a destiny. "The seed is the word of God" (Luke 8:11). If you wish to reap a different destiny in any area of your life in the future, you need to plant new, different seeds today. Seeds grow into plants, and plants grow fruits, and the fruits spread more seeds.

The most fertile soil in the world is found in the human mind. No matter what one desires, it is not until the idea-seeds are planted in the garden-mind with nurturing emotion that they will come forth. To get a high quality of change, we must choose the highest quality seeds and provide them with an abundance of carefully selected nutrients. Those idea—seeds tended with the greatest emotion will grow fastest and most abundant, perhaps even crowding out or overcoming weaker seeds. Strong emotion gives nourishment to thought seeds. Strong emotion sets seeds into vibration.

When you have an emotional thought, whether that thought is positive or negative, it will begin to materialize in your life. That is why it is so important to keep your mind focused with emotion on the things you desire, and off the things you fear. When the emotional desire for a thing is so intense that it illuminates every fiber of your being, then it shall be fulfilled.

As long as one nurtures the seeds of joy, achievement and destiny, these things shall follow in abundance; however, if the poisonous prickly weeds of doubt and fear are allowed to take possession of the garden, they too shall follow. Poisonous prickly weeds grown in the garden-mind lead to negativity, hopelessness, inferiority complexes and mental illness.

Growth, maturity, and reproduction are patterns in Nature. Planting demonstrates how things produce after their kind — it is the Law of Production in action. Use this knowledge now to begin cultivating within your garden-mind the seeds of exceptional health.

THE FOUNDATIONAL LAW

1 Daily, as you arise, and also before you sleep, picture yourself in perfect health, happiness and harmony. Picture yourself radiantly alive. Hold this picture with emotional desire in your conscious mind for 30 unbroken seconds. This will plant a seed. By consistent focus this seed will grow. The power and effervescence of superior health, happiness and harmony will eventually come forth.

2 Begin to trace health challenges (effects), whether they be addictions, illnesses, etc., to their "causes." Record the answer to the following question in your journal: "What is the true cause of my foremost health challenge?"

THE LAW OF PRODUCTION

The Law of our Fate
We choose our wealth.
Love brings love,
Health brings health.

Like produces like,
An effect resembles its cause.
Things produce after their kind,
It's one of the basic laws.

A smile brings a smile,
Peace brings peace;
And never will
This spiral cease.

As you sow,
So shall you reap.
Carefully choose
Which seeds you keep.

Abundant seeds
In the soil spread.
Fertile plants
Will grow when fed.

Things do follow
After their type.
You'll reap your crop
When the time is ripe.

For a future is found
In every seed.
It's "cause and effect"
...with godspeed.

The Law of Production,
The subtleness of mind;
Success breeds success:
Each creates its kind.

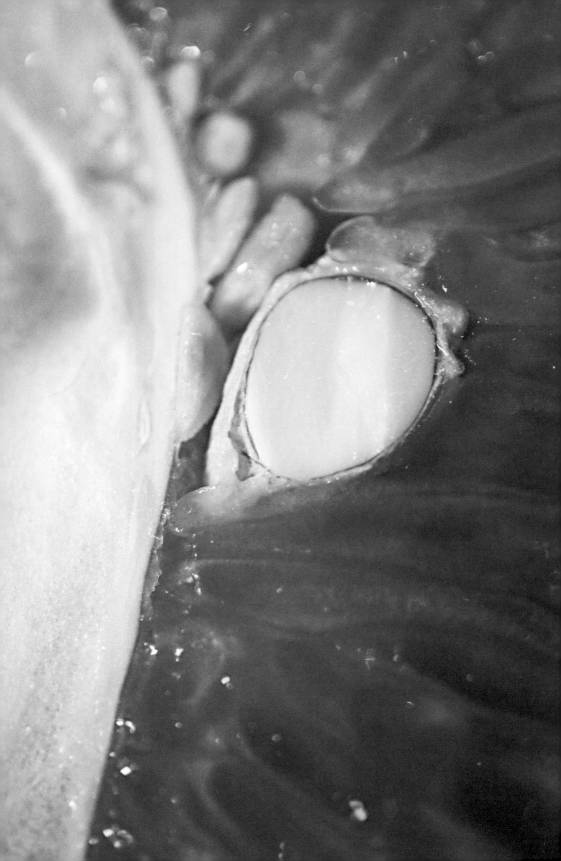

THOUGHTS ARE THINGS

"ALL DESTINY BEGINS WITH THINKING."
— *Percival*

"THE ANCESTOR OF EVERY ACTION IS A THOUGHT."
— *Ralph Waldo Emerson*

"WHEN ANY OBJECT OR PURPOSE IS CLEARLY HELD IN THOUGHT,
ITS PRECIPITATION, IN TANGIBLE AND VISIBLE FORM IS
MERELY A QUESTION OF TIME. THE VISION ALWAYS PRECEDES
AND ITSELF DETERMINES THE REALIZATION."
— *Lillian Whiting*

"WE BECOME WHAT WE THINK ABOUT."
— *Earl Nightingale*

You are not what you think you are, rather, what you think, you are.

Thoughts are things. Thoughts are seeds. Everything you do or think is a cause set in motion. Every thought sent fcrth is a never-ending vibration spiraling its way across the universe and returning to us what we have sent with interest.

Thoughts are energy. Energy pulsates; it sends ripples into the fabric of time and space, affecting all things.

Thoughts objectify themselves. Thoughts turn themselves into physical "objects." You magnetize into your life whatever you hold in your thought. The more often you think about something, the more quickly it will appear in your reality.

Thoughts are the foundation of everything you become. Everything you have in your life right now was once a thought in your mind. Thoughts shape your being and character. Everything, which happens to you, which you attract into your life, is a product of your thinking. This means you are 100% responsible for your life and death, and nothing outside of you can bring illness upon you.

Thoughts are felt. Negative thoughts produce acid throughout the entire tissue system. Thoughts of envy, jealousy, fear and resentment send waves of retentiveness and tension throughout the body. Those with a tendency to hoard typically suffer from constipation. Thoughts are things; they have a physical component.

Your subconscious mind cannot tell the difference between an emotional thought and an actual event. Your body reacts to an emotional visualization just as if the event actually happened! Do you remember times when you thought of something so intensely that your body tensed or relaxed as if you were actually there in the event again? Notice what changed...only your thoughts. Yet, you physically felt different by thinking stressful thoughts.

People who live with stressful thoughts are apt to become ill. Anxiety quickly weakens the whole body. Negative thoughts alone can create havoc throughout the entire nervous system. However, strong, pure and happy thoughts build fortitude and beauty. The natural body is a sensitive, finely-tuned instrument that responds readily to the thoughts it is repeatedly presented. Habits of thought will produce their own effects (good or bad) upon the body.

We must aim to nourish a youthful spirit that can never die. Youth is not a time of life, but a quality, a trait of character, a state of mind. Thoughts of fear, pain and grief age the body. On the other hand, thoughts of joy, beauty and triumph enliven the body. Positive thinking will do wonders and help keep us young.

What the mind thinks, the body expresses. You have the potential of having the body you want. The power of thought (through the aid of the subconscious mind) has control over every cell of the body. You can restructure and rejuvenate your body by rethinking yourself, by grasping on to a healthier vision of yourself. Send down a different body plan to your subconscious mind. With consistency, your body and experience will follow suit.

As a child, you come into the world unafraid and limitless, able to express yourself freely and naturally. Youthful freedom and joy are still with you in your mind. When you choose freedom and joy, you automatically have them!

Your mind is your first-mover. All actions, results, and forthcoming realities we experience in our lives begin with creations in our minds. All these "effects" are derivatives of thought causes. Your life's conditions are the effects of those thought causes.

The "heads I win, tails you lose" scenario is always of one's own making. The prisons people find themselves in are always first in their minds.

You are a creator of circumstance, never a victim of circumstance. There is no such thing as a coincidence. You are at the cause of all effects. We live in an orderly universe governed by definite laws. Everything happens for a reason. You have something positive to learn from each experience. To reach spiritual fulfillment, first you must understand this law.

"Where your thinking is, there too, is your experience" and "As a man thinketh in his heart, so is he" (Proverbs 23:7) are two wise sayings. Successful individuals become successful because they acquire the habit of thinking in terms of success. If you think successful thoughts, you will achieve success. If you think healthy thoughts, you will become healthy. Being healthy is a function of thinking healthy thoughts. Sound physical health begins with a "health consciousness" produced by a mind that thinks in terms of prosperity and dismisses all thoughts of illness and negativity. Empowering thoughts lead to wholesome patterns of behavior. Physical illnesses are essentially psychological in origin in the respect that if the mind is thinking unhealthy thoughts this leads to unhealthy actions which leads to an unhealthy diet and lifestyle.

It is your own habits of thinking which give you mastery in any field of achievement. Thought seeds procuce after their own kind; it is a simple law. The way you think about things determines your level of success in any given area. One cannot think of failure, and then succeed. One cannot plant the jimson weed and get tomatoes.

Life-mastery requires mind-mastery. Mind-mastery begins with one discipline: Keep your mind fixed upon the things you desire and off the things you do not desire! Mind-mastery means using your will to control which thoughts and pictures you are allowing to dominate the computer screen of your conscious mind. It means focusing your conscious mind only on those thoughts and pictures that elevate you to divine heights.

Your ability to take control and selectively monitor the thoughts you allow to dominate your conscious mind determines how successful you will be in any endeavor. By undertaking the process of monitoring your thoughts and transmuting those thoughts into the empowering spectrum of life, you become enlightened.

The Cause Of Negative Thoughts

But how do we get control of our minds? How do we make sure that our dominant thoughts are positive?

Many people think limited, negative thoughts because they think they have to. They have thought negatively for so long that it has become comfortable for them. They know not the cause, nor the effect, of their thinking.

One cannot think negative thoughts and achieve positive results. Negative thoughts are destructive.

Remember: to achieve different results, we are going to have to think and do things differently. To eliminate negative thoughts, open your mind to a new understanding of what causes them. The primary causes of negative thoughts are the following:

Cause 1: Living with love withheld in the past or present. Many of us did not receive enough love from one or both parents when we were children and we carry these feelings of lack into adulthood. Some of us are living in situations right now where love is withheld and/or conditional. To reverse these situations, we can start by freely forgiving our parents, because they did the best they could, with what they had, where they were. Holding on to past injuries serves no purpose in creating a successful future. By applying **Lesson 1: The Principle Of Life Transformation**, we can begin receiving more love from those around us by becoming more loving ourselves and by expressing that love unconditionally.

Cause 2: Enduring destructive criticism in the past or present. Associating with those who criticize spoils the climate of our life. It is imperative to disassociate from people who have the tendency to make us feel inferior — this is absolutely critical to achieving excellent health. We are going to learn more about this in **Lesson 24: The Power Of Association**. The habit of replaying destructive criticism in the mind can be overcome by applying the Law Of Substitution (described below).

Cause 3: Ingesting too many acidic, phosphorus-rich foods or not ingesting sufficient alkaline, calcium/magnesium-rich foods. Food has a profound impact on the way we think, feel and behave as you may discover through your own experiences in applying the diet plan described in this book. Flesh foods, as well as nuts and seeds (including rice and other grains), are high in phosphorous (and other acid-forming minerals) which has a contracting and acidifying effect on the body. These effects are reflected in our state of mind. Alkaline, calcium/magnesium-rich vegetables (especially green-leafy vegetables) calm and relax our bodies and supply magnesium to the brain. We are going to learn more about the effects of flesh foods in **Lesson 8: Food And Karma** and how to balance the high-phosphorus foods, such as nuts and seeds, in **Lesson 14: Alkaline And Acid**.

Cause 4: Ingesting excessive cooked and processed foods (food degraded by heat and flame). Cooked and processed foods have lost their energy and vitality, thus causing us to feel less energetic and alive. A physical state of low energy is associated with negative thoughts and emotions, whereas a physical state of high energy is associated with positive thoughts and emotions (see **Lesson 7: The Sunfood Diet**).

Cause 5: A dietary lack of long-chain omega 3 essential fatty acids in our brain tissue leads to neurological imbalance and, potentially, depression. Oily fish (such as cod) contain long-chain omega 3 fatty acids; however, fish and fish oil is polluted today and eating fish is becoming more and more ethically and environmentally unsound. Hemp seeds and flax seeds, and especially their oils, contain medium-chain omega 3 essential fatty acids. A healthy body converts these over to long-chain omega 3 to form fresh brain tissue at a rate of approximately 3%. Some people convert at less efficient percentages due to health challenges, genetics and metabolism — sometimes the conversion is 0%. While 3% may be enough to keep us healthy, 0% is definitely not excellent. We can double the conversion factor to 6% if we consume hemp seed or flax seed and their oils with coconut oil (a great idea). We can also get the long-chain omega 3 fatty acids from the same place fish get it — algae. Purslane (a wild herb) and blue-green algae from Klamath Lake (a popular healthfood store item) contain long-chain omega 3 fatty acids. Also, golden algae can be dried and pressed for its raw oil which is super-high in long-chain omega 3 fatty acids. This algae oil is called DHA and is essentially a vegetarian form of fish oil. Marine phyto-plankton (the basis of the food chain) is now available as a superfood; it contains two long chain omega 3 fatty acids including DHA and EPA.

Cause 6: A lack of the amino acid tryptophan can lead to depression. In metabolism, tryptophan is transformed along with vitamin B3 into a compound called 5HTP, which along with vitamin B6 is then transformed into the neuro-transmitter serotonin, our primary stress-defense shield and buffer against depression. Tryptophan is found in raw, high protein foods such as hemp seeds, pumpkin seeds, bee pollen, spirulina, blue-green algae, chlorella, goji berries, wolfberries, maca root, cacao, etc. Tryptophan is heat volatile and is therefore corrupted in the cooking process. Meat and fish, though they originally contain tryptophan, lose much of this vita amino acid during the cooking process.

The Law Of Substitution

Once you know the causes of negative thoughts, you can purge them more effectively and use the Law of Substitution to totally eradicate them from your life. To remove a cloud of negativity from your mind, eliminate the causes mentioned, then just relax and substitute positive thoughts and habits in their place. The Law of Substitution is essential to mind-mastery.

Consider the words of Brian Tracy in his book Maximum Achievement:
"The Law Of Substitution: This is one of the most important of all mental laws. It is an extension of the Law of Control. It states that your conscious mind can hold only one thought at a time, and that you can substitute one thought for another. This "crowding out" principle allows you to deliberately replace a nega-tive thought with a positive thought. In so doing, you take control of your emotional life. This law is your key to happiness, to a positive mental attitude and to personal liberation. It can charge your relationships, your conversations and the predominant content of your conscious mind. Many people have told me this

law alone has changed their lives. Your conscious mind is never empty; it is always occupied with something. By using the Law of Substitution, you can replace any negative or fearful thought that may be troubling you. You can deliberately substitute a positive thought in its place."

One thought will always dominate your conscious mind. Sovereignty is never held in suspense.

Thoughts circling and spiraling on a self-destructive tangent always lead to failure. Negative thoughts always lead to negative emotions. You can delete these types of thought patterns immediately from your mind before they arise. Substitute these thoughts by rigorously holding to the beautiful visions of your goals or past successes. Vividly impress in your garden-mind all your desires, and remove all forms of limitation, fear, and doubt. Do not make one concession to any negative thought patterns. Negative thoughts dissipate your power.

The key to life-long happiness is to systematically purge negative emotions from your life — to eliminate anything that triggers negativity or stress in your psyche. A garden-mind encumbered by negative thoughts repels health and prosperity. Purging negative emotions is not optional, it is necessary to achieve a vibrant state of health. This means you have to get away from negative friends, associates or relatives as soon as possible. You cannot let their negativity dissuade you from your greatness.

When you eliminate negative emotions you automatically become a truly healthy individual. Your major health goal should be to keep your mind consciously focused on health and to substitute all unhealthy thoughts with healthy ones. You can tell how powerfully you desire health by how willing you are to focus your mind on the health you want to manifest, and off of the illness, doubt and weakness you wish to avoid

Beautify Your Thoughts

Beautify your thoughts. Thoughts are the headwaters of action, life and manifestation. Make the headwaters pure and the stream of life will flow in a vortex with pure intention.

With the diet information contained in this book, you will be renewing your body, but first you must beautify your mind.

A healthy diet will help you achieve a healthy mind and life. But, even the best change in diet will little help an individual who is unwilling to alter their negative thoughts. In fact, one can never alter their diet beyond a certain degree until the thoughts change first.

Consider the wise words of James Allen in his classic book **As You Think**, "A change of diet will not help those who will not change their thoughts. When our thoughts are pure, we no longer desire impure food."

To beautify your mind, guard against negative thoughts. Thoughts of detriment, disappointment, and depression rob your body of its vibrancy. Any thought of negativity, worry, or doubt diminishes your power; these thought types will alter the future against your favor. Build a fortress around you of positive thoughts and high-energy which repels even the most subtle infusions of negativity.

Use your garden-mind creatively to rethink yourself. You can change what and how you think about things in your mind and achieve incredible results. You can change what you imagine (the content of your thoughts) and how you imagine it (the size, color, volume and tone of your thoughts).

You can accelerate the realization of your mental pictures by writing your thoughts and ideas down. Think on paper. Success philosopher Mark Victor Hansen says: "Don't just think it, ink it." This gives your thoughts more substance. It adds a reality to them making them more likely to manifest. Writing down your thoughts, ideas, worries, expenses, etc. allows you to let go of those concepts and releases more room and energy for other things.

You can also accelerate the realization of your mental pictures by eating lightly or fasting. This allows you to think and visualize with incredible clarity.

Master your thoughts. Keep in mind that a single thought can revolutionize your life. A single thought can make you prosperous beyond belief. Make yourself a powerful magnet by focusing your thoughts consistently on prosperity and happiness. Dwell only upon thoughts of health. Be cheerful by entertaining only cheerful thoughts. Your destiny is within your own hands. You choose the seeds,

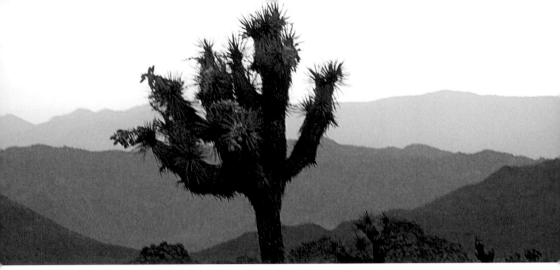

The fabled Joshua Tree stands alone with one thought only:
To be pulled forth towards the Sun with joy.

plant them and harvest the crop. You are the gardener of your future, you are the forestal of orchards to come.

The greatest seed of all — your limitless potential — is with you at all times. Nourish this seed of your divine greatness through concentration of thought. There is no limit to who or what you can be.

One thing is certain in life, you have to think — thought is the very essence of the life experience. Since you are going to be thinking anyway, you may as well think incredibly positive thoughts! Great thoughts produce greatness. Perfect thoughts produce perfection.

THOUGHTS ARE THINGS

1   Get a clear picture on the computer screen of your mind of the primary achievement you wish to have, then continuously think about how to achieve it. What specific actions do you need to take? Record the achievement you have chosen and at least 5 specific steps to achieve it in your journal.

2   For 21 straight days use the Law of Substitution to push out negative thoughts from your mind. Replace them with positive thoughts of your goals, aspirations and the greatest successes of your past.

THOUGHTS ARE THINGS

Thoughts are things and powerful things —
Incredible things they are.
A thought alone
Can send a stone
To a superabundant star.

A thought once thought
Exists and ought
Be revered as such by you.
What you are today
Is the result I say
Of what you perceive as true.

The thoughts that are in your head
Tell all, about who you are.
And if those thoughts don't uplift you,
You'll never get too far.

A thought once thought
Is felt and ought.
To soothe the joints and muscle.
The thoughts in your mind
Should be of a kind
To alleviate Life's stressed hustle.

A thought creates many changes
In your body's biochemistry.
The best action you can take
Is to choose those thoughts carefully.

Your body can't tell the difference
Between experience and state of mind.
The real secret is to control
The interpretation of what you find.

A thought once thought
Is real and ought
To be considered an action.
The thoughts you think
Should be the link
To your greatness and satisfaction.

A thought never heard
Is one-third a spoken word
And one-ninth of a word written down.
Think on paper,
For ideas are safer,
When before your eyes they are found.

Translate an idea into riches
Or other material things.
A thought creates the nest
From which the sparrow sings.

Animals think many thoughts,
That's why humans think they're dumb.
The difference is animals think
Just to have some fun.

Thoughts are things and powerful things
When attached to emotional desires.
Thoughts have carried the fairest of kings
And crumbled the greatest empires.

The thoughts that rule your mind
Say who you are to you.
Rule your thoughts and you shall find
You created you anew.

What you dwell upon grows,
What you think about shows!
Trust your instinct
Think the thought
Live the life
You've always sought.
Strike out boldly with your plans unfurled,
For a thought alone can move the world.

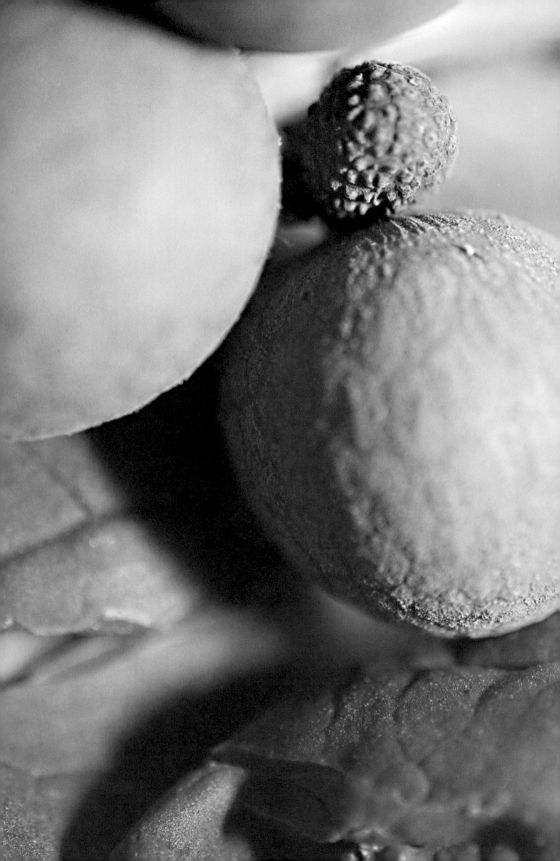

4

BELIEFS

"IF YOU BELIEVE THAT YOU CAN DO A THING, OR IF YOU BELIEVE YOU CANNOT, IN EITHER CASE, YOU ARE RIGHT." — *Henry Ford*

"BELIEFS ARE PREARRANGED, ORGANIZED FILTERS TO OUR PERCEPTIONS OF THE WORLD." — *Anthony Robbins*

A belief is a habitual pattern of thinking about yourself and the world. A belief is a template of thoughts.

Your mind functions on the Law of Belief: whatever you believe with confidence becomes your own self-fulfilling prophecy. Believe it, and it will come to pass. "If thou canst believe, all things are possible to him that believeth" (Mark 9:23).

The power of belief is overwhelming: no matter how right or how true something is, if you believe you can't do it, guess what?...you can't.

Expectations

Your expectations in any area of life are dependent upon your beliefs. Whatever you believe to be true in terms of health, wealth or spiritual growth will be reflected in your expectations about those areas. The world conforms to your expectations. You receive what you expect to receive.

You are where you are and what you are because of the beliefs you have about who you are. You are healthy or unhealthy, successful or unsuccessful, happy or sad because of the beliefs you have about yourself in those areas.

If you keep believing what you are believing, you will keep achieving what you are achieving. If you keep doing what you are doing, you will keep getting what you are getting.

We have, as part of our mind, a filter container called the Reticular Activation System (RAS). The RAS contains our belief system. It sensitizes us to certain types of information from our environment that we are tuned in to taste, smell, see, hear and feel.

Our experience of an event is not the actual event itself, but a representation of the event after it has been run through the RAS filter of our belief system. Because there are billions of pieces of information coming into our sphere every moment, our belief system determines what we are going to allow to enter our awareness — if it did not filter this out, we would be overwhelmed and surely driven insane by too much information!

We do not experience things as they really are! We experience things only through a filter and that filter determines what information will enter our awareness and what will be rejected. If we change the filter (our belief system), then we automatically experience the world in a completely different way.

From this understanding about the RAS, we may realize that little in the universe is absolutely known because what we think is real is actually only a reflection of our beliefs in that area. Two insightful sayings state: "You don't believe what you see, rather, you see what you already believe" and "Seeing is believing? No, believing is seeing." Complete objectivity, in any field, may be impossible. We see that "objective science" is most often subjective (as we shall explore in **Lesson 9: Origins**)!

We do not know how the world really is; we only know what our beliefs are about the world. Our perceptions create our reality. The reality of our day-to-day lives consists of an endless flow of perceptual interpretations that we, as individuals who live in a specific society, have learned to hold in common with other individuals.

The world we think we see is only a view, a collective description of the world that we create through our belief systems. Accepting this fact seems to be one of the most empowering things one can do.

The "reality" of our world is not as real, or as "out there," as we believe it is. Reality is only a description. That which is held in our minds as the real world is merely a description of the world; a description that has been developing within us from our first moments. Overcome the illusion — the world may be a far different place than we believe now.

Your beliefs determine what you consider real. To believe that the world is only as you think it is now, is funny! How many times have you had a belief in your life that turned out to be wrong? To be totally false? How did those beliefs affect your life? Your potential? Remember, it is our beliefs that shape and create our reality, so we must choose resourceful and empowering beliefs for ourselves and others.

An individual's true beliefs are discovered by what they do, not by what they say. What you truly believe is determined by the actions you take. You always act and think in a manner consistent with your beliefs. This is true even if your beliefs are totally irrational and ridiculous. If you believe any "thing," then that "thing" is true for you.

Your beliefs affect your physical body. They shape how you look. The cells are constantly changing and reformulating themselves based on the thought template provided by your beliefs. The mind carves the body. The physical body is nothing more nor less than the beliefs we have about it. Not only do the beliefs themselves create the body we have, but the beliefs also induce the actions. The derivative actions have their effect too! The actions of diet, exercise, rest, play and joy all have their influence.

The question is not: "What should I believe?" The question is: "What is useful for me to believe?" Beliefs are either effective or ineffective. They either help the achievement of our goals and spiritual desires or hinder them.

Each mind is a great power in this world. The only thing limiting anyone is their self-limiting beliefs. Holding onto poisonous beliefs shuts out all of the abundance life has to offer.

Change your beliefs about what you deserve and you will attract a whole new reality around you. You can do this by creating a belief paradigm that allows you to live to your highest health potential — physically, emotionally, mentally and spiritually in a manner which honors all life forms.

As young children we possess a perfect mind and a perfect memory. It is through limiting beliefs that this potential is dampened. When you overthrow limiting beliefs, you will be returned to a perfect mind and a perfect memory.

At any given time you may regain your extraordinary potential by identifying (in writing) all your disempowering beliefs and dissolving them in oceans of new knowledge and wonder. Simply refuse to limit yourself in any way. Ideally, we should proceed as if limits to our abilities did not exist.

When we have eliminated our own limiting beliefs, then we automatically help those around us eliminate their limiting beliefs. This is another aspect of The Principle of Life Transformation, a change of beliefs on the inside of your mind produces a change of beliefs in other minds.

One of the greatest gifts we can give to another is our own strong belief in their potential. By influencing their belief system, we help them achieve their true potential — which makes everybody better off. I attribute much of my success in life to the influence of my Aunt Dee-Dee, who consistently instilled confidence in my abilities. Perhaps the greatest gift one can bestow upon another is to instill confidence by saying: "I believe in you. You are something special. You can do it!"

BELIEFS

1   You have beliefs about how you look, what is a good weight for you, how much you should eat, what types of foods you should eat and how much you should exercise. What are they? Write them down in your journal. Ask yourself: "How can I immediately and powerfully improve or replace these beliefs and enjoy the process?" Write down the answers to this question for each belief, and act upon them immediately.

2   Identify five limiting beliefs in writing in your journal. Replace each limiting belief with a one-sentence empowering belief. For example, if your old belief was "I am too fat," change it to "I am daily making choices which make me look excellent."

3   Tell all the special people around you that you believe in them. Tell them how special they are to you. Sincerely help and support them. By the universal karmic law (the Law of Reciprocity), what you send out will come back multiplied. This is the way to receive the belief and support you deserve.

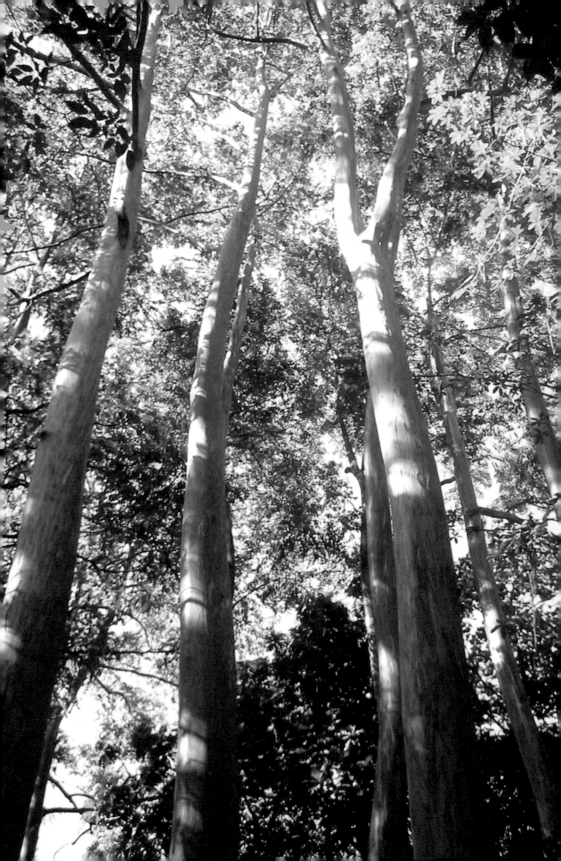

5

GOALS

"GREAT DREAMERS' DREAMS ARE NEVER FULFILLED,
THEY ARE ALWAYS TRANSCENDED." — *Alfred Lord Whitehead*

"HUMAN BEINGS, YOU AND I, ARE GOAL–CENTERED ORGANISMS.
WE ARE TELEOLOGICAL IN THAT WE ARE MOTIVATED BY PURPOSES,
BY DESIRED END STATES. WE ARE ENGINEERED MENTALLY
TO MOVE PROGRESSIVELY AND SUCCESSIVELY FROM ONE GOAL
TO THE NEXT, AND WE ARE NEVER REALLY HAPPY UNLESS,
AND UNTIL, WE ARE MOVING TOWARD THE ACCOMPLISHMENT
OF SOMETHING THAT IS IMPORTANT TO US."
— *Brian Tracy, Success Philosopher*

"SUCCESS IS TAKING ACTION TOWARDS YOUR PERSONAL
GOALS EACH DAY." — *Jim Rohn, Success Philosopher*

"FEELING LISTLESS? MAKE A LIST!" — *Anonymous*

Imagine a beautiful garden with brilliant Sun, crystalline water, friendly insects and rich soil ripe for the planting. A garden, perfect in every respect, except, there are no desirable seeds present because you have not planted them. The only seeds sprouting are those weeds and shrubs planted by others, or by the wind and birds. Yet you continue to tend and cultivate those haphazard plants with your resources. This perfect garden, containing none of your own seeds, is what your mind is like when you have no definite goals. If you have no crop to nurture to an edible state, you drift along with the vagaries, whims and goals of others.

If you are not working to achieve your own goals, you are always working to achieve another's goals. Everything you do, every day, is actually for the achievement of goals. What you may want to ask yourself is: Are they my goals? And: Are they worthwhile goals?

The mark of a winner is intense goal orientation. Napoleon Hill called this: "definiteness of purpose." It is a direction you have selectively chosen for your life.

Few realize that a major cause of stress (the great destroyer of health) is having no clear goals, no future to await you, no plan to get somewhere in life. Setting goals allows us to chart the course of our life and control where we are going. The more control we feel we command over our future, the less stress we feel.

The very first step before you begin a journey is an undiminished decision as to where you are headed. If you are determined to manifest the dormant powers within you, first get clear about what you want and where you are going. Decide. Dedicate yourself wholeheartedly to getting there. Chart your course; it is much easier to travel with a map.

If the success you seek is extraordinary, then you must begin immediately to set extraordinary goals. As long as you are going to dream, dream great dreams. As long as you are aiming for prosperity, go for it all! Spectacular success is always preceded by spectacular goal setting and mental preparation.

Release all limitations today! Set enormous goals! If your daily goal is just to make it home, eat unhealthy foods, watch TV and go to sleep, you will achieve that. If your daily goal is to make it home, exercise, work on your favorite projects all night and wake up in the morning with an abundance of energy, you will achieve that too.

Set goals which challenge your brain to think in new directions. Set too many goals. Set 6,000 goals. Set so many goals it will take you a lifetime to achieve them!

And when you achieve a written goal, draw a star or checkmark next to it. Keep track of your progress. Completing and checking off a complex, challenging goal gives one an amazing boost of satisfaction. Your own self-image will become more positive and confident as you check off each accomplished goal.

Work on yourself like a work of art through goal setting. Sculpt your character, physique and future. Plan and determine the final masterpiece in advance. Set down your personal goals with tremendous clarity and intensity.

Set your goals, then plan how you are going to achieve them. Proper planning prevents poor performance.

Consider the following ratio:
Planning to action = 1:5 (1 day of planning is worth 5 days of action).
Prevention to recovery = 1:5 (1 day of prevention is worth 5 days of recovery).

The more you plan, the more effective your plans will become, and the more you can get done in less time. The more you prevent, the healthier you become, and the less time you need to ever spend on recovery.

Within his book, **Maximum Achievement**, Brian Tracy has outlined twelve steps to achieve goals:
1. Develop an intense desire to achieve your goals.
2. Develop a strong belief in your goals.
3. Write down your goals.
4. Determine how you will benefit from achieving your goals.
5. Analyze your starting point.
6. Set deadlines to achieve your goals.
7. Identify the obstacles that stand in your way.
8. Identify the additional knowledge or information you will require.

9. Identify the people whose cooperation you will require.
10. Make a plan to achieve your goals.
11. Visualize the achievement of your goals.
12. Persist until your goals are achieved.

The present does not spring from the past. The present springs from the future — your vision of the future. To predict the future, assess what is happening in your life now, develop a strategy to reach your goals and create the future.

Humans have the divine ability to visualize, to see the future before it happens. We literally create the future through visualization. Positive, vivid mental pictures activate all of the laws of the universe and send things, people and circumstances to us in harmony with those pictures.

You can go only as far as your vision permits. A common practice in sports psychology is to visualize oneself reaching a goal. In your life you can employ this technique to expand your vision.

To expand your powers of visualization is to recreate the world. Through your imagination you can fly out amongst the stars, scale the majestic mountains of the world, enjoy the lush abundance of the tropics. Your imagination is the key to a brilliant life. Just as you can visualize amazing landscapes, visualize your goals clearly and consistently and they will begin to manifest now.

When goals are visualized creatively, the rest of life is assured to be intensely interesting and endlessly exciting. This is because the sharper and more vivid a visualization, the quicker it will manifest.

Those who think about visionary goals, who use their garden-minds to erect fantastic visions of beautiful orchards, brilliant island vacations, perfect days and radiant relationships, are living the most — they are getting the most enjoyment out of life.

A written goal describes clearly what we are seeking. Writing down a goal is making our desires known to the universe and starts the flow of abundance towards us. When we set down our visionary goals on paper, we give reality to them and solidify their entrance from the realm of pure potential into our lives.

Those who set goals are those whc achieve them.

Anthony Robbins cites a famous goal study in his book **Unlimited Power**: "A study of the 1953 graduates of Yale University clearly demonstrates the power of goals. The graduates interviewed were asked if they had a clear, specific set of goals written down with a plan for achieving those goals. Only 3 percent had such written goals. Twenty years later, in 1973, the researchers went back and interviewed the surviving members of the 1953 graduating class. They discovered that the 3 percent with written specific goals were worth more in financial terms than the entire other 97 percent put together...The interviewers also discovered that the less measurable or more subjective measures, such as level of happiness and joy that the graduates felt, also seemed to be superior in the 3 percent with written goals."

When you take action by actually writing down your goals and reviewing them regularly, you dive into a strong current that will carry you to distant places. Unseen forces will come to your aid.

Writing down a vision, idea or goal makes it a commitment. It tells the subconscious mind what you want to do. It compels the subconscious to figure out how to make your vision become reality. Remember: "Don't just think it, ink it." The more often you write down your goals, review them and get into the habit of working on them, the quicker they materialize in reality.

You are capable, at any time in your life, of doing what you dream. Everything you have in your life right now is only a duplication of what you subconsciously believe you deserve. Many people are afraid to pursue their most important dreams, because they feel they do not deserve them or that they will be unable to achieve them. You can decide now, at this very moment, that you will avoid this trap. You can decide right now that you will change your destiny. Once you have written your goals on paper, you automatically override thoughts of unworthiness and failure.

Think about your goals continuously. When your goals are clear, all the laws of the universe conspire in your favor to help you. Whenever you feel things are going badly, think about your goals! Uplift yourself by thinking about, visualizing and feeling your goals!

To achieve your goals, you must become the type of person who can achieve

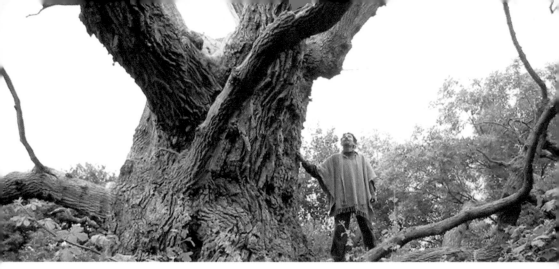

Like a great strong oak tree, goals put our feet on the ground and our imagination into the stars. Goals allow us to manifest an extraordinary destiny.

those goals.

When I first started promoting a raw plant-food diet and lifestyle years ago, I was not the type of person who could bring this information to an enormous audience. But, in the process of my own transformation, goal setting and goal achievements, I became a different type of person: a person brave enough, happy enough and successful enough to take this information to the next level.

How you will achieve your unique goals is not always clear. In the same way, when you begin a garden you do not completely understand all of the implications involved. The garden's growth reveals the full manifestation of the goal. Like a tree that draws nourishment into its trunk, and transforms it with the assistance of Sun energy into whatever it needs (leaf, bark, branch, root, stem, sepal, petal, fruit or seed) to fulfill its destiny, so too will you draw in knowledge and, with the assistance of focused energy, transform it into whatever you need to achieve your goals.

You can learn everything you need to know to accomplish your goals along the way to their achievement. The key is to keep taking action. Action attracts the knowledge you require and makes all things possible.

I tell listeners in my seminars: "Leap and the net appears." Use The Trial and Success Method: Learn from your past mistakes and adjust your behavior accordingly to achieve your goals — treat your past as a school, a vast resource to learn from to better yourself. Maxwell Maltz called this "Psycho-Cybernetics" in his well-known book of the same title. When the mind has a defined target, it can focus and direct and refocus and redirect until it reaches its intended goal.

Remember: The greater your goals, the greater the challenges which await you! Andrew Carnegie said: "Anything in life worth having is worth working for." When you set greater goals, you will face greater challenges. When you set the goal to reach an extraordinary level of health, people will oppose you! Peers may criticize you; family and friends will descend upon you; strangers will try to discourage you. You have to leverage your mind to handle these situations, maintain your focus and enjoy the process!

At the bottom of it all, the final goal is that people just want to be happy. When all else is detoxified away, the pursuit of any goal is about achieving happiness.

To achieve the highest levels of health, maintain your happiness no matter what you are doing. Set happiness as your highest goal and organize your life around it. All beliefs, ideas, goals and activities that diminish your happiness also limit your potential. There is something in Nature that always attempts to guide you towards growing and achieving the greatest levels of happiness if you simply tune in, listen to and act upon your intuition.

Always remember to keep your happiness or harmony of mind as your number one value and all else will fall into place. The best way to make others happy is to be happy yourself. Your own happiness allows you to fully enjoy the abundance life has to offer. As long you choose your own peace of mind as your guiding principle, you will never make a bad decision on the way to achieving your dreams.

It is the possibility of having a dream come true which makes life most interesting! Get excited about your goals. Get excited about waking up in the morning! Become an irresistible force of Nature moving rapidly towards each set goal.

As your goals begin to materialize, you will enjoy life more, you will become more confident, you will set into motion an upward spiral of ever-increasing achievement.

As you work diligently toward the achievement of your goals, you may discover the beautiful truth that, as you fill your spirit with positive thoughts, rewards and exciting challenges, all weaknesses are automatically eliminated. Consider the story of business philosopher Cavett Roberts (whose success audio tapes I highly recommend). By middle age, Cavett's health was failing and he was given a death sentence by doctors. He quit his job as a lawyer, moved to sunny Arizona, started selling real estate and got so busy succeeding and achieving his goals that he forgot to die. He lived into his nineties, and outlived all his doctors!

No matter what your station in life at the present time, you can change your future in a moment with one powerful action. The actions you take, or do not take, each day shape your destny. Each action or non-action is taking you towards a conclusion, a goal. Remember, you are always heading towards goals. The question is: Whose?

We are journeying entities, traveling in the garden of life, drawn to those destinations that are in harmony with our dominant thoughts. Goals are like orchards filled with ripe fruits, they pull us toward them. They breathe in new fragrant sensations into our being. They activate our imagination.

We are designed to set and achieve goals with the content of our life being the wonders we observe along the way.

The ultimate quest has no ending, and that fact gives it incredible value. The true value is not what we get, but what we become along the way. We journey to a goal, and then realize the journey is the goal.

GOALS

1   Set a health goal to continuously act upon the information contained within this book. Record this goal in your journal.

2   In your journal, write down 100 goals that you want to attain within the next year. Review them daily.

3   Take your top 5 goals for this year. For each goal write a sentence fulfilling each one of the 12 steps for goal achievement outlined by Brian Tracy earlier in this lesson.

4   Continuously write down additional yearly goals and long-term goals in your journal. 100 goals is a starting point. My goal is to have 6,000 goals!

5   Consider writing down your goals with different colored inks. The human mind tends to remember words that are written in color better than it remembers words written in black. You may even choose to use crayons!

6   Check off each goal as you achieve it.

THE VISIONARY

The beauty of the world,
Under sunshine, mist, snow
Settles upon dreams
Which nestle and grow,
In the slumbering visions
Of the secret and wild,
The supernal gods
In the feral child.

Vision — the strength,
It shapes and seeks:
The glide of the pen,
And a voice who speaks
To the mass of minds
Or a single face, with
Eloquent, astral, eternal grace.

Your vision is the promise,
You shall one day be.
Your ideal is the prophecy,
You shall one day see.

Nourished by seeds,
Of divine inspiration,
You become as great,
As the finest creation.

That which you love,
Shall come upon you.
That which you need,
Shall find its way too.

Vision — the master,
It guides and creates.
It plans for perfection,
And clearly states:
"The dreamers are the saviors
Of the world."

Those who cherish:
A beautiful vision,
A lofty ideal,
Have but one decision:

Inspire the dream,
To expand and rise.
Nourish that truth
Without compromise.

For those with visions
Of truth and right,
Even alone,
Have strength and might.

With a cluster of sparks,
The air of 'rudition,
That which is nourished,
Will come to fruition.

Vision — the power,
It molds and makes.
Hold it true so long
And evermore it shapes,
The reasons, minds, and the wills
Calling forth a thousand joys,
Disposing of a thousand ills.

Cherished in secret
Yet coming to pass,
Vision — the calm
In a pool of glass.

Tempest tossed souls,
Wherever you be,
Rest under the wing
Of the visionary.

In the Ocean of Life,
Isles of Bliss lay smiling.
The Sunny shore of your ideal
Awaits your arriving.

Keep your hand firmly poised
Upon the helm of thought.
Hold true to the vision
And you'll find what you have sought.

THE VISIONARY'S EPILOGUE

To humanity:
The seekers,
Never forget
Your dreamers.
Their ideals
Must never
Fade and die.
They live forever
And carry us high.
See in them
What you shall know.
Take from them
Some seeds to sow.
For musician, poet, painter, sage —
You are the architects
Of the golden age.

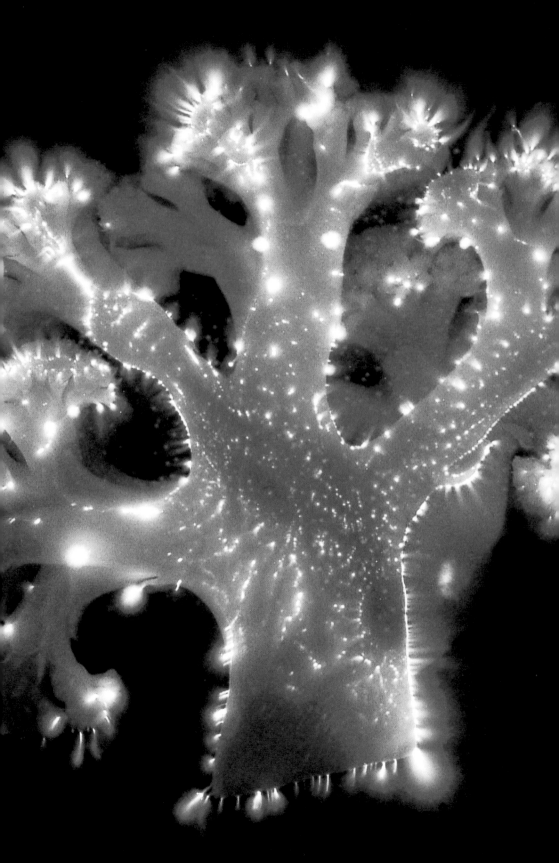

6

FAITH

"JUST AS A GREEN SPROUT NEVER SPRINGS FROM SEEDS THAT
HAVE BEEN SCORCHED BY FIRE, SO NO VIRTUES WILL ARISE
IN PEOPLE WHO HAVE NO FAITH." — *Dasadharma Sutra*

Have you ever wondered why an electron spinning around an atom nucleus does not run out of energy? How does it operate in perpetual motion? The answer coming from the foremost progressive scientific minds is that the electron continually dips into the well of infinite energy and potential called the "zero-point energy." The zero-point energy animates the universe. It provides life-force and organizing principle to all living things through the superconductive properties of monoatomic elements inside living cells which transform or reduce aspects of zero-point energy into this dimension.

Through the great principle of faith we can tap the zero-point energy and draw forth any tangible item or intangible idea into the physical world. Faith is a superconductor that allows us to consciously tap into the cosmic, divine energy. Faith allows us to create things in the material world.

Faith is the ability to have trust in powers greater than yourself, to confidently stride into the unknown, and to believe in your own abilities — no matter what.

Faith is the fountain word; it is the principle of achievement. Faith promises all things; and it fulfills all things. To employ faith is to call upon the divine power and set it into action. "According to your faith be it unto you" (Matthew 9:29). Success philosopher Napoleon Hill described faith as the "élan vital" that gives inspiration. The power of faith becomes tangible as renewed cells and tissues, or in newly created things. Faith is the basic channel of Nature through which all things manifest.

Faith is essential to success. A lack of faith is essential to failure. Every belief we hold requires faith because we can never know anything for sure. Without faith, confusion, distraction and inner uncertainty set in — leading only to failure.

"I would show unto the world that faith is things which are hoped for and not seen; wherefore, dispute not because ye see not, for ye receive no witness until after the trial of your faith" (Ether 12:6). Spiritual power overrides all. You can have, do and be anything you want if only you dare to reach for it in faith. The divine power will make sure your faith is true by testing your faith. The stronger your faith and clarity, the quicker you will set yourself into the divine time flow where one is always in the perfect place at the perfect time.

If you are doing the work you were meant to do, then you can command that everything you require, whether known or unknown, will be there at the precise time you require it. What stops this process from occurring is doubt. What starts this process occurring is faith. Basically, all you need are two things: a goal and faith, and you will get where you are going.

The opposite of faith is fear and doubt. Doubt stops the full expression of your life potential.

The doubter can and shall never obtain anything. The abundance of the world is forever closed to the doubter. A doubter can never know truth, can never make a determined act. Doubt is pernicious as it destroys the climate of success. If you be anything, be not a doubter. Only through faith are things granted. Faith is the one command that overrides doubt.

Embrace faith and you automatically master fear. Faith is the one power against which fear cannot stand.

Strong faith creates a positive attitude. Success seems to be connected with attitude. If your attitude is strong, powerful, attractive and graceful, you can achieve any success you desire!

What the people need more than anything is faith: faith in themselves, faith in their fellows, faith in the power and goodness of Nature, faith in the healing powers of raw plant foods, faith in the divine powers.

All the greatest beings who have ever strolled through the Earth's gardens have been people of transcendent faith. Every one of them had a tranquil attitude and a calm belief in the helpful powers of invisible forces. These forces are always available to everyone!

Those who desire health must have faith, for those who have faith have everything.

Doubt

Forever clashing with the wise
Is the spirit that denies!

And to that Power never reposing,
Creative, healing
Doubt is opposing!

Doubt is a liar,
A burden endured.
From the gilden path,
Many are lured,
In treacherous compassion,
With flame-twisted word,
The mind becomes clouded, and —
Eden lies obscured.

FAITH

Plant the seeds of faith in the s x individuals you associate with most often. Support them with faith; teach them to support themselves with faith. Tell them, without condition, that you believe in them, that you know they can succeed in anything, that you know higher powers will come to their aid.

Open your journal and look at the top 5 yearly goals established in the Action Steps at the end of **Lesson 5: Goals**. As you read them, do the following:

A) Write down all doubts that immediately come into your mind as you review each goal.

B) Resolve to dismiss away any doubts you may have associated with each goal by writing down in your journal the following statement: "I have total faith that everything in the universe is perfect. I have total faith in the magic and mystery of goal setting. I continuously manifest anything I choose. I am activated and inspired by faith."

C) For each of your top 5 yearly goals, write down exactly why you will faithfully persist until you achieve them.

D) Create a discipline to replace any thoughts of doubt or fear with faith. Daily affirmations or prayers are helpful. Meditation on faith is wonderful. Journaling or writing your doubts and fears down removes them from your consciousness and helps dispel them. Remember: as long as you are doing it, never doubt it.

• Now that you have reviewed the fundamental information shared in the lessons thus far, it is time to reveal to you the magic secret. In this next lesson, we are going to discuss an unprecedented health and consciousness-transforming discovery. You are now ripe, through your own exposure and your own seeking to make a dietary choice. You are now at that moment when you can make a leap of faith into a powerful stream of new information.

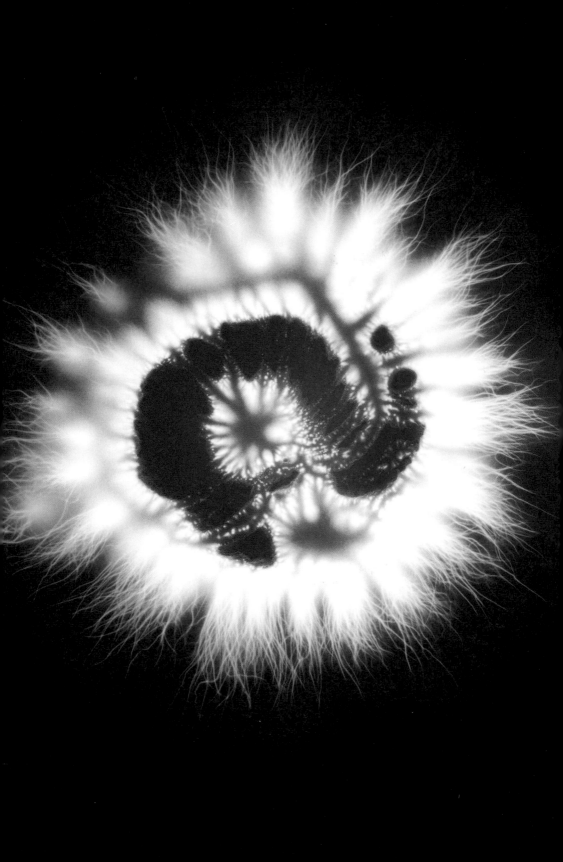

7

THE SUNFOOD DIET

"And God said: Behold, I have given you every
herb bearing seed which is upon the face
of the earth, and every tree, in which is the fruit of
a tree yielding seed, to be your food." — *Genesis 1:29*

"Kill neither men, nor beasts, nor yet the food
which goes into your mouth. For if you eat
living food, the same will quicken you, but if you kill
your food, the dead food will kill you also. For life
comes only from life, and from death comes always
death. For everything which kills your foods, kills your
bodies also. And everything which kills your bodies
kills your souls also. And your bodies become what
your foods are, even as your spirits, likewise, become
what your thoughts are. Therefore, eat not anything
which fire, or frost, or water has destroyed. For
burned, frozen, or rotted foods will burn, freeze and
rot your body also." — *The Essene Gospel Of Peace, Book I
translated by Edmond Bordeaux Szekely*

"WHEN MANKIND WAS CREATED,
THEY KNEW NOT THE EATING OF BREAD,
KNEW NOT THE DRESSING IN GARMENTS;
ATE PLANTS WITH THEIR MOUTH LIKE SHEEP;
DRANK WATER FROM A DITCH." — *Sumerian Tale*

"HANUMAN WAS A MONKEY OF THE WOODS, HE DID
NOT DESIRE FAIR WOMEN AND HE ATE NO COOKED FOOD."
— *Hanuman is the monkey god of India featured in the tale
of the Ramayana from which this passage was quoted.*

"PIOUS MEN EAT WHAT THE GODS LEAVE OVER
AFTER THE OFFERING. BUT THOSE UNGODLY,
COOKING FOOD FOR THE GREED OF THEIR STOMACHS,
SIN AS THEY EAT IT." — *Bhagavad Gita*

"THERE IS AMONG THE INDIANS A HERESY
OF THOSE WHO PHILOSOPHIZE AMONG
THE BRAHMINS, WHO LIVE A SELF-SUFFICIENT LIFE,
ABSTAINING FROM EATING LIVING CREATURES
AND ALL COOKED FOOD." — *Hippolytus, Rome, 225 AD*

"I AM MUCH MORE INTERESTED IN A QUESTION ON
WHICH THE 'SALVATION OF HUMANITY' DEPENDS FAR MORE
THAN ON ANY THEOLOGIANS' CURIO: THE QUESTION OF
NUTRITION." — *Friedrich Nietzsche, Ecce Homo*

"IT CAN BE SAID THAT THE GREATEST SINGLE CAUSE OF
DEGENERATION IN MAN IS THE USE OF FIRE IN THE
PREPARATION OF FOODS." — *Arnold De Vries, The Fountain Of Youth*

"WHY ALL THIS COOKING WHEN THERE IS REALLY NO COOK LIKE
OLD SOL? COOKED FOOD IS DEAD FOOD — AND REMEMBER,
THE WHITER THE BREAD THE SOONER WE ARE DEAD! EVERY ATTEMPT
TO IMPROVE ON NATURAL FOOD MUST PROVE A FAILURE, AND
NATURE WILL REACT AT FIRST ACUTELY TO ANY INTERFERENCE WITH HER
BENEFICENT LAWS OF HEALTH. AND IF WE CONTINUE TO DISOBEY
HER LAWS BY DRUGS OR EVEN SURGERY, THE SYMPTOMS MAY DISAPPEAR FOR
A WHILE ONLY TO REAPPEAR IN CHRONIC OR FATAL DISEASES...
MAN IS THE ONLY CREATURE THAT COOKS HIS FOOD, AND HE IS MORE
SUBJECT TO DISEASE THAN ANY WILD CREATURE THAT DINES ON
UNFIRED FOOD. TRADITION, GLUTTONY, AND INCREASING DESIRE FOR
STRONG STIMULANTS HAVE CAUSED MAN TO PREFER COOKED FOOD, WHICH
HAS SERIOUSLY WEAKENED HIS DIGESTIVE ORGANS.
THIS IS BECAUSE COOKED FOOD CAN BE SWALLOWED
SO EASILY WITHOUT CHEWING, WHEREAS THOROUGH
MASTICATION IS ESSENTIAL TO GOOD HEALTH."
— *Dugald Semple, The Sunfood Way To Health*

"YOUR FOOD DETERMINES IN A LARGE MEASURE HOW LONG
YOU SHALL LIVE — HOW MUCH YOU SHALL ENJOY LIFE,
AND HOW SUCCESSFUL YOUR LIFE SHALL BE."
— *Dr. Kirschner, Live Food Juices*

What we eat deeply and radically affects the way we think, feel and behave. We are what we eat, and we eat what we are. Food affects every aspect of our being. Food is the foundation of our physical body. If the foundation is stable, all that is built upon it will be stable. Everything you physically are was once the air you breathed, the water you drank and the food you ate. The colloidal mineral structure of your body is built out of the foods you have eaten. If there is an alteration in the food, then it is reflected in the look and function of the body. Improve your food choices and you dramatically improve the foundation upon which your body is built.

Success is an accumulation of practicing fundamentals each and every day. And eating is a daily activity of vital importance that cannot be overlooked. A consistent habit of making excellent food choices is an absolute necessity for a successful life.

From average to exceptional is just a slight edge. The proper diet gives you a slight edge and a hundred times more. When you give your body incredible food, it will function incredibly.

To achieve your mission on Earth, you need excellent health and a supreme physical support system to get you there. Excellent dietary habits support your body and mind on the path to reaching amazing goals.

When your diet is pure, the planet freely bestows its wealth upon you. Diet is the mysterious key to life-long massive abundance. Diet is the key to the natural way of life. A wonderful life requires a natural diet rich in Sun-grown foods eaten in their pristine raw state.

If we think about it logically, when we arrived on the planet, we had no tools, clothing, or fire. How did we live? What did we eat? There must be some original diet, a diet we were biologically designed for, a diet that is the optimal diet for humankind.

Simplicity

"SUCCESS IS NOTHING MORE THAN A REFINED STUDY OF THE OBVIOUS."
— *Jim Rohn, Success Philosopher*

"Whatever must be proven is already doubtful."
— *Professor Arnold Ehret*

Simplicity is now, has always been and will forever be, the key guideline of success.

The fact that there is more confusion, conflicting opinions, and false information concerning the field of diet now available than ever before is proof that there must be some simple truth beneath it all. There are always many opinions, but only one truth.

In science there is a principle called Ockham's Razor. This principle tells us that, amongst competing theories, the simplest is most likely to be true.

Natural Law is simplicity itself. A great axiom states: "Once you are complicated, you are ineffective." A great reason for my success and the success of others on The Sunfood Diet program is its incredible simplicity. Whatever simple reasoning cannot ascertain is nonsense and should be dispensed with. Nothing vital is complicated.

There is a poetry, a powerful truth, in simple facts. The simpler things are, the easier it is to live. Foragers/gatherers were the original affluent society on Earth. The best things in life are free, for life depends on simplicity. The worst things in life are paid for with wasted life-force energy, for death depends on confusion.

People confuse things in direct proportion to their simplicity.

Anytime, if you feel you are being overwhelmed with information, simplify. Just get back to basics. All the greatest sports coaches the world has ever seen taught basics. Simple basics practiced over and over make enormous improvements in the long term. Here are the basics of nutrition: RAW PLANT FOODS.

Cooked food was not here when we first appeared on Earth.

Raw plant food is truly the most perfect food for human consumption.

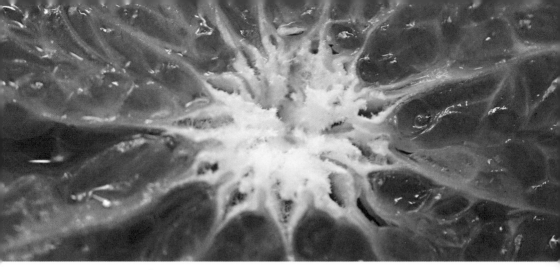

**Citrus fruits display the radiant sun energy they have
alchemically transformed into edible magic.**

The structure and function of humanity's teeth, jaw, digestive canal, sense organs, instincts of the young, psychological aversion towards killing, emotional feelings towards animals, as well as the cause and cure of disease and unhappiness, all demonstrate that humans are biologically and primarily raw-plant eaters — primarily consumers of sweet, non-sweet, and fatty fruits, as well as green-leafed vegetables. (See **Lesson 9: Origins** and **Appendix A**.)

Do you know the power of getting energy solely from plants? Every whole plant food is a symphony. The absorption and organization of Sunlight, the essence of life, takes place primarily in plants. The organs of the plant are therefore a kind of biological accumulation of Sun energy. Eating plant foods transfers the vital Sun energy directly to you, undiminished.

Raw plant foods are massively abundant. 99.99% of all food on Earth is raw plant food. In the grand scheme of things, cooked food is nonexistent, and animal food for omnivores and carnivores is minimal as the plant-eaters (mostly insects) are by far the dominant creatures on Earth.

Eating raw plant food provides you with an unlimited variety of food choices. There are so many raw plant foods on this planet that you could taste something new every single day for the rest of your life and still not even come remotely close to trying 1% of what is here on Earth! For instance, there are over 500 varieties of avocados. And there are at least 80 varieties of persimmons! There are even over 300 varieties of durian!

Raw plant foods fall into fourteen major categories:

1. Fruits: Fruits are raw plant foods that contain the seed within themselves for the reproduction of their kind. Fruits may be sweet, non-sweet or fat-dominant.

2. Leaves: Leaves contain life-giving chlorophyll pigments, and are the best source of alkaline minerals. Many herbs are green leaves.

3. Nuts: Nuts are the reproductive agents of certain trees. They are fat-dominant foods.

4. Seeds: Seeds are the reproductive agents of plants. Depending on the type, they may be protein-dominant or fat-dominant. Grains are seeds.

5. Legumes: Legumes include all peas, beans and peanuts, and are often sprouted before consumption. They are protein-dominant with the exception of peanuts which are fat-dominant.

6. Flowers: Flowers are the sexual organs of plants.

7. Green sprouts: Green sprouts appear when sprouted seeds, or legumes, reach a certain point of growth and shoot forth green leaves.

8. Roots: Roots are the below-ground portion of plants.

9. Shoots: Shoots are young plants spread by underground runners from their parent plants.

10. Bark: The outer, protective layer of trees. Inner barks are occasionally used as foods or for teas.

11. Sap: The life-fluid of a tree. Maple syrup comes from maple water, the sap of the maple tree. Bee propolis is made from tree sap.

12. Stems: Stems are the fibrous, structural pieces of plants.

13. Water vegetation: Sea vegetables are sea plant leaves containing bountiful minerals drawn in from the ocean, and up from the ocean floor. Spirulina and algae of all types are included in this category.

14. Mushrooms: A non-chlorophyll fungus that grows primarily in darkness, and is not directly nourished by the vibrant Sun energy, yet plays a critical role in recycling biological materials in old trees and the soil. Mushroom extracts can be an outstanding source of medicine (e.g. reishi, cordyceps, maitake, etc.)

What Is The Sunfood Diet?

The Sunfood Diet Success System is really The Raw-Food Diet Success System. I use the term "Sunfood" because it implies raw-plant food grown under the vivifying influence of direct Sunlight in a wild, natural state. "Sunfood" has a refreshing, majestic quality to it. "Raw food" is ambiguous — "raw food" could mean anything raw.

The Sunfood Diet is a diet of abundance. The Sunfood Diet Success System demystifies The Raw-Food Diet, and presents a program that allows anyone to achieve the goal of succeeding with a raw plant-food diet.

Of all the raw plant foods on Earth, The Sunfood Diet requires that 80%+ of your food choices contain a balance of green-leafed vegetables, sweet fruits and fatty plant foods. The other 20% can contain any of the fourteen kinds of raw plant foods mentioned above, or other foods that you feel are appropriate for you. This diet is not about denial, it is about success and achievement. The idea behind The Sunfood Diet is to eat at least 80% raw plant foods, and then move forward in your life from there.

Benefits Of The Sunfood Diet

Every so often in history an idea comes along that revolutionizes everything that follows it. The discovery of raw-food nutrition is one of those ideas. The implications of raw nutrition on humankind are immense.

We do not just need information to achieve success, we need transformation. The Sunfood Diet rebuilds you at the most fundamental levels and transforms you in a most profound way. The Sunfood Diet is peerless. Once an individual enters its field, every other power opens up.

A diet of raw plant food puts you in touch with a new vital power. In the source of every vital power lies an endless abundance. A diet of raw plant food presents a whole new paradigm of health, wealth, success and possibility. Since The Sunfood Diet is in alignment with a natural way of life, it brings with it beauty, happiness, long-life and prosperity.

We know that the more perfectly clean your body, the more perfectly it will radiate your super-natural powers. The first things to evaporate in a toxic environment are the super-natural abilities provided to us at birth. These powers are possessed by wild animals, and formerly by humanity. As soon as the body begins to be poisoned, the powers slip away. In any biological degeneration, the higher powers fade first. However, your natural superior abilities have not been totally destroyed by improper food, they are only dormant and are capable of rebirth, regeneration and resurrection.

One of the greatest values of The Sunfood Diet is that it opens you up to the idea that many of your other deep-seated beliefs may be totally false. The effects of adopting The Sunfood Diet disassemble your view of the world. Once you experience that eating cooked and artificially-grown food immediately detracts from the normal functioning of your body, you will begin to question many other aspects of your belief system. So, The Sunfood Diet acts like a battering ram crumbling away the stagnated belief systems of your mind. It allows you to grow in new directions you never would have predicted. You will be ready to try new things and to test new approaches to life's daily challenges.

As we learned in **Lesson 4: Beliefs**, we do not know what life really is; we only know how we represent life to ourselves. When you naturalize your diet, you automatically tune into a different energy band of life. You allow more information from your higher self to penetrate your conscious mind. And what you consider reality will change. Naturalizing your diet aligns and strips away chemical debris and toxins from the endocrine glands allowing insights from infinite intelligence to flow more clearly into your thoughts.

Different foods fuel different perceptions of the world. Eating raw plant foods automatically tunes you in to a positive, prosperous energy band of life. In Nature, there are potions, mixtures and solutions with which anyone may safely stimulate their minds to tune in to inspirational thoughts. Nature's stimulants cannot be improved upon. Nothing can compare to the aristocratic taste of a ripe cherimoya, nothing can touch the rush from fresh watermelons in the summer, nothing even resembles the energy derived from a meal of jackfruit, there is no substitute for the prosperity found in cacao beans (raw chocolate).

Raw nutrition attunes you to the forces that surround us, permeate through our bodies and that make up the essence of our existence. When you eat raw plant foods, your instincts become stronger. Your intuition becomes more reliable — clearer — and decision-making becomes effortless. In my own experience, I go with my intuition every time; I have learned the only thing we have which is not an illusion is our intuition.

During the process of undertaking The Sunfood Diet, you will experience moments of instantaneous change. I recall one afternoon, several years ago, when my cousin and I were juicing citrus fruits and feijoa (pineapple guava) at a former home in San Diego. We were in the middle of drinking a pitcher, when we both simultaneously exclaimed, "I can see better!" And we could see better. My vision permanently improved that day.

During the process you will also experience subtle change. Over time the subtlety builds, and one day you will wake up profoundly transformed. *In general, food choices have a cumulative effect on the body.*

The digestion of cooked food takes more energy from the body than any other activity. You could run a marathon and still be walking and talking. However, an hour after a Thanksgiving dinner, guess what?...you are asleep! We know that all success is about transmuting energy. This message is about transmuting the energy used in digestion into achieving our goals.

On The Sunfood Diet you need less sleep. I used to sleep 8 hours a night. I was the type of person who had to sleep 8 hours. Since adopting The Sunfood Diet, my sleep needs decreased to 3 hours at a minimum to 6 hours at a maximum. On the average, judging from the information I have gathered, the people following this diet will, after a couple of years, experience a decrease of 2 hours of required sleep each night. In one year, that is an additional 30 days worth of extra time to accomplish goals and make a contribution to the planet.

The amazing thing about The Sunfood Diet is that it is something you can physically do. You do not have to think too hard about it, you can just do it.

After you have made the commitment to radically improve your diet, you subconsciously reinforce in your mind that your life has meaning and that striving for extraordinary health is worth the effort. You have made a commitment to really living life.

The strongest factor about The Sunfood Diet is that it compels you to live naturally and in harmony with the Earth.

If we pollute the planet after we eat with food packaging, then we truly are not living in harmony with the Earth. Eating raw fruits, vegetables and other plant foods is the solution to world pollution. Landfills are filled with products directly or indirectly related to cooked and processed foods, such as: packaging, wrappers, bags, old stoves, microwaves, etc. One of the most startling revelations I experienced on this diet-path was that I stopped producing trash! My life has become more harmonious with the Earth.

By following this diet, you may one day find yourself in your garden or home planting seeds and growing plants. The home of the Sunfoodist is often surrounded with radiant plant life. Eating raw foods truly reconnects you to the fabric of life.

True progress in the field of nutrition has been made in this world. Solutions have been found. The confusion of nutrition is the most perplexing challenge humankind has yet faced. The Sunfood Diet brings us closer to solving the confusion of nutrition by simplifying our dietary essentials and presenting a balanced nutrition program consisting of raw plant foods, allowing any single person to achieve an extraordinary level of health.

Ayurveda, Traditional Oriental Medicine & Macrobiotics

When people believed in the "Earth is flat" paradigm, every university taught its students that the Earth was flat. Every scientist and professor could "prove" to you that it was flat. Those scientists and professors were not lying to you — they just did not know. It took a few distinctions put forth by a few noble minds to dissolve away the basic assumptions of all those schools of thought. This is how knowledge moves forward — indeed, it is the only way that knowledge has ever moved forward.

The "Earth is flat" paradigm only allowed human understanding to proceed to a certain level, and no further. In the same way, diet systems such as ayurveda (from India), traditional Chinese medicine (and its macrobiotic offshoot) only allow human health to proceed to a certain level, and no further. The ancient systems have been dulled down over many thousands of years and no longer contain real vitality; the purpose of these systems was to help the average person reach good health. The purpose of The Sunfood Diet Success System is to help an average person become an extraordinary human being who experiences superior health, who encounters the highest forms of life and who unlocks dormant powers. New distinctions have now surpassed the old system paradigms.

My goal has been to draw forth the best elements from ayurveda, traditional Chinese medicine, macrobiotics and other systems and apply them to the

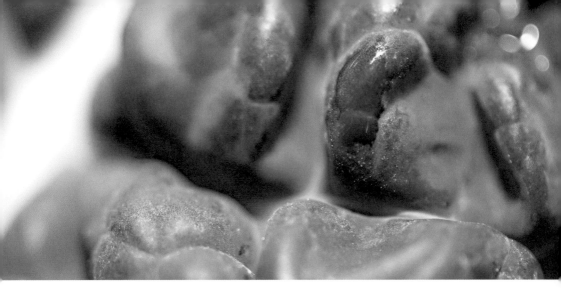

The power of living chlorophyll — it keeps the entire planet alive and well.

Sunfood approach. Special information involving individualizing diets based on ayurvedic and yin/yang balancing insights is beyond the scope of this book. These are explored in my seminars, retreats, DVD programs, websites, other books and are well described in Dr. Gabriel Cousens' books: **Conscious Eating**, **Spiritual Nutrition** and **The Rainbow Green Live-Food Cuisine**.

The insights on body-typing and nutritional balance coming from the ancient dietary systems and my own experiences with internal cleansing, tuning into food instincts and eating a total raw-food diet have convinced me that the original creators of these systems were raw-food eaters. The original systems were certainly much more pure than they appear today.

Throughout its long history up to this day, the presence of raw-food diets has appeared in India. Many yogis currently living in the Himalayas eat only raw plant food or raw plants and raw milk, following in the spiritual traditions of their ancestors. During the Zhou Dynasty in China, it was recorded that: "The tribes in the east were called Yi. They had their hair unbound, and tattooed their bodies. Some of them ate their food without it being cooked by fire." This account continues on by describing tribes to the north, south and west who did not eat cereals and who ate their food raw. From these accounts we know that raw-food diets were present in ancient China. This evidence again corroborates the concept that the original creators of the ancient systems could have been raw-foodists.

Cooked Food

After many years of careful study and investigation on the subject, I am convinced that the "the great change" which came over humankind occurred when humans took the power of fire into their own hands and began experimenting with eating cooked food.

Exactly when and where humans acquired fire is truly a mystery. Fire allowed early humans to begin to control their environment and spread out into more inhospitable places. Those with fire eventually overcame or passed it along to those without it. Whether it was the open flame or the tribal oven formed of red-hot stones paved into an oval hollow in the ground, fire became part of every tribe on Earth. But fire is a double-edged sword; unless one is careful with its power, it can turn on its master.

The world was given for us to turn into a paradise. To make this happen, cooked food needs to be understood for what it is, its consumption minimized, and its use eventually removed or specialized in the human diet (for purposes of dietary balance, herbal medicine, etc.).

The assumption behind cooking is that the original form of Nature, as it exists, must be altered in order that it may be reformed to a new artificial form. The truth is that the original state is always superior. The beauty and taste sensation of a wild blueberry cannot be improved upon!

The raw-versus-cooked distinction is the most important insight in the field of nutrition and one day will be the leading topic of nutritional conversation and science.

Cooking alters organic molecules. When those molecules are ingested, they become part of the tissues. Thus cooking alters the tissues at a fundamental level.

When food is cooked it always becomes less than it was before, never more. Fire is a destroyer; it never creates anything. If you took a flame-thrower to this book, would it become more or less than it was before? Cooking only takes away. Eating cooked food is like spending millions of dollars on a brand new mansion, then burning it to the ground before you move in!

Understand: you are water — magnetic water. Everything you swallow must be broken down into a liquid to nourish you. The first thing to go with cooking is the water.

Cooked food is dense. It leaves a toxic ash, or residue, in the body after it has been processed as fuel. Over years and decades, this debris accumulates in the form of mucus and is deposited throughout the tissues. Eventually, the toxins reach a crisis level and clog and poison the system leading to heart attacks, strokes and cancer. Many illnesses arise out of the toxic residues left by cooked foods.

One of the primary ways your body experiences the world around you is by the food you eat. What does the body sense when one puts a charred piece of animal flesh inside it? The body feels death, pain, fire, destruction.

A cooked seed will not grow. Cooked food has no life-force energy. Cooked food has a lower spiritual energy.

People on a standard cooked-food diet go through life in a weakened condition with their vitality much below par, but they are not aware of this because they have never known anything different. They have no reason to believe their vitality and health are not what they should be. They cannot miss what they never had. People are falling day by day to weaker levels, while believing they are attaining a high standard of living.

Eating cooked and processed foods makes one groggy, affects moods, lowers one's level of awareness and interferes with the body's optimal vitality. A poor diet results in toxic residues that have a long-range effect on longevity.

The nutritional properties of foods are degraded by the process of cooking. Heating converts foods into foreign substances, some of which harmful. Just like chemical-tobacco smoke, or boil-brewed alcohol, these substances have no connection with the body's natural needs.

Cooked food is addictive (there really is no softer way to phrase it). An addiction is a desire for a substance that has no connection with the true needs of the body. Certain cooked food behaviors have all the marks of a physio-chemical addiction. This is a strong statement, but I think, as you experiment with eating more and more raw plant foods, you will find an interesting truth in it.

People are not truly attached to many of the cooked foods they eat. They eat them for flavor or fun. I have found with most people that there are usually 5 or 6 cooked foods that they are actually addicted to and have trouble releasing. These usually include: bread, baked potatoes, coffee, potato chips, corn chips, tofu, candy (cooked chocolate), cigarettes (not a true food) and/or fish. Typically these foods are attached to emotional anchors. When these foods are removed, emotional feelings come up to be detoxified out of the body. One may feel uncomfortable for the moment (as these feelings are released), but feel much better in the long-term. (More on this in **Lesson 10: Detoxification.**)

Cooked Food And The Environment

Cooking led to the animal and seed diet. The most frequent way people interact with animals is by eating them. The most frequent way people interact with seeds is by eating them.

The animal and cooked-seed diet led to grain farming which is stripping the fertile Earth of its minerals. Grain crops are collected, processed, cooked, fed to animals or eaten, and eliminated into the sewers and waterways of civilization. Erosion wears down unstable grain fields, washing minerals away. Farms are turned into deserts; jungles are turned into rice paddies. One way or the other, the soil minerals wash down and end up at the bottom of the ocean.

Eating raw fruits and vegetables radically improves the mineralization of the Earth as it encourages the planting of trees. Trees reach down 20 or 30 feet (6 to 9 meters) — sometime much farther (I have been told that wild grape vines reach down as far as 500 feet [150 meters])! Trees elevate the groundwater table and draw minerals up into their stems, leaves, flowers and fruits. This plant matter then eventually falls to the topsoil increasing the mineralization of the soil for more vegetation to grow. Deciduous trees, which drop their leaves each year, strongly mineralize the topsoil.

The cooking of food is by far the biggest waste of resources on planet Earth. Viktoras Kulvinskas, in his classic book **Survival Into The 21st Century**, reports that cooking destroys 85% of the value of food. When I first realized this,

I was staggered. But I did not understand the full implication of this fact. You see, if 85% of the food value is destroyed in cooking, then, also destroyed, is 85% of the time, labor, resources and energy that went into creating the foods. So this idea of eating raw plant food impacts all agriculture, all business, all the economies of the world, all politics.

Massive abundance is the true law of life. There is no shortage of food on Earth! I know a date-farmer friend who informed me that, "The most vigorous date palms yield over 600 pounds per tree per year. One date palm planted at birth could supply a person with practically their entire lifetime supply of food." Probably everyone would agree that eating only dates would not be ideal, but it does give us an idea of how much food can come from just one tree! There is an infinite amount of food on this planet!

When I was a student at the University of San Diego, I had a job in customer service at the campus bookstore. One day a nun came up to my counter and we began talking. She described her recent trip to Haiti. Apparently, each year she had been spending at least 3 months in Haiti helping the impoverished children. She told me that Haiti had been deforested decades before. I asked her how that happened, expecting the answer to be overgrazing, or too much wood demand for building homes and shelters. Actually, neither was the case. She told me that Haiti had been deforested because the wood was being used for cooking!

Most people who live in first-world countries with gas stoves and electrical ovens have no idea that the other 90% of the planet is cooking with wood. Cooking is a major reason for deforestation. In Africa, the tropical forests of the mountain gorilla are being cut and cleared for cooking wood. Similar tragedies are happening on nearly every continent.

In third world countries, the cooking of food exposes people to the hazards of inhaling wood smoke or emissions from biomass fuels, such as cattle chips (dung). Emissions from wood and biomass fuels are major sources of air pollution in the home and are the number one source of air pollution outside the home (even eclipsing fossil fuels). Studies have shown that cooks inhale more smoke and pollutants than the inhabitants of the dirtiest cities.

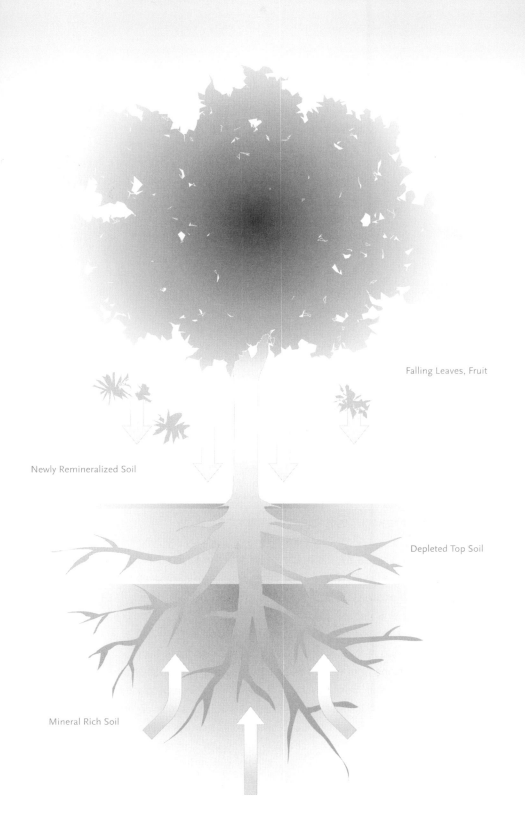

Falling Leaves, Fruit

Newly Remineralized Soil

Depleted Top Soil

Mineral Rich Soil

Overcoming Disease

"TREAT DISEASE THROUGH DIET, BY PREFERENCE,
REFRAINING FROM THE USE OF DRUGS; AND IF YOU FIND
WHAT IS REQUIRED IN A SINGLE HERB, DO NOT RESORT TO
A COMPOUND MEDICAMENT." — *Baha'u'llah*

"NO MATTER FROM WHICH ANGLE WE VIEW HEALTH AND
DISEASE, WE CANNOT ESCAPE FROM BEING ENTANGLED IN THE
CONCLUSION THAT INTRACTABLE DISEASE IS AS OLD AS COOKERY.
DISEASE AND COOKERY ORIGINATED SIMULTANEOUSLY."
— *Dr. Edward Howell, Enzyme Nutrition*

Every living organism is vibrating at a certain metabolic level. If the internal energy of the organism drops below a certain level, then the immune system is compromised. Illness is an energy crisis in the body — the body no longer has enough energy to hold together its integrity. Purifying the body through balanced, mineral-rich, raw-food nutrition raises the energy vibration, thus increasing the immune system.

Chronic disease has two true causes: toxemia and demineralization. Toxemia is an accumulation of spiritual, emotional, mental and physical-waste-mucus residues in the organism. Demineralization is a lack of major minerals (i.e. calcium, magnesium, sulfur, potassium, iron, iodine, etc.) and trace minerals (zinc, selenium, manganese, copper, etc.)

To combat disease by attempting to destroy germs is an incorrect approach. Germs are found everywhere; they enter and exit the body all the time; every day. They co-exist symbiotically with the human body. Only when the human body is toxic and demineralized do germs become threatening. As the saying goes: "The microbe is nothing, the terrain is everything."

Chemical drugs and medicines do not heal, they only cause harm. All chemical drugs and medicines, with the exception of aspirin, have been (and still are) tested on innocent animals. Remember the foundational law? Things produce after their own kind. The torture and suffering of animals in useless attempts to find cures for diseases does no good, actually it can only do bad — it only produces more of its own kind: more torture and suffering...more disease.

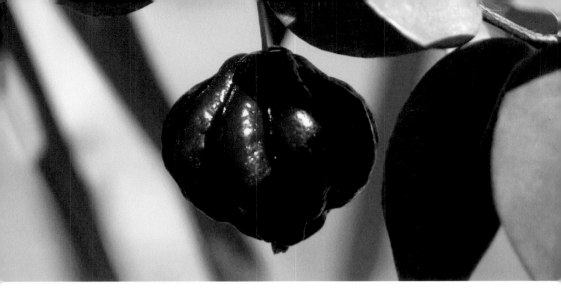

If you find yourself suddenly aware of new food choices grabbing hold of you, then please throw a fruit and raw-food party and experience the best day ever!

True therapeutics involves releasing the power within each person to heal. It is not the disease that must be stopped, but the poisoning of the body by an unhealthy lifestyle. For a complete healing to take place, the body must experience: laughter, love, joy, fresh spring water, fresh air, mineral-rich nutrients, yogic movement and a new-found desire to learn and keep the mind active.

Relaxation is also a factor in overcoming disease. More people die on Monday morning than on any other day of the week or at any other time. Stress accelerates illness as it causes the eliminative organs and the muscular system to constrict and hold onto toxicity and metabolic waste. Stress also causes us to use up certain minerals such as calcium, magnesium and zinc more rapidly. A proper diet will help immensely as certain foods (such as green-leafy vegetables) help to remineralize and open up constricted muscles, and certain other foods (such as juicy fruits) help to flush out the toxicity.

The emphasis here with diet is on removing the physical residue, on cleansing through proper diet. Once the physical body (the anchor) is put in tune — all the other bodies (mental, emotional, spiritual) line up and begin to cleanse as well. It is simple. It is real. It works.

A pure raw-plant diet assists the body's cleansing efforts in the most natural way by eliminating any toxicity from entering the system and by simultaneously moving toxicity through the lymph and blood and out of the body through the eliminative organs (the bowels, kidneys, liver, skin, sinuses and lungs). A purification of the diet enforces a self-healing and a radical, whole-body rejuvenation.

As you apply the health and diet system in this book, you may find that the common cold, flus, fever, grogginess, etc., are all actually efforts by the body to eliminate physical waste; they are symptoms of a body in the process of healing itself. When you have mastered this health and diet system, you will have overcome the major illnesses. You will no longer experience colds, flus, fevers, etc. They will all be looked at as part of a past and unusual way of life.

Enzymes

"ENZYMES ARE SUBSTANCES THAT MAKE LIFE POSSIBLE. THEY ARE NEEDED FOR EVERY CHEMICAL REACTION THAT TAKES PLACE IN THE HUMAN BODY. NO MINERAL, VITAMIN, OR HORMONE CAN DO ANY WORK WITHOUT ENZYMES. OUR BODIES, ALL OUR ORGANS, TISSUES, AND CELLS ARE RUN BY METABOLIC ENZYMES." — *Dr. Howell, Enzyme Nutrition*

Enzymes are vital to all life processes. They are catalysts for all reactions in the body. They are a counterpoint to the vital Sun energy in the body — they are transformers directed by hormones amongst a terrain of vitamins, minerals, carbohydrates, fats and tissue proteins.

There are three classes of enzymes:
- **metabolic**
- **digestive**
- **food**

Metabolic enzymes operate in all the cells, tissues, and organs and are an essential part of every biological activity.

Digestive enzymes are produced by, and appear in, the alimentary organs. They help digest carbohydrates, fats and proteins. Amylases are enzymes that digest carbohydrates. Lipases are enzymes that digest fats. Proteases are enzymes that digest proteins.

Food enzymes come enclosed with all whole raw foods in their proper proportions. These enzymes are there to help digest the food (or to help ripen or decompose the food if it is not eaten). Many food enzymes are destroyed at 118 degrees Fahrenheit (47.8 degrees Celsius). The dehydration of food below 104 degrees Fahrenheit (40.0 degrees Celsius) does keep most enzymes intact. Freezing and refrigeration hinders enzymatic activity. Freezing food destroys at least 30% of its enzymes and can destroy up to 66% or more of its enzymes. Fermented raw foods, including seed cheeses and raw sauerkraut, have a very high enzymatic activity and thus they have been used by natural health pioneers, such as Doctor Ann Wigmore, to accelerate healing and disease recovery.

Food enzyme shortages, sooner or later, result in physical degeneration and disease. When the digestive enzymes present in the body are insufficient, the body draws upon its reserves of metabolic enzymes from the major and minor organs and glands, weakening one's overall vitality. It takes ten metabolic enzymes to form one digestive enzyme.

Just because the dangerous effects of cooked and processed foods are not felt immediately does not mean they are not damaging. Humans have not adapted to cooked food in the way people assume. How can an animal, such as a field mouse, that has never eaten cooked food in its genetic history, be captured, fed cooked food and still live? Did it instantaneously adapt to cooked food? Just because one can chew up something, swallow it and live long enough to tell others about it, does not mean one has adapted to it. White bread, for example, has only been around for the last 100 years. People eat white bread en masse and they are still alive. Does that mean humans have adapted to white bread? Cooked and processed foods have a cumulative effect on the body. The enzyme potential decreases over time. Once the enzyme potential is diminished beyond a certain threshold, the body wears out and inner vitality is lost.

After presenting a host of evidence demonstrating that all living creatures have a fixed enzyme potential which can be (and usually is) prematurely exhausted, Dr. Howell in **Enzyme Nutrition** writes: "Humans eating an enzyme-less diet use up a tremendous amount of their enzyme potential in lavish secretions of the pancreas and other digestive organs. The result is a shortened lifespan (65 years or less as compared with 100 or more), illness and lowered resistance to stresses of all types, psychological and environmental."

The generational introduction of substances foreign to the organism causes enzymatic adaptations to appear in the digestive fluids even though no struc-tural physiological adaptation occurs. Different races of people throughout the world have developed enzymatic capabilities foreign to other groups in order to help digest their traditional cultural foods. These "enzyme mutations" are the body's way of accommodating itself to foreign food substances.

The enzyme mutation in a northern European person might give her/him an enzymatic capability to metabolize raw cow's milk, whereas a Mediterranean person may lack such an enzyme mutation, but possess an enzymatic ability to metabolize raw goat's milk. This capability would last until the person began to exhaust their enzyme potential. If the person drank the milk pasteurized, or if they over-intoxicated themselves with those substances (even if raw) then, over time, they would greatly weaken their enzyme potential, and no longer be able to tolerate such foods.

Even with enzyme mutations, the excessive intake of animal foods is undesirable to the physiology of the human digestive apparatus. The shape of the teeth, jaw, width of the lips, shape of the cheeks, esophagus, stomach, duodenum, and colon, are not suited for an excessive intake of animal foods (see **Lesson 9: Origins** and **Appendix A**). Enzyme mutations come about as part of the Law of Vital Adjustment outlined by Professor Hilton Hotema in his book **Man's Higher Consciousness**. The body's Vital Adjustment to foreign substances taxes the system and is always accompanied by a Vital Reduction in the body's overall health and energy level. After a degeneration has occurred, the Law of Vital Adjustment can also work in reverse, as foreign substances are eliminated from the body, a Vital Increase occurs; the body is always capable, over time, of re-adjusting to its natural state because the underlying original biological design is still the same.

Genetic enzyme mutations in accordance with the Law of Vital Adjustment caused by generations of unnatural feeding have turned the human digestive fluids into an anomaly in Nature. The enzymatic activity in the human mouth and digestive system is far out of sync with anything in Nature.

Consider again the writings of Dr. Howell, in his landmark work **Enzyme Nutrition**: "The digestive enzymes of civilized humans are infinitely stronger and more concentrated in enzyme activity than any of the metabolic enzymes — more concentrated than any other enzyme combination found in nature. Human saliva and pancreatic juice are loaded with enzyme activity. There is no evidence that wild animals, living on natural raw diets, have digestive enzyme juices even remotely approaching the strength of those found in civilized human beings."

Dr. Howell has demonstrated, through what he calls The Law of Adaptive Secretion of Digestive Enzymes (a manifestation of the Law of Vital Adjustment), that animals eating raw diets have no enzymes in their saliva, but they begin to when fed a heat-treated diet. Dogs taken away from their natural raw diet and put on a cooked-food diet had enzymes show up in the saliva in about a week. The opposite is true as well. When one returns to a natural raw diet, the frenzied enzymatic activity in the saliva eventually disappears.

Personal experience and review of some of the enzyme literature including **Don't Dine Without Enzymes** by Viktoras Kulvinskas and Dr. Howell's other enzyme book: **Food Enzymes for Health and Longevity** indicates that allergies to raw foods may be connected with enzymes. Some people are allergic to oranges or strawberries, or some other plant foods. These foods may actually contain enzymes that are like keys that unlock poisons the body has stored in locked "boxes." The allergy is actually a release of a toxicity. If these foods are introduced slowly, and in small amounts, each "box" is opened and a little more toxicity is released. Once all the "boxes" are open, the allergy may simply disappear.

Dr. Howell also uncovered a connection between enzyme deficiencies in the diet (cooked food) and a decrease in brain size and weight. This connection should be clearly understood by those interested in maximum brain performance and in maximizing human potential.

Proper nutrition is the basis of mental power. The nutriment of the brain cells is derived from the blood corpuscles perpetually being pumped into them by the action of the lungs and heart. If the food stream is devoid of enzymes and impure, then the heart valves will be out of gear, the stomach will become disordered, the liver will be corrupted, the lungs will become congested, and the brain will be starved, drugged, and poisoned, while all the thoughts that germinate therein will be inappropriate and out of harmony with the Earth.

Thoughts of failure, world-weariness, morbidity, despair and sorrow are all associated with states of low energy and enzyme depletion in the body caused by eating the wrong food. Low energy deeply affects the state of mind. If every mental disorder is accompanied by a physical disorder (psychosomatic illness), then it must also be true that every physical disorder (enzyme deficiency) is accompanied by a mental disorder (which can be healed by an enzyme-rich diet).

Recommendations For Rapid Results

Before continuing on with more specifics on raw foods and health, I want to provide you with specific foods, juices and recipes to try now so that you may begin getting immediate results. Applying these suggestions demonstrates first-hand how raw plant foods work.

All these foods, juices and recipes help detoxify our bodies while providing us with excellent nutrition. All ingredients should be raw and organic!

For Increased Energy
Blend:
5 oranges
3 tablespoons of flax seed oil

Peel the oranges, but maintain the nutritious white pith. Flax seed oil may be found in any natural food store. Blend the oranges and flax seed oil together. Do not bother removing the orange seeds as they are nourishing and contain anti-fungal qualities. Drink slowly. The fat in the flax oil allows the sugar in the oranges to release slowly over time. This provides excellent energy over several hours. This is a particularly beneficial blend to drink before a business meeting or as a starter in the morning.

For The Flu Or A Cold
Blend:
4 oranges
6 figs
1 medium-sized papaya

Peel the oranges, but maintain the white pith. Remove any stems from the figs (figs should be soft and ripe). Skin the papaya and remove all seeds. Be sure all fruits are at room temperature — putting cold refrigerated food into the body can shock the immune system. Place all items in a blender. Add spring water if necessary to thoroughly blend all ingredients. Drink this blend three times throughout the day; abstain from other foods. Oranges and papayas are alkaline fruits which provide excellent calcium and are rich in vitamin A (beta-carotene) and vitamin C (which, among other things, is an antioxidant). Flus and colds are typically caused by too much toxicity in the body, leading to a weakened immune system. These fruits help cleanse the gastro-intestinal tract of toxicity and simultaneously nourish the body. Figs are especially excellent mucus dissolvers and are ranked with an acid-binding value of 27.81 (one of the highest ratings of any food) in Ragnar Berg's Table in the book **Mucusless Diet Healing System**.

To Alleviate Stress or Anxiety
Juice:
5 leaves of kale
1/2 head of green cabbage
1/2 head of loose-leafed lettuce

Process all ingredients through a juicer. Drink 30 minutes before an event that has you nervous. If stress and anxiety is persistent, drink one juice in the morning, and one in the evening. Kale, green cabbage and loose-leafed lettuces together provide a sodium-potassium balance that keeps us centered. Also, these three contain an abundance of alkaline minerals, especially calcium — which has a calming effect on the body. Lettuces have a soporific quality and can even induce sleep when taken in large quantities.

Or...
Breathing:

Oxygen is a food. Stress and anxiety are associated with shallow breathing. Relieve stress by taking 10 deep breaths in the ratio of 1:4:2 as described in **Lesson 22: Breathing (Pranayama)**, Action Steps.

For A Sore Throat
1/2 lemon
1 tablespoon of fresh ginger juice or raw ginger powder
6 ounces (0.2 liters) of spring water warmed up to 96° Fahrenheit (36° C).

Mix ginger into the water. Squeeze lemon into the mix. Lemon is an excellent cleanser. Ginger works as an antibiotic and an expectorant, helping to relieve the sinus cavities and lungs of mucus. Drink this mix 4-5 times a day until symptoms disappear. The old home remedy also included 2-4 tablespoons of raw honey.

Or, if you are more active, try...
Juice:
3 apples
1 lemon
1 slice of ginger root

Peel the lemon, but maintain the white pith. Put all contents in the juicer. If desired, warm this drink to 96° Fahrenheit (36 C). The apples are "soft" on the throat and provide you with sugar as fuel. Apples also contain pectin, which forms a gel in the intestines that helps remove toxins while simultaneously stimulating a bowel movement. A bowel movement drains the lymph system, allowing lymphatic tissues throughout the body, including the tonsils in the throat, to alleviate any swelling. Drink this juice 3-4 times a day until symptoms disappear.

For A Headache
Juice:
4 ribs of celery
4 ounces of fennel
1 apple
1 orange

Peel the orange, but keep the white pith intact. Process all ingredients through a juicer. Drink immediately. Fennel is a wonderful, cooling, licorice-tasting herb. The ancient Greeks and Romans used fennel to treat migraine headaches. Fennel thins the blood and in women builds healthy hormones (progesterone) which can help balance excessive estrogen. This allows obstructions — which place pressure on the blood vessels (headaches) — to flow on and be removed by the kidneys. Celery and apple are provided to maintain a sodium-potassium balance in the blood. The orange is added for its alkalinity and calcium.

For Back Pain
Juice:
1 head of dark-leaf lettuce
1 head of broccoli
2 apples

Process all contents through a juicer. Drink once in the morning, once in the evening. Back pain is associated with a high level of sodium (salt) and phosphorus (acid) in the tissues. The high calcium content of the lettuce and broccoli immediately loosens constricted tissues. The high potassium content of this drink provides a mineral balance against sodium. The apple is provided to sweeten.

Or...
Salad:
1 head of lettuce
1 large collard leaf
1/4 head of green cabbage
1 ounce (30 ml) of organic stone-crushed, cold-pressed extra virgin olive oil
1-2 avocados
10 strawberries

Mix together and toss into a salad. Eat this salad twice each day: once for lunch, once for dinner. The high-calcium content of green-leafed vegetables loosens constricted tissues. Most back pain is associated with an acid condition of the body — calcium counteracts and neutralizes acidity. The strawberries are included because they contain organic salicylates, which are the basic ingredient of painkillers, such as aspirin.

For An Upset Stomach Or Ulcer
Juice:
1/2 head of green cabbage
2 ribs of celery
2 apples

Cabbage is rich in beta-carotene, vitamin C, sulfur, selenium and especially the amino acid glutamine. Studies done by Dr. Garnet Cheney, who at one time headed the Cancer Division of Stanford Medical School, revealed the value of glutamine in healing ulcers. Dr. Cheney administered 1 quart (1 liter) of cabbage/celery/carrot juice a day to 65 ulcer sufferers. Within 3 weeks 63 of the patients were healed and 2 retained only minimal symptoms. I learned this one from Jay Kordich "The Juiceman" and have recommended it with success to many people over the years.

Or...
Salad:

1/2 head of green cabbage
1/2 head of purple cabbage
2 small avocados

Dice up the cabbage. Mix in the avocados. The sweet fat of the avocado is very soothing on the delicate mucous linings of the stomach and intestines.

Constipation

Constipation is caused by fecal matter that collects in the colon, dries out and is difficult to move. Constipation indicates that a person has been eating too many cooked foods which are devoid of water and too few raw oils which lubricate the digestive tract. To prevent constipation in the future, drink plenty of high quality water with lemon and a mineral-rich salt when the stomach is empty, also eat chlorophyll-rich fibrous foods (green vegetables) with oil (flax seed, olive, etc.) as a dressing. This will softly broom and sweep the intestines alleviating this condition. Apples and pears may be added to help stimulate a bowel movement.

If suffering from constipation, try the following:
Lemon Water:
1 quart (liter) of spring water
1 lemon
2-3 pinches of unheated sea salt or rock salt

Constipation may be caused by dehydration. This may be brought on by stress, overexertion or overexposure. Eating too much sugar can cause excessive urination and lead to dehydration and constipation. Drinking 3/4 to 1 quart (liter) of spring water containing the juice of 1 whole lemon with salt the first thing in the morning can stimulate a bowel movement and alleviate this condition.

Or...
Juice:
2 handfuls of parsley
4 ribs of celery
2 apples
1 pear

Process all contents through a juicer. If the constipation is more difficult, drink 12 ounces of this green-leafy vegetable juice first thing in the morning. Add more parsley to this mix if constipation persists.

For A Hangover
Juice:
1 head of romaine lettuce
1 stalk of broccoli
1 handful of spinach

Process all ingredients through a juicer. Drink immediately. Alcohol destroys the B vitamins. Romaine lettuce, broccoli and spinach contain excellent quantities of the B complex, including thiamine (B1), riboflavin (B2), niacin (B3), pantothenic acid (B5), pyridoxine (B6) and folic acid (B9). I used to be quite a "social drinker" before I became a raw-foodist. As I began eating significant quantities of raw foods, I no longer would feel hangovers after a night of drinking with friends.

Or...
Fruit:
1 cantaloupe

Eat one whole cantaloupe. Cantaloupe is, overall, the richest fruit in B vitamins. Remember to buy organic foods and eat all the way to edge of the rind to get the maximum nutrition available in the fruit. Melons contain most of their vitamins and minerals near the edge of the rind.

Boost The Immune System
Juice:
2 cloves of garlic
1 slice of ginger
1 handful of parsley
4 pears
1 ounce (30 ml) of organic stone-crushed,
cold-pressed, extra virgin olive oil

Process all ingredients through a juicer, except for olive oil, which can be stirred in with a spoon, or blended into the juice. Garlic and ginger are natural antibiotics that assist the immune system. Parsley is rich in iron to build strong red-blood corpuscles. Pear contains pectin which will stimulate a bowel movement, helping to drain the lymphatic system of toxins. Olive oil provides excellent monounsaturated fats the body needs to build strong white blood corpuscles. In my own diet, I include a habanero pepper in my immune system juice, you may want to try adding some hot pepper.

For Depression
Fruit:
Berries

To break a bout of depression, eat one or more trays of berries in the morning for breakfast daily for 5-6 weeks. Eat them on an empty stomach and avoid other foods until 12 noon. Berries are an incredibly balanced food and their moderate sugar content does not jar the nerves. Spells of depression are often associated with moments of low blood sugar and poor food choices. Eat mildly-sweet fruits such as berries throughout the day to keep the blood sugar up. If one is too sensitive to sugar or fruit, one can eat combinations of seeds (pumpkin, hemp) and vegetables to maintain energy without stimulating the body with sugars. Avoid dried fruit binging, complex carbohydrates (baked potatoes, french fries, breads, cakes, cookies, rice) and alcohol as these can cause erratic blood sugar fluctuations.

Consuming 300-600 milligrams of algae oil (DHA) could also be helpful in nourishing neurological tissue. Vitamin B12 is helpful for depression as well.

THE SUNFOOD DIET

1 Begin today by treating yourself to luscious fruits and beautiful salads. Eating raw foods has a cumulative effect. The more raw foods you eat over time, the better you feel. The ess cooked foods you eat, the better you feel. Do your best to increase your raw food intake and specifically decrease your cooked food intake each day. Visit a raw-food restaurant!

2 Cut out five cooked foods from your diet today. List them in your journal. Notice the difference this decision makes in your life. Become more discerning in your food choices.

3 Seek out a source for organic (pest cide-free), mineral-rich foods. Support organic farmers by purchasing their higher-quality foods.

4 Invest in a juicer for you and your family.

5 Invest in one or more raw-food recipe books.

6 Check out our web-site at:

   www.davidwolfe.com
   ...and peruse the latest and greatest goodies in the field of raw food!

   Special Note: Raw plant foods (from herbs to fruits and everything in between) are the single most effective antidote to anxiety, depression, disease, fear, immobility, insomnia, pain, stress and worry!

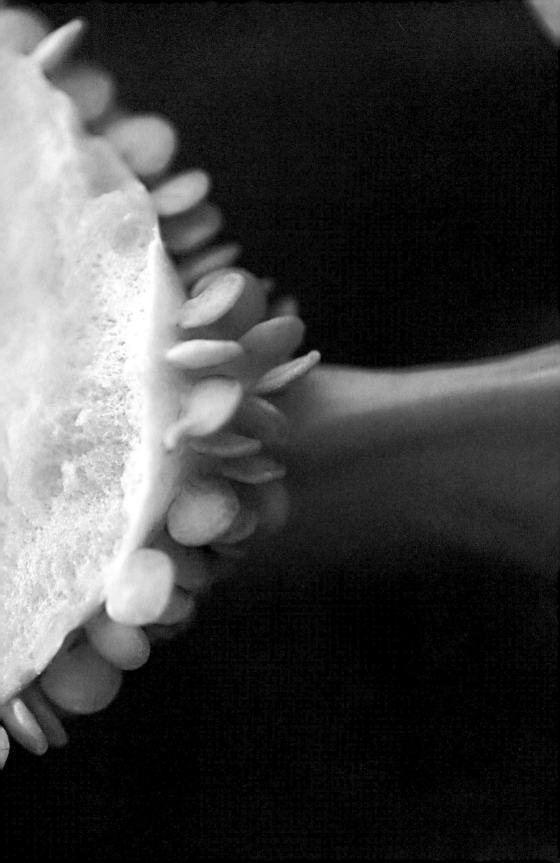

8

FOOD AND KARMA

Things don't just happen, things happen which are just. The universe is governed by a karmic law.

Karma is the total effect of an individual's actions and conduct during the successive phases of existence. The greater karmic forces include:
1. Individual karma
2. Past-life karma
3. Collective karma

All the things we have done or have not done in our lives add up to form our karma. Karma is energy. Your karma is what we actually are. What we are is all the thoughts and emotions we have released into eternity up until right now. Life is a mirror that magnifies. What we see out there is only a duplication of what we are inside. The vibrations we send forth are magnified by life and returned to us.

As we have discovered in **Lesson 3: Thoughts Are Things**, thoughtfulness is a key attribute of super-success. The most thoughtful people draw all "effects" back to their "causes." They take full responsibility. They are aware of the karma associated with their thoughts and actions.

If we involve ourselves in the pursuit of discordant desires, then truly a karmic web is woven to capture us. We place our lives in jeopardy by our own discordant passions, pursuits and blind ignorance of cause and effect.

A tremendous amount of destruction is caused by negative emotions and attitudes directly resulting from the karmic consequences of taking in negative karma (energy) through food.

Genesis 9:4 states: "But flesh with the life thereof, which is the blood thereof, shall ye not eat." Leviticus 3:17 describes: "It shall be a perpetual statute for your generations throughout all your dwellings that ye eat neither [animal] fat nor blood." Throughout history, many great religious leaders, spiritual teachers, yogis and many of the world's religions have recommended a vegetarian diet, and they have done this for a good reason. The karmic consequences of haphazardly eating animals without appreciation and respect diminishes the spiritual powers while raising the emotions of fear and doubt in the mind.

If one exploits the animals and the Earth — the subtler truths of life will remain hidden — that is the fact, simple as that. The enslavement, torture and death of animals for food, leather, wool, cosmetics, toiletries, down, medicine, etc. is leading humanity's fate to an ever-more perilous position. The mass destruction and exploitation of animal life is causing chaos in the spiritual world. Every animal exploited leaves a karmic ripple in the fabric of time that must eventually return back.

We should take only enough for our needs, otherwise the plants and the animals we have harmed would turn against us and cause us disease and misfortune. A thoughtful person is aware of this and strives to appease them, so that when the opportunity arises, the plants and trees, the worms and birds, and the rabbits and coyotes will send forth a positive vibration to help that person along.

In his book **Diet For A New America**, John Robbins describes in detail the correlation between eating animal foods and disease. Heart disease, the number one killer in the United States, is directly attributable to eating animal fat and protein. The incidence of cancer has been statistically correlated to the consumption of animal-derived foods. Colon cancer and other diseases of the digestive tract are directly related to the overconsumption of animal foods and the underconsumption of raw plant foods. Environmental toxins accumulate in animals, especially in animal fats. All the toxins being poured into the atmosphere end up being collected in the tissues of animals. Eating those animals, whether they be insect, fish, or mammal, will give one a strong dose of toxins. In his book, Robbins mentions that meat contains 14 times the pesticide level that an equivalent amount of commercial plant food would contain; dairy products contain 5 1/2 times as much. The more animals people eat, the more likely they are to experience all sorts of health problems. That is a fact. The opposite is true as well. The more raw plant foods people eat, the more likely they are to experience all sorts of health benefits.

Some intellectual types have forwarded the argument that plants actually have a higher consciousness than animals and should therefore not be eaten. What this argument does not understand is that animals are simply transformed plants, thus eating animals brings along with it the karma of the plants they have eaten, plus their own karma. For karmic purposes, one does not have to kill plants, but instead simply eat their leaves, fruits and the other edible portions that do not harm the plant. In the case of leaves, many times a plant thrives better when its leaves are trimmed, and this actually associates a slightly positive karma to eating those leaves.

What I have discovered from my experience in the field of the raw-vegetarian lifestyle is that the whole question of carnivorism, omnivorism, vegetarianism, veganism, raw-foodism and fruitarianism comes down to dietary fat. Good wholesome fat in our foods, not just protein, is essential to good health and longevity (as we shall discover in **Lesson 11: The Secret Revealed**).

Fatty foods are associated with strong karma. Humans could be primarily frugi-vores when they derive their fat from fruit (or other plant sources). Humans could be omnivores when they derive their fat from animal sources. The truth is: we have been given a choice. I find that fascinating. The whole question is: From where are you going to get your fat? Which fat source has the least side-effects and is the most natural to eat? Of course, fatty fruits — the magic ingredient of The Sunfood Diet. For ethical, karmic and health reasons, I recommend you get most of your dietary fat from fruits, such as avocados, Sun-ripened olives, durians or olive oil (hemp seed might also be considered a fruit here as it is the only seed that does not contain enzyme inhibitors).

Fatty fruits have the most positive karma of all foods aside from mother's milk. All fruits with viable seeds have a positive karma. Green-leafy vegetables have a neutral energy associated with them. Hybridized or seedless fruits have a slightly negative karma, because their reproductive purpose has been eliminated.

Hybridized vegetables (carrots, beets, potatoes) have a negative karma asso-ciated with them (more details will be given on hybrid foods in **Lesson 16: Hybrid Food**). Not only are carrots, beets and potatoes hybrids and not capable of growing wildly, but also they are roots that, if eaten, are typically killed. (Special note: the nubs at the top of carrot and beet roots should not be eaten or juiced as they contain enzyme inhibitors; if these nubs are planted, they may root and the plant could survive).

Consider the following chart (on the opposite page). Use the chart to increase the karma of your daily meals. By following the chart to guide your food choices, you will be eating neutral karma foods daily to stay grounded. Between positive and negative karma foods is the area of the green-leafy vegetables. When one wishes to pass negative karma foods into a positive karma body, one must pass through the area of the green-leafy vegetables (eat negative karma foods with green-leafy vegetables). As long as the overall karma of each day's meals is positive you will begin to attract beautiful events and experiences into your life.

The level of the food on the chart from positive, neutral, and negative corre-sponds to the energy (positive, neutral or negative) of the karmic seed planted by eating that food. Raw foods have more karma than cooked foods. Cooking actually degrades energy and moves both positive and negative karmic foods to a more neutral level. Cooking degrades the energy in food and mitigates

POSITIVE KARMA

Mother's breast milk

Fatty fruits

Dehydration

Sweet fruits

Non-sweet fruits

Raw plant foods prepared with Love

Greens picked by the leaf

Seaweeds

Onion and garlic bulb *(root-ball viable)*

Milk given freely

Neutral Karma

Flowers

Greens picked by killing plant *(green sprouts)*

Onion and garlic bulb *(root-ball killed)*

Hybrid seeds *(rice, wheat, legumes)*

Coconut

Tree nuts

Seeds

Hybrid roots *(carrots, beets, potatoes)*

Eggs, insects, fish

Cooking

Milk taken from enslaved animals

Animal muscle

Organ fat

Blood

NEGATIVE KARMA

the karma. That is why people are better off, for karmic purposes, eating cooked flesh, than raw flesh and worse off eating dehydrated fruits than raw fruits. Cooking animal foods introduces a mitigating factor which disrupts and delays the karmic consequences, but eating animal flesh raw is not only dangerous, it has more intense karmic consequences.

Many people have adopted vegetarian and vegan lifestyles, yet they still face health challenges because they have not grasped the distinction of "Sun-cooked" versus oven-cooked food. By cooking food energy is degraded. By switching to The Sunfood Diet (a wide variety of raw plant foods) they will experience higher levels of health, happiness and harmony.

Fruit

> "WITH ALL THE TIME THAT HUMANS HAVE BEEN AROUND, I CAN'T
> BELIEVE THE EARTH IS NOT COVERED WITH FRUIT TREES YET!"
> — *Steve Adler, raw-foodist, alchemist*

Aside from mother's milk, fruit is the only food which possesses a powerful positive karma. "Only fruits make you pure in thought, word, and deed." Fruits deserve special attention.

Fruits are the glowing visions of the plants and trees. All other things being equal, a diet rich in fruit is most conducive to the completeness of bodily development and perfectness of symmetry and beauty.

Even the Eskimos eat fruit! Berries — especially blueberries — grow abundantly in and around the tundra areas of the far north.

Eat wild fruits. Give fruits away. Send positive affirmations out to everyone you find before you each day. Compliment them. It will help them out immensely and it will come back to you in many positive ways as well.

Fruit vibrates at a frequency to attract our attention. Fruit is the means trees have invented for traveling from one place to another. When you are attracted to, and eat, fruits, occasionally a seed will be carried within you to a fertile ground. Fruits are the pregnant embryos of the trees.

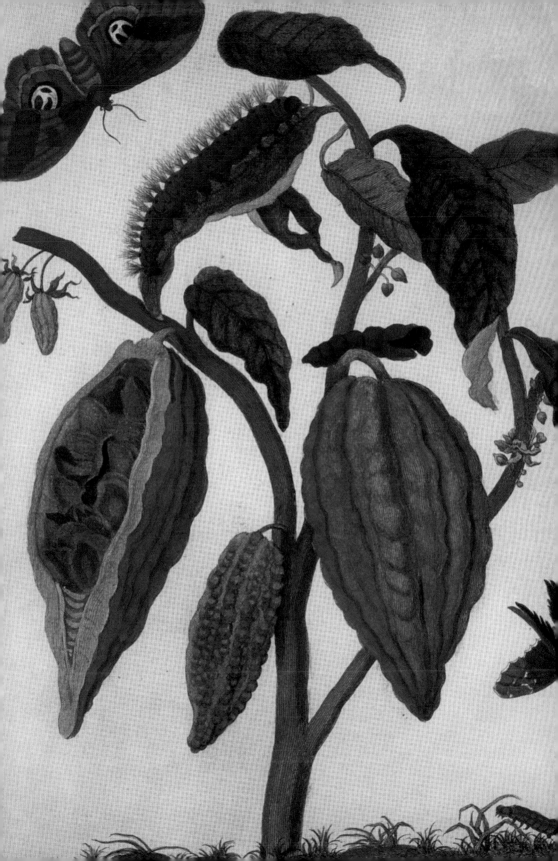

NATURE'S MASTER PLAN

Invest your Life
In every fruit,
Whose secret is unknown.
Your destiny
You shall see
In the fruit trees you have grown.

Eat the fruit and launch it far,
Out the window of a car!
Spread more Life,
As much as you can:
Fulfill Nature's master plan.

Our fate is aligned:
With the fruit of the vine,
With the fruit of the tree,
With fruit that grows
Next to the sea.

Love your food,
It all begins
With a fruit seed simply sown.
Nothing by chance;
It's a reflected dance of
Fruit seeds that you've thrown.

Fruit is your food —
Dispel each myth.
Align your fate, entwine it with:
Sumptuous fruit,
The deepest tan.
Fulfill Nature's master plan.

A fruit tree,
For those who see,
Is greater than any throne.
Its enchanting wealth
Can't be found
In any castle made of stone.

Fruit reveals the truth:
It frees the best in you.
Doing what you do best
Is best for Nature too!

Fun and family,
Life without need,
Spreading the vibrant, vital seed.
This is Life, at its most.
Bring enchantment to every coast.

Propagate fruit
Far and wide.
Let Earth flower
On every side.

Take the seed
And hurl it far,
'Till it reach
The farthest star.

A call to you
As woman, man:
Fulfill Nature's master plan.

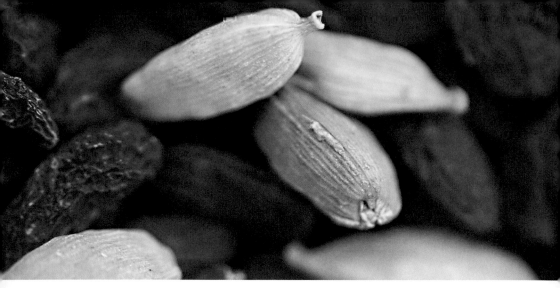

An unlikely combination of goji berries and cardamom —
each contains dozens of viable seeds.

Karmic Sense

This world is meant to be, among other things, a sanctuary for all forms of wildlife. It is my duty as a Sunfoodist to protect, preserve and defend all animals and plants, making no exceptions. I have personal convictions to uphold. All creatures are here with us as companions. Loving innocent life is a high frequency of being. The Jain religion tells us, "Harmlessness is the supreme religion."

Every chicken killed, every calf stripped away from its mother, every fish plucked from its school, every monkey tortured in a cage is a burden of pain upon total humanity and weighs heavy on the karmic scales.

The factory-farming techniques of present-day civilization have created a frightening karmic debt and health danger for anyone still consuming flesh foods — especially if eaten raw. Factory-farmed animals are injected with, sprayed with, and fed antibiotics, artificial hormones, chemicals of all kinds, and genetically-modified foods; these toxins are present in the flesh when the animals are slaughtered; they are passed directly into the body of the flesh consumer. Factory-farmed animals are kept in darkness and squeezed together in inhospitable cages. They are fed the most outrageous and unnatural foods imaginable. In the book, **Mad Cowboy**, former cattle rancher, Howard Lyman details that mad cow disease stems from the feeding concoctions of dead cows and other animals in the factory farms to the living cows. When those living cows are slaughtered and eaten, they pass the mad cow disease on to humans.

When one eats the flesh of tortured animals, or the milk of dairy cows, or eggs from factory chickens, one also ingests the fear, the pain, the exhaustion and the sorrow of those beings. These energies manifest within the consumer in the form of negative attitudes, depression and illness.

All the animals one has killed or eaten begin to form an ensnaring trap. Even done unconsciously, it does eventually catch up to us. Going 100% raw-vegan, even if only for a time, has the power to recall the karmic vibrations we have released into the world in ignorance and error (100% raw-vegan means letting go of all animal-derived foods and products from our lives). With deep desire we can correct our errors and throw off our past mistakes.

Just as you cannot make others happy while being unhappy, one cannot heal while inflicting hurt. Hurting animals to try and find a way to heal only inflicts pain, and never heals anything. This exposes the logical fraud of animal experimentation (vivisection).

All pharmaceutical medicines and drugs, with the exception of aspirin, are tested on innocent animals (read Hans Ruesch's book **Naked Empress** for information on this subject). Modern technological medicine represents a warfare against life. Pharmaceutical medicines and drugs are always harmful to you, the planet and to innocent animals.

I will not cite animal experiments in this book because I am morally and ethically opposed to them. Animal experimentation (vivisection) is unnatural, unscientific, and always leads to destruction. I feel very strongly on this subject. Animals are beautiful creatures. I have an overwhelming obligation to save as many animals as possible from torture and death.

Once we know that we thrive on a 100% raw-vegetarian diet, then there no longer remains any reason to exploit animals. What incredible knowledge this is!

Eating raw plant food is a guiltless lifestyle. No pollution is created peeling fruit and throwing away vegetable leaves. Little, if any, packaging is thrown away. Little water is used to clean dishes and utensils. No animals are exploited to present delicious foods to us. Eating raw plant food is the only "win-win" dietary solution.

Living without the death of animals weighing on your spirit, increases your aliveness. Your aliveness is reflected in your physical body, which takes on a more perfect beauty and a new type of positive energy.

Every thought sent forth into action is a never ending vibration which whisks its way across the universe bringing us back a magnification of what we sent forth. By fulfilling a natural diet rich in raw plant foods, and by allowing only positive thoughts to govern our minds, only glorious vibrations will emanate from us and all earthly conditions will begin to sway positively in our direction. It is in this way that a new destiny is shaped for our lives.

The Sunfood Diet beautifies the body, mind, emotions and spirit. Following this diet gives you glimpses of life in the state of instant karma: when an idea is thought, it is automatically transformed into actuality. After you adopt The Sunfood Diet, an amazing synchronicity will occur. Seemingly unrelated events will coincide for you to help you along in your growth and enjoyment of life! The more "raw" you are, the more you will experience synchronicity and serendipity. A 100% raw-vegetarian diet maintains you in that state of instant manifestation indefinitely. Remarkable coincidences become common place. Extraordinary circumstances begin occurring daily.

Remember: Virtue is rewarded in this world. Natural Law makes no false judgments. The karmic scales of all our deeds are constantly being weighed out. The universe is governed by laws — even if we do not know what they are. A true coincidence does not exist; everything happens for a reason.

FOOD AND KARMA

1 Set a goal to adopt a vegetarian diet. Decide to let go of animal-based foods. Start by going one day without flesh foods (i.e. no chicken or fish), then go three days, then five days. Simultaneously eat more green-leafed vegetables, juicy fruits and avocados. If you really need motivation, visit a slaughterhouse.

2 Next, set a goal to adopt a vegan lifestyle. The vegan lifestyle makes choices for foods, clothing and other items that are not derived from animal sources.

3 Make a record in your journal of everything you eat in one week. You can start today and record everything you eat this week. Compare your food choices to the Food And Karma chart. Where is your overall balance? Are you developing a positive karma based on your food choices?

4 Read John Robbins' book **Diet For A New America**, Howard Lyman's book **Mad Cowboy**, and Jeremy Rifkin's book **Beyond Beef**. If you have teenage children, have them read the book **Fast Food Nation** by Eric Schlosser.

5 Dedicate some time in your schedule to enjoying cats, dogs, rabbits, birds and other animals. Discover the truth behind vivisection (animal experimentation). Watch the video **Lethal Medicine**.

6 Keep in mind that karmic energy may be balanced in other ways than from eating. Planting produces favorable karma. If one eats coconuts, tree nuts and seeds, one should also plant coconuts, tree nuts and seeds to balance the karma. Consider donating to or becoming a member of our non-profit Fruit Tree Planting Foundation **(www.fruittreefoundation.org or www.ftpf.org)** an organization founded to plant 18 billion fruit trees on the Earth!

THE CELESTINE LAW

A celestial being,
A cosmic seeing.
New vision of Life
Now grasped;
False views of Life
Now dashed.
The glow of eye
Then seen,
The when, how, why
So keen.
The secret in this time
Revealed:
We choose which destiny
To wield.
For what you give out
Comes back!

.

Something has been
Keeping track.
Lest we should
Ever forget
What you give is
What you get.
When you throw off
The karma inside,
By giving more
Than you can hide,
Your life-force
Will grow ever stronger,
And you may even live
A little longer!
Remember this secret,
So true,
And you will see Life anew.

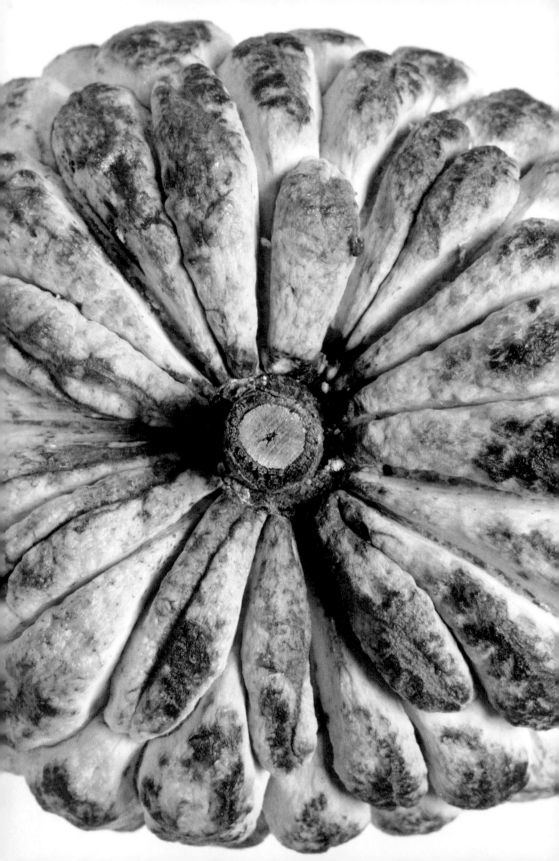

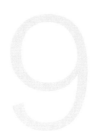

ORIGINS

EVOLUTION: A Monkey's Perspective
(Author Unknown)

"Three monkeys sat in a coconut tree
Discussing things as they are said to be.
Said one to the others: "Now listen, you two
There's a rumor around that can't be true,
That man descended from our noble race.
The very idea is a great disgrace.

No monkey has ever deserted his wife,
Starved her babies, and ruined her life.
And you've never known a mother monk,
To pass her babies on to another,
Till they scarcely knew who is their mother.

Here's another thing a monkey won't do:
Go out at night and get on a stew,
Or use a gun or club or knife,
To take some other monkey's life.
Yes, man descended, the ornery cuss,
But brother, he didn't descend from us."

Introduction

Life is a mystery, so grand, so vast.
Origins are hidden, deep in the past.
Worn out, eroded,
Are they
Hopelessly unsuited?
Nothing is more fantastic,
Is anything more farfetched
Than slates of fossil stone
Which reality once etched?

Any philosophy of diet leads, typically, to a philosophy of human origins. It seems reasonable that the diet humanity originated on, should be the diet that best suits us or at least point us in the correct direction. From research and experience we see that primitive diets do actually work because they are simpler, more natural and the body has less confusion to contend with. Primitive peoples have more robust jaws and more beautiful teeth, which is reflective of their superior diet. But even primitive diets do have their limits. They contain cooked foods and animal foods that will only allow consciousness to reach a certain level within a certain parameter of positive energy.

Some argue that humans have actually adapted through evolution to cooked foods and animal foods, yet the thousands of gastro-intestinal and related diseases (which do not afflict natural creatures eating their natural diet) are positive proof that humanity's food choices have not been optimal.

This lesson challenges many of the false assumptions underlying the theory of evolution. It exposes some of the dangers of "raw-food evolutionary diets" and "paleolithic diets" and describes that these diets, like all diets, have their faults. With the theory of evolution proved faulty, all dietary systems based upon it must be reevaluated.

This lesson demonstrates that the form, function and food choices of every plant and animal are not primarily determined by evolution or adaptation over time. But that each organism has a form, function and food category ordained by design. When we humans follow our dietary design, the results are extraordinary.

This lesson also demonstrates concepts in lateral thinking and may be particularly interesting for those of a "success consciousness" who are always looking for unique intellectual angles and ways to think things differently. Understanding this lesson is not entirely necessary to succeed with The Sunfood Diet. Those who find the information here to be less than essential may move forward to **Lesson 10: Detoxification**.

Those who choose to study this lesson will find that many scientists and researchers have shattered the glass towers of evolution where hypotheses are based on hypotheses and fact and fiction are mingled in an ever-deeper confusion... the evidence of which I present.

Objectivity?

The challenge presented to all explorers of the microcosm and macrocosm is not to confuse the observed with the mind of the observer, not to construct a picture of external reality, which is only a mirror of the thinker. Can this challenge be overcome?

No one could accurately describe what happened on planet Earth yesterday, let alone what happened 100,000 years ago! History books and media consist of what is believed to have happened in the past, not of what actually happened in the past.

The whole field of darwinism/evolution is based on the critical assumption that life is shaped by the outer environment. This generated the sociology of "the environment" as determining the character of living beings. And yet, in a pure sense, what is life? Life is the unfolding of the inner potential. Potential is fulfilled by action, just as a seed, with its inward certainty of bursting life and future fruit generation, is fulfilled by action through water, soil and Sun. The environment does not determine the inner potential — it can only help or hinder its expression. The physical world of Nature is in reality the materialization of the inner spiritual potential of all living things. The inner world creates the outer world (**Lesson 1: The Principle Of Life Transformation**).

Science Or Philosophy?

"As the creation myth of scientific naturalism, darwinism
plays an indispensable ideological role in the war
against fundamentalism. For that reason, the scientific
organizations are devoted to protecting darwinism
than testing it, and the rules of scientific investigation
have been shaped to help them succeed."
— *Phillip Johnson, Darwin On Trial*

Today's one-sided, fatalistic science includes philosophical deductions that are not science and are not supported empirically. The scientific observation of the world is simply empirical study. However, today's science implicitly contains philosophical deductions (loaded with ideas about the ultimate existential meaning of the universe, such as notions of how life began, what life is, etc.) not supported by empirical proof.

For example, implicit in darwinism is the "common ancestor" idea, which sounds great to a materialistic mind, but is not supported by the fossil record. The common ancestor idea contains science (quantifiable similarities between species) and the philosophical deduction that they share a common ancestor — which has not empirically been shown.

Utilitarianism?

There is no evidence that the Earth's biological history or "evolution" (as it has been termed) is a mechanical process of increasing fitness and utility over time.

What of "survival of the fittest"? The philosopher Nietzsche pointed out that survival of the fittest happens, but is meaningless most of the time, because the vast majority of organisms do not fight, do not kill for food and do not compete for territory in such a way that cause competitors to die out.

The utilitarian aspect of the darwinian theory is quite subjective. The utility of an "adaptation" is relative to the use sought to be made of it. A species without feathers has no need of feathers. A feather which gradually evolves would be a positive disadvantage over the "millions of years" necessary to perfect the feather. Furthermore, how did this process start? For an "adaptation" to be utile, it must be ready; while it is being prepared, it is inutile. But if it is inutile, it is not darwinian, for darwinism says evolution is utilitarian.

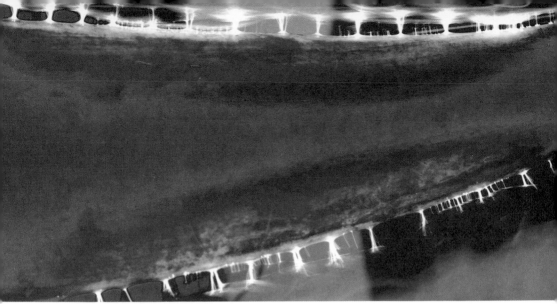

Can evolution explain <u>every</u> aspect of every food? Observe the stunning color, energy, chemistry and power revealed in this Kirlian photo of aloe vera.

Why is it that the "lower" forms (e.g. the horseshoe crab), those which are simpler (less fit?) have not died out, and have not yielded to the principle of evolution? They remain in the same form they have had for vast expanses of the fossil record. Why do they not "evolve" into something "higher?"

The Fossil Record

The most conclusive refutation of evolution is furnished by paleontology. Simple probability indicates that fossil records can only be test samples. Each sample, then, should represent a different stage of evolution/adaptation, and there ought to be "transition types," not particularly of one species or another. Instead, what we find, in the actual fossil record, are genus forms (a genus is a collection of related organisms usually including several species) that have not developed themselves on the fitness principle, but appear suddenly and at once in their definite shape; that do not thereafter evolve towards better adaptation, but become rarer or finally disappear, while quite different forms arise again.

The mathematician Mandelbrot in his casebook **The Fractal Geometry of Nature** (about Chaos theory) describes two types of quantity variations recognizable in Nature:

    1. *The Joseph Effect.* This means persistence: despite an underlying

randomness, the longer a quantity grouping has experienced a condition, the likelier it is to experience more of that same condition. The Joseph Effect means that a certain genus of species, despite erratic conditions, may persist through countless eons, essentially unchanged.

2. *The Noah Effect.* This means discontinuity: when a quantity changes, it can change arbitrarily fast. Quantities can change instantaneously. They do not pass through all intervening points on their way from one point to another. The Noah Effect means that a quantum of species may instantaneously alter form and function.

Consider how Mandelbrot's observations are mirrored by Stephen Gould (quoted from **Darwin On Trial**), developer of the evolutionary "punctuated equilibrium" theory which attempts to explain away the embarrassing fact that the fossil record is devoid of transition types:

"The history of most fossil species includes two features particularly inconsistent with gradualism:

1. *Stasis.* Most species exhibit no directional change during their tenure on earth. They appear in the fossil record looking pretty much the same as when they disappear; morphological change is usually limited and directionless.

2. *Sudden appearance.* In any local area, a species does not arise gradually by the steady transformation of its ancestors; it appears all at once and 'fully formed.'"

All that we see about us impels us to the conviction that again and again profound and extremely sudden changes take place in the forms of living plants and animals. These changes are of a chaotic, cosmic or divine origin and may be beyond human understanding.

Similarly, all active beings (including those reading this now) have striven towards their fulfillment by turning points or "epochs" in their lives — not by gradual evolution. Think about the events of your own life and decide which is a better description: a series of significant turning points or gradual evolution? The origins of the Earth, of life, of the free-moving animals, are such turning points or "epochs" of change.

Quantum physics is telling us things do not change slowly over time — they make quantum leaps. We jump from one level of experience to another.

Evolutionists never demonstrate what a smooth transition is — they never define it. A transition of macro-form should be demonstrated somewhere in a long sequence, say 50, 30, or at least 10 successive fossils in transition. Yet, with all the billions of fossils on Earth, no one has met this simple criteria for a fossil sequence.

We also do not find any genetic mistakes (one-shot mutations which failed) in the fossil record which is impossible if random mutation through natural selection (trial and error) is true.

By far the most abundant fossils in the world are the 14 types of ammonites — little shelled snail-like ocean species which, as far as we can tell, have existed essentially since life began on Earth. Literally billions of these fossils have been found, but never have there been discovered any transition types, or smooth transitions, between any of these 14 types.

The first treatise that described that the basic forms of plants and animals did not evolve step-by-step, but were suddenly there, was given by Hugo de Vries in his work **Mutation Theory** in 1886. He described that we can clearly see (through scientific/utility analysis) how the "impressed living form" works itself out in the individual samples, but we cannot see how the "die was cut" for each whole genus. We cannot see how the genus appeared. Origins remain hidden from us.

We cannot ascertain how the Homo genus (Homo habilis, Homo erectus, Homo ergaster, Homo neanderthalis, archaic Homo sapien, Cro-Magnon, Homo sapien, Homo sapien sapien) appeared, yet it was suddenly there in the fossil record.

Evolutionists continue to argue the tired line that humans smoothly transitioned from one form to another, and assume modern Homo sapiens arose merely 100,000 to 200,000 years ago (based on the present questionable dating system). In December 1997, **Discover** magazine reported the findings of a Spanish team working in Gran Dolina, Spain who uncovered an 800,000 year-old skull with remarkably modern features. The discoverer, Juan Luis Arsuaga Ferreras, stated, "It is so surprising we must rethink human evolution to fit that face." Discover magazine stated: "The Gran Dolina face is 800,000 years old and yet distinctively ours. It is almost that of a modern human."

The evidence is showing and will continue to show that all the Homo forms have existed together for thousands — or millions — of years without the gradual evolution through common ancestry concept.

The Homo life-form, like every other, originated in a sudden appearance or mutation (the Germans have the great word w*andlung* meaning "instant trans-formation") of which the "when," "how" and "why" remains a secret. There exists somewhere in the recesses of time a sharp frontier on the hither side of which we see Homo as a completely formed type, endowed with a certain bodily struc-ture, walk and posture that has not materially altered up to the present day. All the ape-like remains (Australopithecus, etc.) and the hominid remains (Homo) found on Earth are still distinctly different, and bridging that gap to find a missing link remains elusive. No missing link can be found. This is because no missing link exists.

The fossil record is actually a liability that must be explained away by evolutionists. Pre-darwinian paleontologists were right on when they cited the lack of intermediaries as a conclusive reason for rejecting biological evolution initially. Stephen Gould has described "the extreme rarity of transitional forms in the fossil record" as "the trade secret of paleontology." Darwin wrote: "Nature may almost be said to have guarded against the frequent discovery of her transitional and linking forms."

Think about it logically, if there were gradual evolution, in the adaptation sense of the word, there could not be specific animal classes, but only a chaos of living singular forms left over from some "struggle for existence." Darwin posed this question to himself: "…why, if species have descended from other species by insensibly fine gradations, do we not everywhere see innumerable transitional forms? Why is not all nature in confusion instead of the species being, as we see them, well defined?" Rupert Sheldrake described the individu-ality of species as determined by individual *chreodes* — each species sits in a chreode or valley that creative Nature settles into amongst the pathway of form outcomes.

Essentially, the species we know today are all stable.

Common Ancestors?

"DARWINISTS ASSUME THAT THE RELATIONSHIP BETWEEN, SAY, BATS AND WHALES IS SIMILAR TO THAT BETWEEN SIBLINGS AND COUSINS IN HUMAN FAMILIES. POSSIBLY IT IS, THE PROPOSITION IS NOT SELF-EVIDENT...WE OBSERVE DIRECTLY THAT APPLES FALL WHEN DROPPED, BUT WE DO NOT OBSERVE A COMMON ANCESTOR FOR MODERN APES AND HUMANS. WHAT WE DO OBSERVE IS THAT APES AND HUMANS ARE PHYSICALLY AND BIOCHEMICALLY MORE LIKE EACH OTHER THAN THEY ARE LIKE RABBITS, SNAKES OR TREES. THE APE-LIKE COMMON ANCESTOR IS A HYPOTHESIS IN A THEORY, WHICH PURPORTS TO EXPLAIN HOW THESE GREATER AND LESSER SIMILARITIES CAME ABOUT. THE THEORY IS PLAUSIBLE, ESPECIALLY TO A PHILOSOPHICAL MATE- RIALIST, BUT IT MAY NONETHELESS BE FALSE. THE TRUE EXPLANATION FOR NATURAL RELATIONSHIPS MAY BE SOMETHING MUCH MORE MYSTERIOUS." — Phillip E. Johnson, Darwin On Trial

Based on the fossil record, the general picture of plant and animal history is a burst of general body forms followed by stasis or extinction. We may hypothesize that relationships between these forms come from common ances- tors, or from ancestors which were transformed by some means other than the accumulation of small mutations or from some process altogether beyond the scope of human understanding at this point.

Neo-darwinism (the present-day evolution philosophy) has chosen the common ancestor idea as the key to understanding the relationship between the great classes of living beings. This is a philosophical deduction based on materialist misconceptions and is not a fact. If neo-darwinists truly wanted to be scientific, they would have to define the common ancestry idea as an empirical fact rather than as a "logical" deduction from material classifications of species.

Primates And Diet

Omnivorous feeding patterns among primates have been used to justify omnivorous eating by humans through evolutionary theories (if chimps eat animal foods and humans evolved from chimps, then humans should eat animal foods). These comparisons are reasonable; but could also be specious, not only

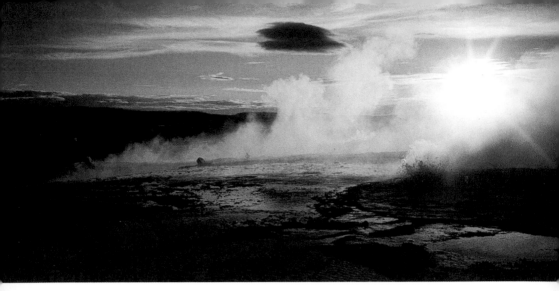

**Who could know or even guess at the great mystery
and majesty that was the ancient Earth?**

because the common ancestry idea is faulty, but because of the objectivity problem.

In his phenomenal book, **L'Homme, Le Singe, Et Le Paradis (Humans, Primates, and Paradise)**, Frenchman Albert Mosseri cites professor Henry Bailey Stevens' insightful observations:

(Translation): "In his study, **Pyramid of Life**, professor Henry Bailey Stevens writes: 'Short term effects appear in tropical monkeys, where humans deranged their natural habitat. Civilization, with its growing demand for monkeys for lab experiments, completely changed their behavior. We must keep that in mind during interpretations. For example, we never saw in the past a monkey kill for food. Now in 1960 Jane Goodall Lawick went on an expedition to live a year with the chimpanzees in Tanzania. The chimpanzees got used to her presence and lost all apprehension. During this period, they had also the occasion to observe her own behavior and diet. They are gifted imitators, so they were able to admire human ingenuity. When she announced that some young chimpanzees in the group killed 4 monkeys, one antelope, and a pig, we saluted this as a scientific contribution. Alas, it was only a deviation due to what our civilization reflected on the chimpanzees.'"

The point here is instructive. Many chimpanzee groups — especially the bonobo chimps (the most genetically similar to humans) — do not engage in hunting behavior. It is equally as likely as any other explanation that the chimpanzees of Gombe (Jane Goodall's research group) and other chimp groups learned their much-publicized killing and meat-eating behavior from humans; probably originally deriving such practices from local human tribes with whom they lived amongst for thousands of years.

Among the more remote anthropoid apes, such as orangutans, we find no hunting behavior. Studies of orangutans have revealed they occasionally eat insects or bird's eggs, but do so initially in their youth out of curiosity and, as adults, due to hunger or specific nutrient needs (i.e. vitamin B12).

Amongst omnivorous eating patterns of some primates we find the folivorous gorilla. No one who looks into a gorilla's eyes — intelligent, gentle, vulnerable — can remain unchanged. Gorillas are a shining example of the raw-plant diet amongst a primate in Nature.

Dr. George Schaller, in his incredible book **Year Of The Gorilla** describes: "I never saw gorillas eat animal matter in the wild — no birds, eggs, insects, mice, or other creatures — even though they had the opportunity to do so on occasion. Once a group passed over a dead duiker without handling the fresh remains, and another time a group nested beneath an olive pigeon nest without disturbing a single egg." Gorillas have been observed to remove insects from vegetation before eating it.

Diet And Evolution?

At its inception, each new genus form is associated with a definite energy and a specific physiological design. Its functioning environment, physical form, social life, physical life (i.e. how to spin a web) and food/fuel choice are pre-determined within a narrow variable range. These are not subject to change and do not (actually cannot) adapt beyond a certain threshold without causing imbalance or illness.

The Homo genus has a specific biological design for food/fuel, as do all other genus forms.

Those who espouse evolutionary diets have as their base tenet the assumption that we have adapted to a specific diet through millennia of certain feeding behaviors. These behaviors vary widely and can never be precisely known. They can only be guessed at, as both frugivorous plant eating and omnivorous feeding teeth-striation patterns have been discovered amongst various fossils in the Homo genus.

To a degree humans have adapted. Enzymatic adjustments or mutations have occurred amongst the different human races to help accommodate foreign foods. For example, Caucasians have the ability to enzymatically breakdown alcohol, whereas Native Americans do not have the enzymes to do so easily (Dr. Bert Vallee and other researchers at Harvard Medical School have isolated 15 different types of alcohol dehydrogenase (ADH) liver enzymes. They discovered that the number and variety of these enzymes vary between individuals and ethnic groups. The number and variety of these "isoenzymes" appear to be genetically controlled).

In spite of enzymatic mutations, amongst all the races, no "macroevolutionary" change has occurred to the human digestive organs (the teeth have not sharpened, the bowels have not de-sulcified and shortened, the liver has not enlarged), even in spite of humanity's recent history of chaotic dietary patterns.

Different races and blood types display patterns of enzyme mutations allowing certain groups to metabolize certain foods, while other groups lack those enzymes. This understanding underlies the blood-type theory. This theory describes that our blood type (of which there are actually more than four different varieties: O, A, B, AB and many other groups and subgroups) exerts a powerful influence on the foods which digest and assimilate well for us. The theory states that Blood type O is for omnivore (an eater of both plant and animal foods).

I am a blood type O and have had no problem eating a 100% raw diet since January 1995, and plant foods only since January 1993. Brian Clement, director of the Hippocrates Health Institute, is a blood type O and has been a vegetarian for over 40 years. Dr. Gabriel Cousens is a blood type O and has been a raw-food vegetarian for over 20 years. There are hundreds of other examples I could site.

In my own experience in counseling people on diet, I have found the suggestions of what foods are agreeable and disagreeable based on one's blood type to be often applicable to cooked foods and rarely applicable to raw foods and raw-food eaters. I have also found that people of blood type A tend to burn sugars (carbohydrates) more slowly and can generally handle more sugars in their diet. People of blood type O tend to burn sugar more rapidly and do better eating less carbohydrates and more fats and/or protein for energy. But these are not rules.

Obviously different blood groups, races, and ethnic groups share different affinities for natural foods (e.g. northern Europeans tend to like green apples, southern Europeans tend to like red apples). Each group has different enzymatic capabilities to digest their traditional cooked staples. So there is a partial truth in the blood-type theory; however, the blood-type theory makes no distinction between raw or cooked foods, nor does it address blood type O's who thrive on a vegetarian, vegan or raw-food diet — indicating a flaw in its reasoning.

If we look closely, we see that eating animal foods (meat, milk, eggs), or ingesting alcohol, requires enzyme mutations present in some groups, and absent in others. This means that these foods were added later in our history on the planet and were not originally present. All the enzymes originally present are still with all of us now and are most amenable to digesting simple plant matter.

As mentioned in **Lesson 7: The Sunfood Diet, Lesson 8: Food And Karma** and **Appendix A**, the structure and function of humanity's dull canines and grinding teeth, the pouchy shape of the lips and cheeks, the elongated digestive canal, the sensitive nature of the sensory organs, the method of nourishment for the young, the pattern of children's development, mental set, emotional feelings, as well as the cause and cure of disease and unhappiness, all demonstrate that humans are biologically and predominantly plant eaters. Humans descend from the natural state into carnivorism when foods, especially fats, are drawn from animal sources (more on this in **Lesson 11: The Secret Revealed**).

Carnivore theorists believe that because an animal can chew something up, swallow it, and live long enough to tell others about it, then that animal is an omnivore. For example, the herbivorous cow has been fed the flesh of other dead cows, mixed in with its feed, for at least a century by the cattle industry. Cows still continue to survive on such food. Yet, an omnivorist would argue that the cow is no longer an herbivore, but is now an omnivore, because it can eat something aside from common grass. Almost any animal, can eat just about any type of so-called "food," and still live, but that does not mean it has "evolutionarily adapted to," or is designed for, that food.

Every natural species can tolerate a vast amount of improper food (fuel). That is why dogs, mice, rats, cats, birds, etc. can tolerate large volumes of denatured, dead and improper food even though they have never seen these types of foods in their genetic history. The cells and tissues composing the anatomy of these organisms always display an amazing degree of resilience, elasticity and buoyancy. However, every living organism can "adapt" itself up to a certain point only, and beyond that point follows illness and degenerative conditions. And every "adaptation" along the way occurs at the expense of a repression of the body's desire to express the inner potential into the outer — each "adaptation" has its price. Professor Hilton Hotema termed this the Law of Vital Adjustment, and later specified it as really the Law of Vital Reduction. This is how the body builds up a tolerance to food and air pollution: the body's eliminative and higher developmental functions must first be weakened before it will submit to inimical foods and environments.

The most amazing thing about human life is that we can discover our form, function, and food choice design and choose to follow it, therefore actualizing the highest potential of our species. That is the purpose of this book. We will discover the specifics of our natural food choice design in **Lesson 11: The Secret Revealed**.

Natural Selection And The Species Boundary

Returning back to the discussion of evolution, we find that natural selection (the primary agent of species creation under the evolutionary theory) is a tautology — it can be made to explain anything. For example, evolutionists claim plant-mimicry among insects is beneficial and will be selected for, but they also claim that warning-warrior colorations, such as insect stripes, are beneficial and will be selected for. Yet if both these hypotheses are true, any kind of coloration on the insect will have some beneficial value and will be selected for. Natural selection cannot make unique predictions, but is used retrospectively to explain everything.

Natural selection, as observed in operation, permits variations only within species boundaries. It operates also to preserve those boundaries. The theory that natural selection has the creative power needed to fuel the changes necessary to turn one species into another is unsupported by the empirical scientific evidence.

The claim of "evolution in action" is simply the observation of local fluctuations of genotypes within a single species. To be more specific, we know certain circumstances favor drug-resistant bacteria as opposed to normal bacteria, or big-beaked birds as opposed to little-beaked birds, or black-peppered moths as opposed to white-peppered moths. In such circumstances, the population of normal bacteria, small-beaked birds and white-peppered gypsy moths may become reduced as long as circumstances adverse to them prevail, but they do not disappear. As circumstances change, their portion of the genome may again come to predominate, and the population can fluctuate back.

How far can a new species vary? Consider this fact: no one has yet bred a new species artificially. Species have inherent biological limits. The hybridization of the beet vegetable is instructive. Wild beets have a sugar content of less than 4%. Hybrids were developed from wild strains which increased the sugar yield to 17%. However, biologists have never been able to get beets of a higher than 17% yield. By breeding high-yield varieties together they often get throw-backs to the wild stocks. 17% is a barrier.

Nature has to economize in one area in order to expand in another area. This is a basic law of compensation which limits variability. This opposes evolutionary theory which suggests each organism has an infinite genetic plasticity which, coupled with mutation and natural selection, can stretch a bacteria into a human given enough time.

The Random Mutation Theory

Let's think logically: natural selection implies the selection of certain traits from a larger pool of traits within a group. Thus, over time, it is a mechanism which reduces biological diversity. Obviously, the diverse natural world itself represents the opposite. The random mutation theory has to provide the favorable characteristics to create diversity. Micromutations, we are told, stem from random mistakes in copying the commands of the DNA's genetic code. To say that such chance errors could construct even a single complex, healthy and functioning organ, such as a stomach or an intestinal tract, is like saying a dictionary could result from a print shop explosion.

Just how the unique bone structure of birds could have evolved gradually through natural selection and mutation from the standard vertebrate design is fantastically difficult to imagine and even more difficult to prove. All micromutations have to appear simultaneously and work together at every step along the way. For instance, the spine and bone structure are absolutely vital to every moment of the organism's existence — even the slightest mistake or variance leads to death.

One eminent scientist of the mid-twentieth century, who concluded the theory of evolution had fallen apart, was the geneticist Professor Richard Goldschmidt of the University of California at Berkeley. In his book, **Darwin On Trial**, Phillip Johnson describes Goldschmidt's now-famous challenge to the neo-darwinists, listing a series of complex structures, from mammalian hair to hemoglobin, which he concluded could not have been produced by the accumulation and selection of small mutations. Goldschmidt described how the idea that an accumulation of micromutations could lead to new organs and species is a mathematical impossibility.

Beyond Natural Selection And Random Mutation

"A very large yet undefined extension may safely be given to the direct and indirect results of natural selection; but I now admit... that in the earlier editions of my **Origin of Species** I probably attributed too much to the action of natural selection or the survival of the fittest...I had not formerly sufficiently considered the existence of many structures which appear to be, as far as we can judge, neither beneficial nor injurious, and this I believe to be one of the greatest oversights as yet detected in my work." — Charles Darwin, **The Descent Of Man**

We know that close contact with other living beings unites patterns of thought, emotion, biological appetites and impulses. And that people do resemble their pets and vice versa. Biological theories have not been able to explain the "Power of Association" scientifically.

Natural selection is the most famous mechanism that can cause biological adjustments in organisms, but it may not be the most important element. Other factors that cause changes in species include: directed mutation and/or geographic morphism.

Experiments have shown bacteria can mutate in beneficial ways, due to directed mutation, without natural selection. Consider the results of the following experiments conducted on E. Coli bacteria. Researchers Dr. John Cairns and Dr. Barry Hall independent of each other confirmed that when bacteria are deprived of certain nutrients, such as the amino acids tryptophan and cysteine, they are able to, under hostile conditions, give rise to offspring which can internally synthesize these nutrients. This is a directed mutation. (See Cairns, J., "The origin of mutants," **Nature**, 335:142-145 and Hall, B., "Spontaneous point mutations that occur more often when advantageous than when neutral," **Genetics**, 126:5-16, September 1990). If simple bacteria can synthesize their own nutrients, imagine what humans can do!

Environmental factors directly affect the structure of living organisms — this phenomena is termed "geographic morphism." Within each landscape, the forms of plants and animals have local characteristics that can be, and often are, picked up by transplants of plant and animal strains and stocks from other landscapes. For example, in the 19th century it was discovered that for any given inhabited area of the world there was an average cephalic index (the ratio of the greatest breadth of the head to its length from front to back) of the human population. More important, it was learned, through measurements on immigrants to America from all over Europe, and on their American-born offspring, that this cephalic index corresponds to the geographical location, and immediately makes itself manifest in the new generation. Thus, long-headed Sephardic Jewish people and short-headed Ashkenazi Jewish people, after arriving in America, produced offspring with a specifically American cephalic index.

From intuitive observation, it is apparent that the landscape exerts an influence on the plant and animal life within its bounds. The mechanism of this influence is beyond our scientific understanding at this time. The source of it, however, we know: it is the cosmic unity of the totality of things, a unity that shows itself in the rhythmic and cyclic movement of Nature.

Embryology

If evolution were correct, then we should find that the embryonic development of animals would replay a synopsis of the whole evolutionary picture. Organisms should start out in life as relatively similar, and then form their differing features later.

In reality, the embryonic patterns represent a mysterious puzzle for the evolutionary theory. Although it is true that different vertebrate types pass through an embryonic stage at which they resemble one another, they develop to this stage very differently. Each vertebrate egg, upon fertilization, undergoes cell divisions and movements characteristic of its class: fish follow one pattern, amphibians another, reptiles another, birds another and mammals yet another.

Embryologists have known for many decades now that vertebrate embryos develop along different lines which converge in appearance midway through the process, then diverge again until they finally develop — in totally different ways — similar organs, limbs and bones.

Darwin thought embryology was a guide to evolutionary genealogy. If this were so, then embryology is telling us vertebrates have multiple origins and did not inherit similar characteristics from a common ancestor.

Are Species Real?

Up until now, I have used the word "species" in its traditional sense (the way neo-darwinists have defined it for decades). The traditional definition of "species" connotes organisms which can breed together. There are major problems with the definition of the word "species." Pleomorphic organisms and all animals and plants which reproduce asexually fall out of the species categorization. This presents an enormous population of living things on Earth and an enormous problem for neo-darwinists. How do we classify such organisms? Another problem with this definition is that extinct populations of fossils do not breed, so we do not know whether they could breed together and do in fact represent one or more species. This also can never be tested. And what of living populations that are genetically identical but cannot breed together, such as varieties of the fruit fly? And what of an offspring of a horse and a donkey (a mule) that is fertile, even though most are not? A bull can be crossed with a bison to produce fertile offspring, and this also violates the definition.

Even defining a species by chromosomal similarities may prove impossible. Italian researchers have discovered a strain of mice with only 16 chromosomes instead of 20. But Silvia Garagna, a zoologist from the University of Pavia involved in the research, has stated: "We have not found a new species. We have just found a new chromosomal race within the mouse species." (**The San Diego Union Tribune**, "Of Mice And Scientists...", Section E-1, December 17, 1996.)

When the definition of "species" is thrown up to the wind, then statements such as "all the species of Galapagos finch have evolved from common ancestors" loses any value.

Claims of new species forming within the present day continue to be asserted by neo-darwinists. In all of the examples they offer, however, what we actually find are two types of situations.

The first type involves blurring the definition of what they have defined a species as and replacing it with a definition so poorly defined that any sub-species variation can be claimed as "speciation." The Galapagos finches are an excellent example of sub-species variations claimed to be different species. Jonathan Weiner, in his Pulitzer-prize winning book **The Beak Of The Finch**, describes researchers Peter and Rosemary Grant's observations that different finch "species" do breed together and produce fertile offspring.

The second type involves chance mutations where the chromosomes suddenly double (as in plants), or change in some other way, but these mutations have never been shown to reproduce themselves into a new species.

The fact that a "species" cannot be precisely defined disassembles the entire darwinian classification system which relies on categorization.

The Fallacy Of Radio-Isotope Dating

> The vertebrate sequence
> A reflection in rock
> Obscured by the ages,
> A frozen time clock.
> But how many years,
> Into the din,
> Dates each fossil
> We're examining?

More than anything else, evolutionists do not like having their dating system challenged. The present dating systems for organic material and rocks are so ingrained into the present scientific consciousness in the fields of biology, anthropology, paleontology, etc., that to question their veracity is bound to raise emotions. As strange as it may sound, radioactive dating — the most crucial leg of the neo-darwinian support structure — is perhaps the least scientific and the most flawed of all evolutionary postulates.

Richard Milton, in his phenomenal book, **Shattering the Myths of Darwinism**, outlines the history of present-day dating systems and their flaws, some of which I have outlined in the section below, along with my own research:

In the 1940s, American chemist Willard Libby developed the radiocarbon method of dating organic materials. His system was based on carbon 14, a radioactive isotope of carbon 12. Carbon 14 begins to decay as soon as it is created at a half-life rate of 5,700 years. When a plant or animal dies, it stops taking in carbon 14 from the land and atmosphere, so the amount of carbon 14 in its body begins to decay, while the ordinary carbon 12 remains the same. All other still-living organisms, argued Libby, still retain the same proportion of carbon 14 to carbon 12. This proportion does not change as long as the organism is still alive, thus it can be determined, based on the proportion of carbon 14 to carbon 12, how long ago the organism died.

Willard Libby made the crucial assumption that the total amount of carbon 14 in the atmosphere has remained constant over time.

Studies by researchers Richard Lingenfelter, Hans Suess, V. Switzer, and Melvin Cook (done independently) have determined the proportion of carbon 14 to carbon 12 in the atmosphere is increasing (see Lingenfelter, R., "Production of C-14 by cosmic ray neutrons" **Review of Geophysics**, Feb. 1963, 1:51; Suess, H., "Secular variations in the Cosmic-ray produced carbon 14 in the atmosphere and their interpretations" **Journal of Geophysical Research**, Dec. 1965, 70: 5947; Switzer, V., "Radioactive dating and low level counting" Science, Aug. 1967, 157:726; Cook, M., "Do radiological clocks need repair?" **Creation Research Society Quarterly**, Oct. 1968, 5:70). Melvin Cook found, at present, carbon 14 is increasing 38% faster than it is decaying. The Earth's atmosphere is accumulating carbon 14.

If carbon 14 levels are increasing, the amount of carbon 14 the animal had before it died will be lower than assumed. This assumption will cause test samples to appear older than they actually are, causing inaccuracies. Also, the carbon-dating system is not usable after 57,000 years because after ten half-lives, very little carbon 14 is left in the sample to examine.

Researcher Melvin Cook has also demonstrated that uranium-lead and potassium-argon methods for dating inorganic rocks are also severely flawed. Cook's findings have been supported by other reputable scientists in the peer-reviewed literature. Funkhouser and Naughton demonstrated the flaws in uranium-lead methods by dating volcanic material known to have been formed in a Hawaiian volcanic eruption in 1801. The dating system showed these new materials to be three billion years old (see Funkhouser, J., Naughton, J. **Journal of Geophysical Research**, July 1968, 73: 4606). In another related study, Professor McDougall of Australian National University found, through potassium-argon dating, ages of up to 465,000 years for rocks known to be less than 1,000 years old (see **Nature**, 20 March 1980, p. 230-232, 12 November 1981, p. 123-124).

Most people do not realize that the four-billion-year-age estimate of the Earth derives exclusively from methods of assessing radioactive uranium decay (and the decay of similar elements). No other dating system presents an age of the Earth even in the ballpark of four billion years.

The uranium-dating system works by tracking lead isotopes formed from the decay of radioactive uranium 238. Uranium 238 decays into lead 206, which is distinct from common lead 204. The half-life of uranium 238 is 4.5 billion years; thus, a sample of uranium 238 should become half lead 206 in 4.5 billion years. From this relation, rocks are dated. The amount of uranium 238 and lead 206 in the sample are compared. The problem with this dating system is that lead 206 can be formed by other processes. While uranium 238 is decaying, it is also releasing neutrons which bombard surrounding particles, including common lead 204. By absorbing neutrons, common lead 204 can be converted into lead 206.

Uranium 238 and other isotopes are not metals in their natural form, but appear as water-soluble uranium oxide which can wash from one place to another, thereby enriching some sites and depleting others, throwing off the dating accuracy yet again.

The problem with radioactive dating is there is no independent means (outside of the radioactivity paradigm) of verifying the ages of samples. Most rock samples, when dated, present a range of dates that appear as a bell curve.

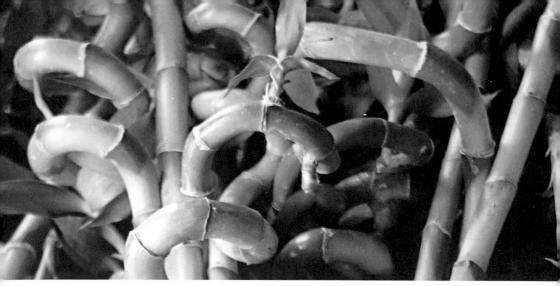

Here visible in bamboo is the *cycloid spiral space curve*
that animates all living things and causes them to levitate against gravity.

Along the curve some ages are too old and some are too young, and ages are chosen subjectively often because they "feel right" within the context. Consider the McDougall study (cited in **Nature**, also see and compare **Nature**, 18 April, 1970; 20 September, 1974; 4 December, 1975; 28 October, 1976), where the "scatter" of dates conducted by different groups of researchers ranged from 0.52 million to 17.5 million years ago for a sample of KBS Tuff rock material used to date the age of the Lake Turkana Man fossils. The dates for rock samples taken from the KBS Tuff were all over the place. The date of 2.6 million years arrived at for the KBS Tuff sample was eventually chosen, to end the whole debate, because it was apparently "reasonable" to the scientists involved.

The assumptions behind radioactive dating cannot be applied to a system that is not understood within the unrestricted world of physics in Nature. When we pull out the dating system and really understand that the entire methodology for dating the Earth, the fossils, and even the Universe itself is flawed, then we may, perhaps for the first time, appreciate the incredible mystery of Life. The Earth may have been here for trillions of years, millions of years, or thousands of years — the truth is... nobody knows.

Raw "Evolutionary" Diets or Paleolithic Diets: Do They Work In Practice?

If humans are truly carnivorous, then, in the natural state (naked, with no tools or traps, and no fire), humans should be capable of, and enjoy, capturing and eating wild game and fish, worms and insects of all types, as well as eggs. Such raw animal-food diets are promoted without any mention of restrictions or parameters of quantity. "Instinktive eating" is one such philosophy as promoted by the staunch evolutionist Frenchman, Guy Claude-Burger.

Eating raw animal flesh is better than cooked animal flesh for a time and people will feel better until the body begins to accumulate the stronger, unmitigated death energy (karma) of the animals in the raw state. This is why primitive tribes usually ate mostly cooked animal foods and did so with respect and understanding of the cycle of karma, life and death.

I have seen people on high-concentration, raw animal-food diets over the long term and have seen lives significantly altered by the negative energy of such foods. I personally believe, based on my experience, that eating a diet consisting of 10% or more raw animal flesh leads to or exacerbates major physical, psycho-social issues including: addictive behavior, emotional imbalances, body odor, cancer, immobility, infertility, and parasite challenges. It is interesting to note that wild chimpanzees, who include animal food in their diet (mostly insects), do not exceed 10% animal food in their nutrition.

Unchecked levels of raw animal-food consumption seems to be associated with a poverty consciousness — a subconscious belief that killing, lack and hardship are laws of life. Repeatedly thinking about demineralized food and deficiency is another facet of a poverty mentality. Thoughts of lack create lack. Thoughts of abundance create abundance. Feelings of fear along with thoughts of lack, deficiency, and doubt lead one to create a reality and diet where those thoughts thrive.

A few people opt for raw-animal food because they sincerely need nutrients, others opt for this approach due to food addictions and an unwillingness to detoxify. They want benefits without detoxification, but do not understand that something for nothing disobeys the karmic law. They replace cooked-food stimulation with another kind — raw-animal food. Eating raw flesh as a significant part of the diet can lead to food obsession. Poignantly, this is also true with a high tree nut or fruit dietary intake.

Typically, on a high raw-animal diet, people become so unbalanced, confused, and filled with negative energy, they (intelligently and intuitively) go back to cooked food to buffer the karmic energy of eating excessive levels of animal foods.

Those who stick with raw-animal foods in high concentrations long enough can get into some troublesome areas. The case of Guy Claude-Burger's wife, Nicole, is instructive. From the Internet I downloaded the following:

"...there was a letter from Montrame which explained (their version) of the reasons and the course of events of Mrs. Burger's death. The letter explained that both Burgers acquired the habit of eating lots of meat during an experimental phase, after they and their friends discovered the beneficial effects of raw meats, particularly for people who suffered from cancers. After some time Mr. Burger developed one small cancer-like melanoma on his legs, which was removed by surgery. He stopped eating meat for some time, then. After some time, Mrs. Burger, who already was in menopause, did get her period again. The reason was cancer. But Mrs. Burger was addicted and couldn't break the habit of eating meat, she didn't believe in her husband's new theory that meat can also cause cancer. She ate it every day and after Orkos stopped delivering it to her, she ordered through other people. One has to know, that she had lots of bad stress during that time. She worked a lot, regularly sleeping only 3 hours per day and her husband was in jail at that time, because of charges of working as a doctor without admission. (These were dropped much later). So Mrs. Burger became sicker and sicker and lost a lot of weight. And then she resorted to conventional medicine. She was treated with chemotherapy and artificial food for gaining weight, containing milk products. Probably caused by that she got pneumonia, from which she recovered when she started Instinkto again, but it was too late, she died some days later. This kind of addiction can happen with all kinds of natural foods, but especially easy with meat and other proteins..."

Eating a meat-based diet, especially a raw-meat diet, can also lead to parasite susceptibility despite claims that parasites in flesh foods are not dangerous (and this is promoted by certain paleo-nutritionists!). Once one is infested with parasites, a "parasite consciousness" is likely to arise. I was once talking to a long-term raw-foodist on the phone and he had a most insightful observation. He said to me, "David... parasites rule the Earth. They have infected the entire population and are bending it towards ever more chaotic dietary patterns so that their consciousness may dominate the world."

The mythology of the "wonderfully healthy meat-eating Eskimo" has been shattered in the past twenty years. Eskimos have the highest suicide rate of any ethnic group on Earth. Typically, they suffer from such severe teeth problems that the pain may be a primary factor that eventually drives them to suicide.

Raw fish is not a safe choice as we move into the future. I have repeatedly seen how raw-fish diets lead to parasite-worm infections and/or mercury poisoning. This is because animals accumulate and concentrate toxicity from the environment and no places are left on Earth that are entirely devoid of pollution. It is especially true with fish, as they live in and constantly filter impure water leaving toxins in their tissues. Because toxicity is channeled to the liver of animals, fish liver oil is likely to contain large doses of PCB's. We must keep in mind that, either we filter out what we are allowing into our bodies, or we ourselves will become a filter.

I knew of a case involving a long-time raw animal-food eater in Hawaii, who was eating up to 5 pounds (2.2 kilograms) of fish a week, discovered he had a mercury level of 16, where 1.5 is considered a dangerously high level. If you or someone you know has eaten large quantities of fish, raw or cooked, please consider testing for mercury.

The truth is that flesh-eating is a habit with karmic consequences and is probably best avoided if possible or in the alternative done safely, rarely and respectfully. Even though human behavior has been more like scavengers eating everything in sight, we appeared on this planet as raw eaters with a specific food design. We are not designed to eat large amounts of raw (or cooked) animal foods and that is why these diets can be inappropriate.

Does biting into a raw fish with its slime, scales and watching eye sound appetizing? Of course not. Does eating bugs out of a garden sound enticing? It would not be a first choice. No one has the propensity to go outside of their home at 3:00 am and chase a rabbit down, kill it, rip it apart and chew it up with their teeth into small digestible pieces. Raw animal foods cannot be eaten in good conscience and in a natural way (without tools) and this is strong evidence in favor of vegetarianism.

Conclusion

As I have demonstrated, radio-isotope dating is inaccurate, "smooth" transitions are riddled with irreconcilable gaps, natural selection cannot form a new species, the fossil record contradicts the darwinian theory, there are no missing links, etc. These truths indicate that the theory of evolution is flawed and predicated on wrong assumptions.

Along with the elimination of evolutionary philosophies sold to us as facts, collapses a major philosophical basis for humanity's indulgent, disrespectful omnivorous and cooked-food diet. Are we supposed to understand the theory of evolution to know how to eat? Such a proposition is absurd on its face. Eating naturally is an intuitive knowledge, a natural propensity. It is easier to sneak up on lettuce than a rabbit. Raw plant food stands as the obvious primary food of human beings.

We arrived on this spinning planet with a design to subsist mostly on raw plant food — and that is still our design now. This fact is proven by the extraordinary results, one will achieve by following The Sunfood Diet program.

ORIGINS

1 For more information scientifically and specifically discounting the theory of evolution, please read **Forbidden Archeology** by Michael Cremo.

2 Exercise your skills in contrary thinking. Write in your journal 10 statements that peers told you were true. These could be statements you still believe are true. After writing them all down, directly below them, reverse the statement and review it. For example, let's say you heard: "Money doesn't grow on trees." You would write down: "Money does grow on trees" and review it. Ask yourself questions: Which statement is true? Is one more true than the other? What are the short- and long-term consequences of believing these statements? (By the way, cacao beans (raw chocolate) were used as money by the Olmecs, Mayans and Aztecs — and they grow on trees.)

EVOLUTION: A MONKEY'S PERSPECTIVE REVISITED

One day the monkeys played
Amongst the trees,
When their fellow appeared
From a canopy of leaves.

"There is a rumor about,
Have you heard?
It's being touted
As the new holy word:

That humans are descended
From our noble tribe.
The arrogance of this
I can hardly describe.

Our joy and laughing,
Our natural bliss,
Is something the humans
Seem to totally miss.

Our zest for life,
Our radiant glow
Is this something
They can ever know?

They claim they've found
The secret design,
But the simple word: "species"
They cannot define.

Where are the transitions
The claims between form?
Nature is ever-changing
Yet stasis is the norm.

Guesses upon guesses
And the ages of rocks,
A blind watchmaker run
By atomic time clocks.

The theory is so boring
And mechanically untrue,
Science can't pollute the Earth
And understand it too!"

The monkey paused,
To stretch and yawn
Took a deep breath,
And continued on:

"Trust in faith and
Common sense
Have no place
In their science.

They don't understand
The reality they picture
Is but a reflection —
Of the thinker.

Divine and regal,
Is the grand-ancient world
The creation riddle
Cannot be unfurled.

Out there is a different place,
Older, greater, deeper by far
Than the twinkling of
The farthest star.

The harm to the Earth
Might be absolved,
But her mysteries
Will never be solved."

They chewed on fruits
In the soft, warm breeze.
As a waft of smoke
Caused a monkey to sneeze.

"Here they encroach
On our Paradise Found
They'll slash and burn this
Place — to the ground.

They don't think
Beyond the fringe
Of the tiny world
They're living in.

They cut then build
Another sharp fence,
When all they need is
Water, leaves... silence.

Materialist obsessions,
The Survival of the fit
Has turned the Earth
Into a fire pit.

And it becomes clear,
The deeper one delves...
That they've brought this
Misery, upon themselves.

Their race is declining
Into brutal passions,
Of which this theory
Is the latest of fashions.

The Earth is weary.
Of misdirection
This theory dies first
By natural selection."

Into the distance
The raindrops poured
Pattering the leaves
Between each word.

"Fancy theories,
Can never express,
The ancient dreams
Of this old forest.

Those splendid secrets
The poetry of facts.
Shouldn't lead them to worry
But simply relax."

The wise monkey grinned
As he declined some food
And all ears turned
To hear him conclude:

"Humans are something,
A different breed,
And compared to them
We have all we need.

You'll never see a monkey
Be hostile or rude,
You'll never catch a monkey
Cooking her food.

So to answer the charge
Of this latest fuss,
Tell them humans have descended alright
But they haven't descended from us."

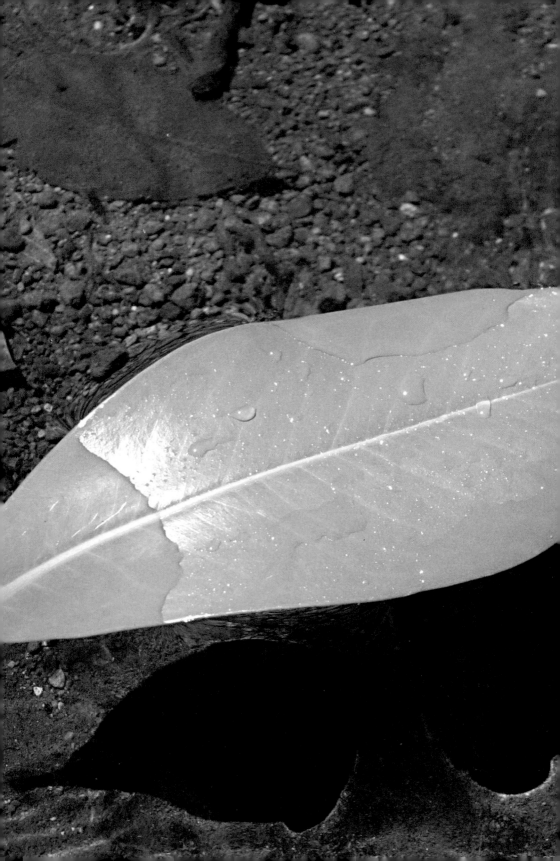

10

DETOXIFICATION

"KNOW THOU THAT THE HUMAN SOUL IS EXALTED ABOVE, AND IS
INDEPENDENT OF ALL INFIRMITIES OF BODY OR MIND. THAT A SICK
PERSON SHOWETH SIGNS OF WEAKNESS IS DUE TO THE HINDRANCES
THAT INTERPOSE THEMSELVES BETWEEN THE SOUL AND THE BODY, FOR
THE SOUL REMAINETH UNAFFECTED BY ANY BODILY AILMENTS.
CONSIDER THE LIGHT OF THE LAMP. THOUGH AN EXTERNAL OBJECT
MAY INTERFERE WITH ITS RADIANCE, THE LIGHT ITSELF CONTINUETH
TO SHINE WITH UNDIMINISHED POWER. IN LIKE MANNER, EVERY
MALADY AFFLICTING THE HUMAN BODY IS AN IMPEDIMENT THAT
PREVENTETH THE SOUL FROM MANIFESTING ITS INHERENT MIGHT AND
POWER. WHEN IT LEAVETH THE BODY, HOWEVER, IT WILL EVINCE
SUCH ASCENDANCY, AND REVEAL SUCH INFLUENCE AS NO FORCE
ON EARTH CAN EQUAL. EVERY PURE, EVERY REFINED AND
SANCTIFIED SOUL WILL BE ENDOWED WITH TREMENDOUS
POWER, AND SHALL REJOICE WITH EXCEEDING GLADNESS."
— *Baha'u'llah, Gleanings From The Writings Of Baha'u'llah*

"THE CONSTITUTION OF MAN'S BODY HAS NOT CHANGED TO MEET
THE NEW CONDITIONS OF HIS ARTIFICIAL ENVIRONMENT THAT HAS
REPLACED HIS NATURAL ONE. THE RESULT IS THAT OF PERPETUAL
DISCORD BETWEEN MAN AND HIS ENVIRONMENT. THE EFFECT OF
THIS DISCORD IS A GENERAL DETERIORATION OF MAN'S BODY,
THE SYMPTOMS OF WHICH ARE TERMED DISEASE."
— *Professor Hilton Hotema, Man's Higher Consciousness*

"LONG-CONTINUED VIOLATION OF THE LAWS OF BEING IS
THE CAUSE OF DISEASE; LONG-CONTINUED PERSEVERANCE IN OBEDIENCE IS
THE ONLY MEANS BY WHICH HEALTH CAN BE RECOVERED."
— *Dr. Herbert Shelton, Hygienic Review*

The Physiology Of Detoxification

In a world given to superstition, we must always get back to basic simple concepts.

Over a lifetime of eating cooked foods, the body gets "silted up." This silt consists of the residues of an improper breakdown of cooked food, the elements of which are spread throughout the body. These obstructions act as blockages in the electro-magnetic circuitry of the body.

Dr. C. Samuel West, chemist and lymphologist, in his amazing book **The Golden Seven Plus One** describes that the primary obstruction in the body of the typical person is protein trapped in the intercellular fluid between the cells. He discovered that: "If the blood proteins cannot be removed from the spaces around the cells by the lymphatic system, they can cause our death within just a few hours."

The whole process of detoxification consists of removing these obstructions from the lymph fluid (intercellular fluid) and washing them out of the body. As your body is lightened of obstructions, your health will rise accordingly.

Within a few hours of eating food, the quality of the blood is changed. Dr. Michael Klaper, in his video, **A Diet For All Reasons**, shows an example of thick, heavy blood drawn from a person on the standard cooked meat and pasteurized milk diet. Surgeons know that the blood is almost immediately thickened by eating heavy foods, making it dangerous to perform surgery. This is one of the main reasons why they will only perform surgery after the patient has fasted on water for at least eight hours. Eating raw fruits and vegetables, and drinking their juices, thins the blood, as does fasting.

The average person has approximately 1.2 gallons (4.5 liters) of blood. But each person has four times as much lymph fluid as blood. Your lymph fluid bathes every cell. Because the blood feeds and draws waste from the lymph fluid directly, the process of detoxification begins as soon as the blood is thinner than the lymph fluid, allowing trapped toxicity in the lymph to diffuse back into the blood to be detoxified. The principle of diffusion states that things move from areas of greater concentration to areas of lesser concentration.

Clean and light foods allow the blood to become clean and light, which in turn allows the lymph to become clean and light. Over a period of years (at least three) on The Sunfood Diet, as the body is purified, it will change from a solid, rigid, weakened condition to a comparatively elastic, fluid and energetic state. Yoga, exercise and massage speed up this process by stimulating the circulation of blood and lymphatic fluid.

As the lymph unburdens itself of undigested proteins, toxins, chemicals and other undesirable elements, the substances flow into the bloodstream. Instantly a poison may be all over the circulatory system before it is filtered out as waste. This is why some may have sudden cold or hot flashes, fevers, diarrhea, rashes, desires for poor foods, tastes of old medicines, mucus discharges and other symptoms, while detoxifying. These physical eliminations also carry with them a variety of emotional releases, such as anxiety, depression and other imbalances. These are good signs — you want those poisonous substances and emotions out of your body. Don't worry about them, embrace them as part of the detoxification process. Other detoxification symptoms may include: bad breath, coughs, cold symptoms, drowsiness, headaches, momentary aches, nausea, unclear thinking and/or weight loss.

While detoxifying, the body makes use of all its eliminative organs: the bowels, lungs, mouth, sinuses, skin and kidneys, thus releases will occur in those areas. The urine, in general, is an excellent reflection of the blood; urine is purified blood. Turbidity in the urine is indicative of toxicity being released from the blood. Clear urine is a sign that the blood is clean at that moment.

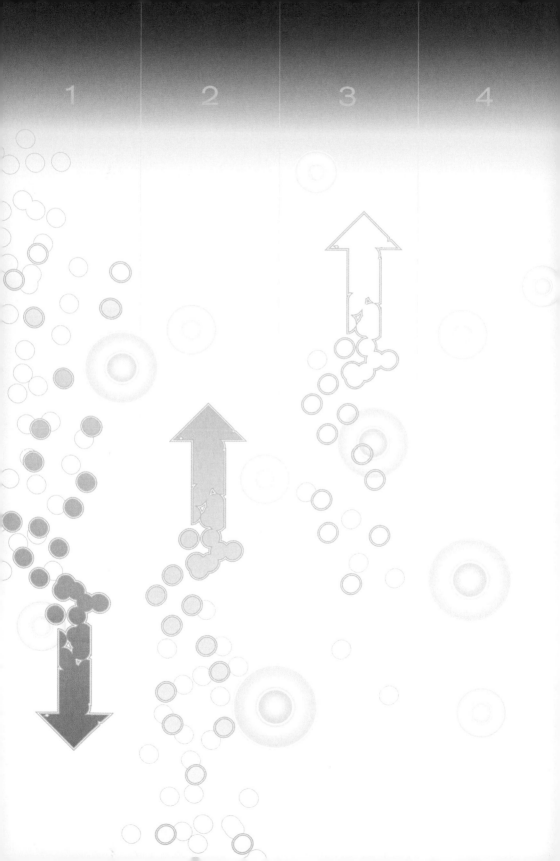

The Detoxification Pressure Gradient

STAGE 1 Intoxication.

STAGE 2 On The Sunfood Diet the blood thins and blood obstructions disappear.

STAGE 3 Detoxification: Obstructions move from areas of greater concentration to areas of lesser concentration.

STAGE 4 Purity. No obstructions.

Blood

Cells

Lymph Fluid

Dietary Obstructions

Remember, as soon as anything cooked enters your mouth, detoxification stops immediately. Symptoms of detoxification will clear up almost instantly upon eating cooked food, as the blood is thickened and the lymph's waste elimination halted. If you feel you are detoxifying too rapidly, you may want to introduce heavier foods to slow the detox process down. Eating lightly cooked foods or steamed vegetables will slow detoxification. Eating more young coconut, avocados, nuts, and seeds with green-leafed vegetables will thicken the blood to a degree that slows detoxification; this will allow you to remain on the raw diet, but also to comfortably detoxify.

During detoxification, blood pressure may increase as thick, soupy materials pass out of the lymph into the blood. This will pass over time on a natural diet as the lymph and blood unburden themselves and normalize. An elevated blood pressure is caused by obstructions in the blood vessels (cooked fat, cooked protein, chemicals), an increased thickness of the blood and/or a constriction of the arteries due to stress, all of which cause the heart to work harder to push blood through the vessels. Nutritionally, the blood pressure can be quickly decreased by adding garlic bulbs and onions into the diet. These foods help thin the blood so as to lower blood pressure.

Healing Through Detoxification

The major diseases and illnesses are diet-related. Detoxification through a raw plant-food diet is a major part of a physical path back to radiant health. If diet is ignored, the maximum benefit of other therapies will not be achieved.

There is no magic pill, but there is a magic process. For you, detoxification can be the greatest event of your life. As you become more aware of your body's true condition, you will intuitively be presented with intelligent plans, renewed strength and energy with which to retrace the steps back to physical perfection. You will be healed naturally through detoxification.

Hering's Law of Cure describes that all diseases retrace their history during the healing process. Specifically, the following pattern occurs:
1. Healing begins deep within and works its way out.
2. Healing occurs from the head down.
3. Symptoms occur in the reverse order from the way they developed.

The process of detoxification is non-linear. It travels in circles and waves and heals you in cycles according to Hering's Law. Depending on your previous diet, you may feel worse before you feel better, as toxicity is washed out of the body. If one is coming from the Standard American Diet (SAD), a powerful detoxification may occur. If one is more purified on a vegetarian or vegan diet and eating organic food, the detoxification may be more mild.

Just as it takes years for your tissues to become encumbered by improper materials, so too does it take years to dissolve and eliminate these improper materials. In general, I have found that it takes one month on a 100% Sunfood Diet to reverse one year on a cooked, toxic diet. So, for example, if one is 45 years young, then it will take 45 months to detoxify the body on a 100%

Sunfood Diet.

Every living organism strives always to remove obstructions and achieve perfect health. When you start removing obstructions from your body, radiant health appears. Obstructions are the residues left over from a lifetime of improper foods, spiritual stagnation and negative thoughts. Illnesses are caused by obstructions of one form or another. Symptoms are caused by the body's attempt to detoxify obstructions. Death is caused by a suppression of detoxification.

When I began to study the psychology and science of physical detoxification, I used myself and my situation as the test of what was true. You must do the same. Listen to your inner voice. Detoxification is a skill. This is an "unwinding" process — seek the best way to unwind yourself out of the old habits. Nurture yourself through this process. Be kind and gentle to your body, mind and spirit.

Success philosopher and author, Og Mandino, used to say that, "You are not a human being, you are a human becoming." You are constantly becoming something different. Remember, the human body is constantly recreating itself out of the air, water, food and thoughts you ingest. Studies show 98% of the atoms in the body are completely replaced in two years. In seven years, 100% of the body is replaced. In just a few years you can completely reconstruct your entire body from totally brand new high-quality materials! It is never too late for anyone. You can regenerate. My friend Shanti Devi says, "It is never to late to live, it is always too early to die."

The body is a self-sustaining, wonderfully regenerating organism that wears out due to high levels of physical, mental, emotional and spiritual toxicity. This toxicity comes through diet, negative thinking, poor quality relationships and disempowering belief systems. Detoxification ("letting go") at all levels heals all things.

The Mucous Lining

Your entire digestive tract and breathing apparatus is lined with a very sensitive, naturally transparent membrane. This mucous lining becomes irritated on a diet of chemicals, pesticides and cooked foods. An irritation of the delicate lining causes sensitivities or allergies.

The mucous membrane is always trying to diffuse impacted mucus and cooked-food residue up from the colon, intestines, and stomach to the less impacted areas of the digestive tract, such as the throat, mouth (tongue), and sinuses, through the simple process of diffusion (the movement of particles from an area of greater concentration to an area of lesser concentration). This is why Professor Arnold Ehret, author of **The Mucusless Diet Healing System** and **Rational Fasting** called the tongue the "magic mirror" because as soon as the body has a chance to diffuse toxins out of the lower digestive organs (through fasting or sleeping) it will do so and mucus will migrate up through the stomach lining, esophagus lining and into the mouth. The tongue will become coated, the breath will turn foul. The coating on the tongue then, becomes a key indicator as to how much constipated mucus has accumulated in the digestive organs.

Constipated mucoid plaque in the intestines is the product of decades of eating improper foods. To achieve excellent health, mucoid plaque has to be flushed out through the colon with the help of raw foods, herbs, colonics and fasting. Even if bowel movements are regular everyday, mucoid plaque can still be present, clinging to the intestinal walls, and should be addressed.

Mucoid plaque also builds up from incomplete bowel movements caused by not fully squatting while eliminating. Sitting on the standard toilet pinches the colon, hindering complete elimination. Consider squatting on the toilet, or purchasing a small footstool which raises the knees into more of a squatting position when sitting on the toilet.

Parasites

By far the greatest variety of parasites afflicting the present population of the Western world comes from animal foods. According to Dr. Hulda Clark, almost every variety of commercial meat available is loaded with parasites of one form or another. Also, parasites are present in tainted water sources. Parasites thrive in an unhealthy body. They feed on excessive toxicity (constipation) in the intestines, particularly cooked starch and decaying cooked animal foods. In that way they are somewhat beneficial; they help detoxify the intestines by breaking down substances the body cannot deal with into waste the body can eliminate. However, when the body becomes so weakened from a toxic lifestyle that the parasites breach the digestive tract and enter the internal organs of the body, major problems arise. Liver flukes, pancreatic flukes, eggs in the brain tissue, eggs in the liver (occasionally mistaken as liver cancer), etc., all have their role in the manifestation of the major diseases.

Freshly picked, raw plant foods typically have excellent microbes and bacteria for our digestive tract. They do not typically have harmful parasites on them, unless picked near contaminated water sources, or grown in soil saturated with toxic fecal matter.

The way to eliminate parasites is to stop taking in animal products of all kinds. Only pure (preferably fresh spring) water should be introduced into the body. Adopting The Sunfood Diet along with herbs, oxygen and taking special care to send "hot" foods through the digestive tract regularly, such as garlic, onions, hot peppers (cayenne), ginger and radishes. will help to eliminate parasites. These foods may be mixed in juices (see **Appendix C: Sunfood Recipes under Molotov Cocktail**), or eaten whole with raw plant fats, such as walnuts. Black walnut hulls have been used as a treatment for intestinal worms for thousands of years.

Colon hydrotherapy will also help flush parasites out of the system. I have worked with people who have passed worms in excess of 1 foot (0.3 meters) in length, and upon passing them, experienced a subsidence of disease symptoms and/or a transformation of consciousness.

Colon Hydrotherapy

Colon hydrotherapy speeds up detoxification. It allows a great amount of toxicity to be flushed out quickly, so we can continue with our daily lives without enduring extreme detoxification symptoms. I recommend beginning The Sunfood Diet and/or any healing regimen with a series of colonics. Colon hydrotherapy is simple, painless and discreet.

Trips to the colon hydrotherapist may replace trips to the doctor. The habit of regularly visiting a colon hydrotherapist will extend your life and increase your health. The raw-foodist Dr. Norman Walker had two series of 6 colon cleanses done every year of the second half of his life... he lived to be at least 109 (some say older). I've found that one colonic every 4 to 6 months has been effective for me — although I am sure that more would do me good. At the initial stages, I would recommend a series of 4 to 6 sessions even if you feel like you do not need it.

The primary goal of colon hydrotherapy is to empty the bowels completely in order for the lymph system to drain. The secondary goal is to remove encrusted mucus (which feeds parasites and poisons the system) from the inner intestinal lining. The third goal is to allow the liver to flush and release. The first time I ever had a colonic done, at the very end of the session, my liver released a deep yellow fluid (a standard colon hydrotherapy machine displays a clear tube which allows one to see exactly what is being eliminated from the colon). I felt a jump in vitality immediately. I later intuitively concluded that what was released was beer residue of some type, because I could never drink a beer again after that moment.

Colon hydrotherapy is a way to keep our colon mechanically operating properly, it is not a crutch to help us eliminate. Good elimination comes from eating healthy raw plant foods, from practicing yoga and from squatting naturally to release.

The growth of healthy bacterial flora can be assisted in the colon by eating raw foods, especially unwashed garden plants (roots in particular), wild plants and/or fermented foods. Probiotics (cultures of beneficial bacteria such as acidophilus, bifidus and bulgaricus) in powder or liquid form will work more effectively to restore harmonious digestive conditions and reverse problems due to an overgrowth of harmful bacteria.

Aside from colon hydrotherapy, you may also speed up the detoxification process by doing enemas coupled with fasting on lemon and fresh spring water or green-leafy vegetable juice.

You alkalinize your body by taking in green-leafy vegetable juices, which increase the blood's electricity. Electricity increases the solubility of the blood. The more solubility in the blood, the more undigested and misappropriated minerals it can suspend, remove and metabolize or chelate. Chlorophyll and the alkaline compounds in green-leafy vegetables combine with heavy metals and foreign chemicals in the body to form salts, allowing the body to eliminate them from the system. I have coached and worked with many people who have overcome mercury and chemical poisoning by eating raw plants foods, especially green-vegetable juice and certain supplements such as digestive and metabolic enzymes, powdered raw vitamin C-containing berries (such as camu camu berry) and MSM (methyl-sulfonyl-methane), a biologically available form of powdered sulfur, as well as a teaspoon of chlorella with a shot of straight cilantro juice drank three times a day.

Liver

Even if the diet is toxic and deficient, if the liver is still functioning at a high rate, the body will compensate for deficiencies through biological transmutation. Louis Kervran, in his fascinating book, **Biological Transmutations**, demonstrates that living organisms have a limited ability to transmutate one element into another alchemically. That is, they can convert organic silica into calcium, or magnesium into calcium, or sodium into potassium, or manganese into iron, etc.

Biological transmutations most often occur in the green leaves and roots of plants. In the human body, such transmutations occur in the liver and intestinal flora (probiotics). To maintain vibrant health it is very important to keep the liver functioning at an optimal level. If the liver function drops below a specific level, biological transmutation stops, and one's health is compromised.

One of the main goals of detoxification is to get the liver clean. The liver can completely rejuvenate itself even if only 10% functional. Fasting on juice or fresh spring water can help the liver deal with an overload of toxicity. Milk thistle seeds eaten whole and raw have been scientifically shown to accelerate healing in the liver. Dandelion and its juice are also beneficial for the liver. MSM (methyl-sulfonyl-methane) powder helps assist with liver cleansing as long as one starts using it slowly; MSM powder should be added to one's drinking water at 1 table-spoon per liter.

One of the best ways I have discovered to increase liver function quickly is to do the following flush (or a more elaborate 14-day program as described in Dr. David Jubb's work **LifeFood Recipe Book**).

Gall Bladder Flush

This flush dramatically increases liver function and bile flow as the bile ducts are a waste release area for the liver. Once cleared, the liver can detoxify itself and excrete its waste properly. This will assist the entire digestive system, and improve overall feelings of health and well-being.

The gall bladder flush:
1. Fast for three days on fresh, raw apple juice (preferably made from organically-grown sour green apples or wild apples).
2. During the evening of day three, suck on 15-20 cassia discs (cassia is a wild pod-fruit possessing powerful laxative qualities) or simply take some laxative herbs such as senna.
3. At 3:00 pm on day four, at least two hours after your last drink, break the fast with six to eight ounces (0.25 liters) of organic stone-crushed and cold-pressed olive oil drank straight.
4. Follow with six to eight ounces (0.25 liters) of freshly-squeezed, organic lemon juice.
5. Rest the remainder of the day. Lie down on your right side. Stay warm. Place a warm castor compress (a towel soaked in warm castor oil) on your abdomen over your liver. Your liver is located on your right side just below your right, front, chest muscle.
6. During the evening of day four, suck on 15-20 cassia discs.

This will flush out "gravel" from the gall bladder and bile ducts, that will be eliminated out in the stool (usually on the morning of day five). The "stones" will be ovoid in shape, and may range in size from smaller than a bell pepper seed to as large as a Brazil nut. True stones consist of foreign cholesterol (from meat and dairy) and starch (some stones may simply be saponified oil). Most people on a toxic diet have anywhere from 300-1500 "stones" of various sizes in their gall bladder and bile ducts.

The Two Selves

In his wonderful book, **The Master Key To Riches**, Napoleon Hill describes that every human being has two sides, two separate entities, two counterparts that become operative at birth. One is a negative sort of person who thinks and moves and lives in an atmosphere of doubt, fear, poverty and ill health. This

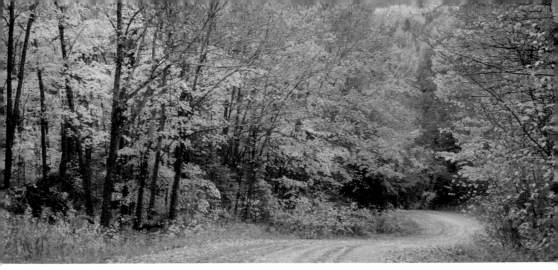

Seasonal cycles and weather patterns allow Nature to clean and detoxify herself. Cold, raw weather should be embraced as it brings clean air and active oxygen.

negative self expects failure and is seldom disappointed. It dwells on poverty, greed, superstition, fear, doubt, worry and physical sickness. The "other self" is a positive sort of person who thinks in dynamic, affirmative terms of wealth, sound health, love and friendship, personal achievement, creative vision, service to others, and who guides one unerringly to the attainment of those blessings.

I wonder if Napoleon Hill ever realized that these two mental selves have their physical equivalent? They have a physical basis in the foods we eat.

The average diet today consists of large amounts of animals (meat), roots (potatoes) and/or seeds (grains or rice), all of which are high in phosphorus and other acid-forming minerals. An overabundance of acid-forming minerals eventually causes an acid condition throughout the body, contributing to anxiety, edginess, irritability and worry — all these are emotions associated with the "negative self."

Cooked animals, fried roots and incinerated seeds leave residues behind which are difficult for the body to metabolize and detoxify. By eliminating these cooked foods, and increasing your intake of green-leafy vegetables and alkaline fruits (olives, figs, oranges, papayas, etc.), you eliminate the physical basis for the "negative self."

After you detoxify your body; when you become a raw-enthusiast; when at last you reach the point of maximum weight loss; when your body has emptied itself of all toxins... that is when your outward appearance will alter. You will literally push out your old persona (your false body) and, as it is purged, you will momentarily take on that appearance. You will see it in the mirror. Some have called it: "the alternating faces of detoxification." It is one of the most stunning revelations one can experience. After that you will be a transformed person.

Rejuvenation

Then the body rebuilds. Your appearance will undergo a radical transformation. Your hair will be thicker and wilder. Facial lines may fade or even disappear. A chalky complexion will dissipate. The bone structure of your face may alter. You will be filled with a youthful vigor. You may appear younger and have people comment on this. You will radiate health and vitality. This entire change of your physiology will stand as proof that extraordinary transformations are possible.

When you begin eating only raw plant foods, when you start to delve deeply back into the plants and animals in Nature far away from civilization, you will see there are no longer familiar features in the world. Everything is new. Everything has never happened before. The world reveals itself and it is incredible.

Your own detoxification process will allow you to take on a wider vision of yourself and your potential.

When you cleanse yourself inside, you will surely find the outside cleansed and made more perfect. You will unfold as if from a dull green bud into a brilliant flower. Imagine a neglected houseplant with brown leaves. If one improves the soil, provides it with the right lighting and water, sends positive love energy to it, then it will dramatically change. So too will an unhealthy person be changed into a healthy person through detoxification, subsisting on living foods and love.

As you lighten the body of obstructions, a joy shall usher forth, such as you have never experienced in your life. You will laugh for no reason.

When one radiates health and vitality, one no longer draws on the vitality of other humans, animals and plants. This is due to one's increased energy which diffuses from areas of greater concentration to areas of lesser concentration. As energy diffuses, it also creates a magnetism which manifests itself, in the form of charisma. A clean body is charismatic.

DETOXIFICATION

1 Ask yourself the following question: How can I celebrate my life and enjoy the process of detoxification, while letting go of toxicity? As soon as your mind comes with the answer, write it down in your journal and act on it immediately.

2 Decide in advance how you will deal with detoxification symptoms. Decide what level of detoxification will be too much for you to handle. Decide now what foods you will use to slow down the detoxification process. Write down your strategy in your journal.

3 In times of a healing crisis, maintain your poise, reread this lesson and fully understand the physiology of detoxification.

4 Read Dr. Norman Walker's book: **Colon Health: The Key to a Vibrant Life**.

5 Call and set up a colon hydrotherapy appointment today. Check for listings in your local phone book or natural-food store.

INSTANT TRANSFORMATION

What if your life was suddenly changed?
How would you feel if your destiny was one day — exchanged?

How long does each moment last?
How would your life be if you rewrote your past?

Could life be more than it seems?
What if you become something more — on the way to your dreams?

Can you undo the things you've done?
Just how and when is a new life begun?

Are such transformations true?
What if you awoke and everything was new?

What would you do or say?
What if your moment of transformation happened — today?

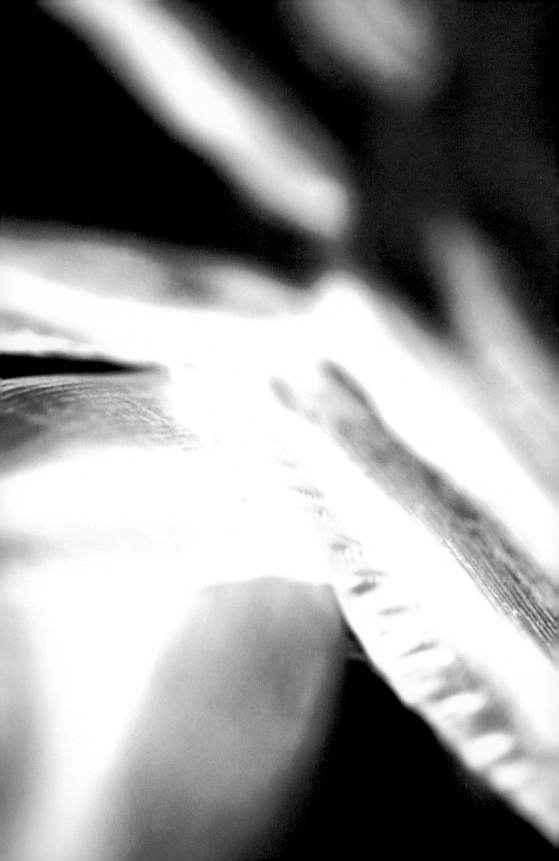

THE SECRET REVEALED

Now that we know we should be eating a diet rich in raw plant foods: What do we do? How do we do it? How do we make the transition? How do we stay balanced? These questions and others will be answered in this and following lessons.

Since beginning my speaking career in 1994, I have become the world's leading voice of raw nutrition. I have spoken to hundreds of thousands of interested people at seminars, retreats, on radio, and on television. I have coached people over many years of eating raw plant foods. Doing this type of work has brought me into contact with many people in North America, Europe and other parts of the globe, who have been successful with raw-food nutrition in the long-term. I do not know of another person who has communicated with as many successful raw-foodists as I have. I feel, through experience, that I know what the challenges are with raw diets, what the solutions are and how we can experience the maximum amount of benefits with insurance for success.

Knowledge, we know, rests not upon truth alone, but also upon the understanding of error. Genesis 1:29 tells us to eat "herbs and fruits" but it does not tell us how much of each or which ones! I know where the gaps are in the knowledge; this book is designed to fill those gaps.

From studying both the successful and unsuccessful I have deduced a startling pattern that I have seen in every single person who has been successful with raw-food nutrition in the long-term. To me discovering this pattern was a revelation; it was like the Sun bursting through after 40 days of clouds and rain. This distinction improved my understanding of nutrition tremendously and tuned me up to an incredible level of balance.

I discovered there are three essentials to raw-food nutrition (actually to any diet) or imbalances will occur. One can eat other foods, but these three

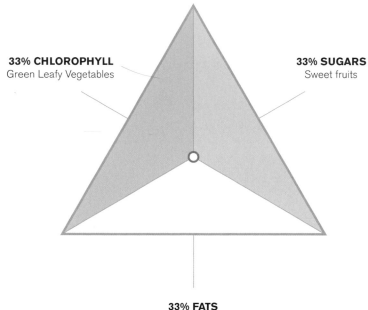

33% CHLOROPHYLL
Green Leafy Vegetables

33% SUGARS
Sweet fruits

33% FATS
Fatty fruits, nuts, coconuts, seeds

elements must be there to achieve harmony. Here is the dietary pattern I discovered:

1. Green-leafy vegetables
2. Sweet fruits/foods
3. Fatty foods

If one of these food classes is missing in the diet for a significant period (ranging from a few weeks to several months), imbalances will occur. In fact, I have never discovered any raw-foodist to have gone more than 2 years with one of these food classes missing.

Every raw-foodist who follows this pattern, whom I have met, has attained a nice dietary balance which helps one advance into the realms of extraordinary health and clarity. As raw-foodists tend to be more in tune with their diet and how it influences each facet of health, and also tend to experiment more with the effects of raw foods on the body, we may conclude that the collective wisdom which has attracted long-term raw-foodists into this dietary pattern brings forth a powerful insight for us all.

I have found this insight of the three food classes to be extremely useful in assisting thousands of people to improve and balance their diet, no matter what kind of diet they were following. I have found, even with people on standard diets, that if one of these three food classes is entirely missing in the diet, imbalances will occur within two years, and often much sooner.

Anyone who makes 80% or more of their diet consist of green-leafy vegetables, sweet fruits/foods and fatty foods (from raw plant sources) will begin to feel a startling level of magic and transformation.

These three food classes balance against each other in the Sunfood Triangle outlined below:

This is how it works: if one eats green-leafed vegetables, for example, then sweet fruits/foods and fatty foods must be eaten in the same day to balance the body. If the green-leafed vegetables one is eating are very stimulating (i.e. kale), then stronger sweet fruits and fatty foods can be eaten to balance. If one is eating green-leafed vegetables that are not very stimulating (i.e. butterleaf lettuce), then less stimulating sweet fruits and fatty foods are all that is needed to balance.

Another example: If one eats avocados (a strong fat), then deeper green-leaves (cilantro), along with stronger types of sweet fruits (such as oranges), may be eaten in the same day to balance.

Another example: If one eats bananas (a strong sugar), then heavier fats, such as nuts (which go well with bananas), may be eaten along with dark green-leafed vegetables in the same day.

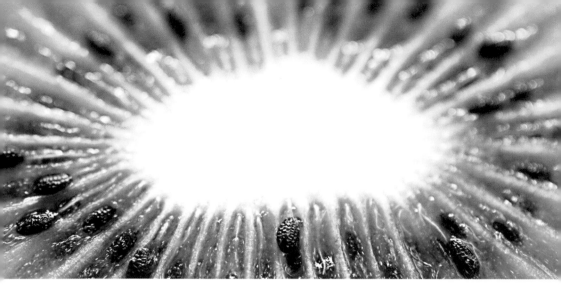

**The radiant kiwi, like citrus fruits, represents the Sun's energy
in edible, botanical form.**

Another example: If one eats cucumbers (a non-sweet fruit), then that individual will remain centered as non-sweet fruits are low in stimulation and are located at the very center of The Sunfood Triangle. This, by the way, makes non-sweet fruits (such as cucumbers, okra, bell peppers, tomatoes, noni, etc.) excellent snack foods.

For optimal results, all three food classes should be eaten each day (unless one is doing a fast or cleanse of some type). All three can be eaten at each meal, or two can be eaten at one meal, with a third eaten later, or all eaten separately throughout the day. Find out what works best for you and your digestion.

I have found that sweet fruits (carbohydrates) as the dominant food in the morning, green-leafed vegetables as the dominant food at lunch, and fats as the dominant food in the evening works rather well.

We must keep in mind that each body has its own biochemical individuality, and that the exact ratios of green foods (protein), sugars (carbohydrates) and fats/oils differs from person to person. Through insights I have gained by working with Dr. Gabriel Cousens (author of **Conscious Eating, Rainbow Green Live-Food Cuisine** and **Spiritual Nutrition**), I now have more tools of specificity in which to design diets for different types of people. However, you can design your own diet, by following your intuition. A good place to start, unless one is going for a desired effect (see **Lesson 13: How To Use The**

Sunfood Triangle), is to eat: 33.3% green-leafed vegetables, 33.3% fatty plant food, and 33.3% sweet fruits/foods by dry weight (total food weight minus water). This puts one at the exact center of the triangle. For example:

Protein	
Daily Menu Item	Dry Weight:
Fats	
0.33 lb (0.23 kg) Macadamia nuts *(18% water)*	**0.27 lb** (0.1 kg)
1 lb (0.45 kg) Avocados *(75% water)*	**0.25 lb** (0.14 kg)
Sugar	
1.5 lbs (0.68 kg) Apples *(84% water)*	**0.24 lb** (0.11 kg)
2.5 lbs (1.13 kg) Oranges *(87% water)*	**0.26 lb** (0.12 kg)
Chlorophyll	
1 lb (0.45 kg) Kale *(65% water)*	**0.35 lb** (0.16 kg)
2 lbs (0.9 kg) Lettuce *(93% water)*	**0.13 lb** (0.06 kg)
Non–Sweet fruits	
1 lb (0.45 kg) Cucumbers	*Not applicable*
0.5 lb (0.23 kg) Tomatoes	*Not applicable*

From this example we can see how balanced this daily diet would be. All the dry weights balance out: fats at 0.52 lb. (0.24 kg), sugars at 0.50 lb. (0.23 kg), and chlorophyll at 0.48 lb. (0.22 kg).

If you would like to work out this type of analysis for certain meals, I have provided the following chart.

Now I do not recommend that you break down every single daily menu as I have here to determine whether you are balancing chlorophyll, sugar, and fats

Water Content of Fruits, Vegetables and Nuts

Fruits	Water	Fruits	Water
Cucumbers	96%	Mangos	83%
Honeydew Melon	94%	Pears	83%
Tomatoes	94%	Raspberries	83%
Watermelons	94%	Blackberries	82%
Bell Peppers	93%	Cherries	82%
Cantaloupe	93%	Lychees	82%
Grapefruit	91%	Nectarines	80%
Okra	90%	Persimmons *(soft)*	80%
Strawberries	89%	Figs	79%
Apricots	87%	Grapes	79%
Tangerines	87%	Prickly Pear	79%
Lemons	85%	Huckleberries	78%
Mulberries	85%	Avocados	75%
Apples	84%	Olives *(Sun–ripened)*	70%
Oranges	84%	Dates *(fresh)*	55%
Plums	84%	Prunes *(dried)*	35%

Vegetables	Water	Nuts/Seeds *(unsoaked)*	Water
Endive	94%	Coconut water	99%
Lettuce	94%	Coconut flesh *(young)*	64%
Asparagus	93%	Coconut flesh *(mature)*	35%
Celery	93%	Almonds	26%
Watercress	91%	Walnuts	25%
Green Cabbage	90%	Macadamias	18%
Bok Choy	87%	Brazil Nuts	15%
Onion Root	87%	Pine Nuts	15%
Parsley	79%	Pine Nuts	15%
Kale	65%	Sunflower Seeds	15%
Garlic Root	64%		

(Sources: Paul, A.A., Southgate, D.A.T., **McCance And Widdowson's The Composition Of Foods**, 4th Revised Edition, London: Her Majesty's Stationery Office, 1978; and various other references.)

properly. This example is simply to identify two simple relationships:

1. A small portion of nuts and seeds balances against a large portion of fruits and vegetables, because nuts and seeds are low-water content foods. (If nuts are freshly picked, or soaked in water, they can be eaten in larger portions, as they will have about twice the water content as is listed in the chart above.)
2. Green-leafy vegetables need to be eaten in significant quantities as they are actually high-water content foods.

The best path is always the simplest path. Balance the three classes in the easiest way possible, by intuition. If you feel low in greens, eat more. If you feel low in fats and oils, eat more. If you feel you have overdone sugar, eat more fats and greens to balance. Just by knowing that these three classes are the essentials, you will have the tools to stay in balance.

Understand that if the quantities of one class are too low, one can go longer than a day, even for many days or weeks or months without requiring much of that food class — but eventually it will catch up. This helps us understand cravings. If one goes without sugar for several weeks, the desire can become great, and the body will grab for sugar however it can get it, raw (fruit) or even cooked (candy or cake). The same holds true for fat. If the body is deficient in fat, the craving will become overwhelming and one will grab for it, raw (avocados or nuts) or even cooked/pasteurized (cheese or ice cream).

Imbalances are caused by consuming one class of food that stimulates the person away from the center of The Sunfood Triangle. For instance, deficiencies may be caused by consuming excessive sweet fruit (sugar), which can run minerals out of the body. Frugal eating, and fasting, often correct deficiencies because they balance one from excessive stimulation and bring one back towards the center of The Sunfood Triangle.

The fear of fruit (too much sugar), the fear of vegetables (too bitter), and the fear of fatty foods (too fattening) leaves one confused and with dietary health challenges. Motivational speaker Anthony Robbins provides a good metaphor for FEAR: False Evidence that Appears Real. Remember my earlier advice: Stop listening to anyone in any field who is not getting the results that you desire. By reading this lesson you have made the decision to dismiss any fears of fruits, green-leafy vegetables or fats/oils.

Chlorophyll, sugar and fat are the three classes of foods that comprise humanity's natural dietary character. The eater of sweet fruits becomes a Sun-worshipping, zesty, clean type. Those who eat green vegetation take on the stoic calmness of that food class. The eater of plant fats becomes a stolid, beautiful being.

Chlorophyll

> "IF YOU'RE GREEN ON THE INSIDE, YOU'RE CLEAN ON THE INSIDE."
> — *Dr. Bernard Jensen*

Green is good. Green is the very center of the rainbow. Green is centering.

Eat green-leafy vegetables for strength. Green leaves are transformed into the structure of the body.

Whether it is green herbs or big leafy vegetables (such as kale) green leaves should be a significant part of the diet. Green-leafy vegetables are our best and most reliable source of fiber.

Fortunately, herbs have become quite popular in recent times. Green-leafed vegetables (lettuce, celery, parsley, cilantro, etc.) are truly herbs, but are so common, they are often overlooked for their healing and rejuvenating properties.

Chlorophyll is the pigment in plants within which photosynthesis takes place. It absorbs the vibrant Sun energy and transforms it into plant energy. This energy is transferred directly to you when you eat chlorophyll-rich foods, such as green-leafed vegetables.

Chlorophyll is the blood of plants, just as hemoglobin is the blood of the body. The difference between the two molecules is that chlorophyll is centered on magnesium, while hemoglobin is centered on iron. Eating green-leafy food is a transfusion of Sun energy to blood energy in the arteries.

Green-leafed vegetables are overall the best source of iron; dandelion, parsley and spinach are particularly high in iron. Greens heal anemia. (Other sources of iron include red-colored fruits, such as cherries, berries, pomegranates and red-flesh figs).

Green-leafed vegetables often do not taste as wonderful as fruits. But eating them nonetheless breaks associations of pleasure with eating, therefore decreasing the possibility of overeating. Green-leafed vegetables diminish the enjoyment in eating and act as a natural stop for us in the eating cycle.

Where does the cow get its calcium for its milk? From green grass of course. Now we are not primarily grass eaters, but this analogy is instructive because it demonstrates that all the minerals a cow is constructed from are present in grass — in simple green grass!

Green-leafed vegetables are always the best source of heavy alkaline minerals: calcium, magnesium, iron, etc. The alkaline minerals in greens balance the acid-forming minerals (sulfur, chlorine, and phosphorus) found in avocados, nuts, seeds, onions, garlic, flesh products, etc.

Green-leafy vegetation is also an excellent detoxifier of the liver, especially wild green vegetation. The calcium, magnesium and iron in deep green and wild green vegetation bind with heavy metals, chemicals and chemical drugs and allow the body to wash them out as salts through the urine.

If green-leafed vegetables, which are high in oxalic acid, such as beet greens, chard, lamb's quarters, rhubarb, and/or spinach are cooked, then the heat-altered oxalic acid can combine with calcium in the body, interfere with iron absorption, and eventually (if eaten in large quantities over a long period of time) form stones in the kidneys. If eaten raw, the oxalates in these vegetables are normally metabolized properly by the body. If one feels kidney pains 3-6 hours after eating these vegetables (even if in the raw state), then they should be avoided.

Alkaloids

Alkaloids are bitter organic compounds which are derived from plants bearing seed. Aspirin, caffeine, cannabinoids (THC, THCV, CBD, CBC, anandamide), cocaine, morphine, nicotine, etc. are all alkaloids. Alkaloids provide the heating quality in hot peppers. Peyote probably contains the most powerful alkaloids that we know of. Drugs such as ecstasy, in their original plant derivation (from sassafras and nutmeg), contain alkaloids as their active agents.

Joshua Rainbow, a one-time fruitarian activist, described in his booklet, **Biotrophic Protocol**, that when alkaloids are introduced into a body with an acidic biochemistry, they neutralize the acid and eliminate acid-induced pain. Alkaloids create a temporary high as acids are neutralized and the blood is alkalized. The alkalizing of the blood tunes one into natural resonant frequencies and insights begin to be drawn in from infinite intelligence — that is until the body's acid-biochemistry begins reasserting itself mostly through the desire for acid-forming foods which makes the blood more acidic and diminishes the alkaloid high. The insights diminish as one is tuned back into the static.

It is because of the effects of alkaloids on the body, that drugs, coffee, and the smoking of marijuana and tobacco, etc. are so popular. The typical body, acidified by a cooked animal-food diet, is actually alkalized or balanced by the alkaloids of these substances and achieves glimpses of resonant states of consciousness.

By eating significantly more green-leafy vegetables, especially wild herbs, one will alkalize the body chemistry and be able to tap into the natural human frequency more easily and more often, without drugs and their side-effects. (Joshua Rainbow believed this could be done with fruits also, but fruits do not contain enough alkaline minerals to produce the effect.) Placing green leaves in an acid body raises the consciousness as the body becomes more alkaline.

One can overcome coffee addictions (coffee is a cooked beverage as it is made by passing hot water through ground, roasted seeds [beans] of the coffee fruit) by drinking fresh green-vegetable juice in the morning instead of coffee. This will stimulate an excellent bowel movement and give the body the alkaloid stimulation it desires.

I know some raw-foodists who smoke marijuana regularly. Even if a person is consuming an all-raw vegan diet, the habit of typically overeating sugar and fat, and undereating green-leafed vegetables (while trying to make up for it with superfoods such as spirulina) leads to a slightly acid and constricted body chemistry — leaving one tuned-out, just a bit. This condition is alleviated by

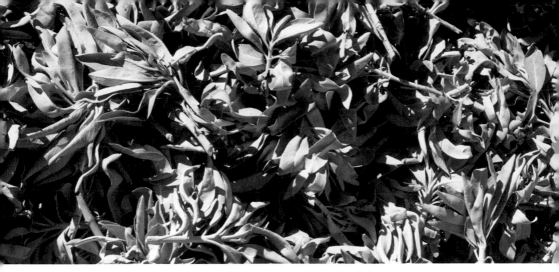

**Sacred white sage contains thujone alkaloids
which are likely the primary source of its magical properties.**

smoking marijuana, hence the desire. The alkaloids in the marijuana smoke neutralize the acid condition, relax the body and tune one into a resonant consciousness. But smoking marijuana actually perpetuates the same biochemistry that created the desire for alkalinity (alkaloids). Because smoking marijuana interferes with the ability of the blood to carry sugar. The more one smokes, the more sugar the body desires. Also, the higher one goes the more acid-forming foods the body asks for (dehydrated crackers, nuts, seeds, olives, avocados) to come down. This cycle can be broken by eating significantly more green-leafy vegetables and wild herbs which alkalize the body, loosen the tissues, and open the mind.

To overcome the desire for cooked alkaloids, one should replace them by eating them raw and/or by eating more green-leafed vegetables and wild herbs. Raw green leaves have the same effect as alkaloid substances, however, their high lasts much longer. By repeatedly introducing significant amounts of green-leafed vegetables and wild herbs we raise the alkalinity of the body and loosen the constriction of body tissues.

Green leaves soothe the nerves and calm the body. Those with chronic back and muscle pains should be sure to eat plenty of green vegetables. Green leaves relieve pain. Green-leafy foods decrease the overall stress of the body and facilitate yoga practices. For those raw-foodists practicing yoga: drink more green vegetable juice for better flexibility.

Consider that the number one cause of death in the western world is heart disease. The heart concentrates magnesium at a level 18 times greater than what is found in the blood. Magnesium is the primary alkaline mineral in chlorophyll. An abundance of green in the diet strengthens the heart. The heart chakra is green (chakras are bodily energetic centers studied in yoga that correspond to the glands/organs [i.e. heart/thymus]).

Sprouts

In my classification, there are two different types of sprouts: seed/legume sprouts and green sprouts.

Seed/legume sprouts fall into the first stage of sprouting; these types of sprouts are protein-dominant foods. As the sprout matures, it begins to form green leaves of one type or another; it has then become a green sprout and falls into the green-leafy vegetable category. So, for example, sprouted wheat is a seed sprout, but as it grows its green blades, and turns into wheatgrass, it becomes a green sprout.

Seed/legume sprouts include: sprouted sunflower seeds, sprouted wheat, quinoa sprouts, mung bean sprouts, lentil sprouts, pea sprouts, soaked peanuts, sprouted rice, etc. Seed sprouts are not essential in the diet. However, if they are eaten occasionally, they can be beneficial because high-quality seeds contain many trace minerals and available amino acids. Also, seed sprouts are therapeutic in the transition from cooked to raw food as they are very high in enzymes and help reverse an enzyme deficiency situation. If overeaten or miscombined (with avocado for example), seed sprouts may create digestive distress.

Green sprouts include: wheatgrass blades, clover, sunflower greens, barley-grass blades, radish sprouts, pea shoots, alfalfa, etc. Green sprouts fit into the category of essential chlorophyll foods. For most people, sunflower greens are the best sprouts of all; they are the "softest" and most nourishing for the body. Wheatgrass often comes from weak hybridized seed strains; quality counts and one should seek out the best quality seed stock available. Other grass seeds tend to be of a higher quality (kamut, rye, barley, oat) than wheatgrass. Grass juice is an excellent transition, detoxification and maintenance food (especially for overcoming heavy metal poisoning). Grass juice may be too harsh on certain body constitution types and should be avoided if too unsettling.

Sugar

Eat natural sugar foods for brain fuel. Cognition is dependent on blood sugar.

Our brains run primarily on oxygen and glucose (or fruit sugar). That ought to give us a clue as to what our natural fuel is. Glucose is the fuel of our being.

The more (mentally and physically) active you are, the more fuel (sugar) you can burn off. The less (mentally and physically) active you are, the less fuel (sugar) you require.

Sugar is the fuel of the human body, but it must be taken in the correct form. Sugar in the diet should come from primary organic raw sources, such as sweet fruits with seeds and/or wild (not orchard-grown) honey.

Refined and processed sugars (e.g. high fructose corn syrup, table sugar, brown sugar) are drugs. Natural sugars are also drugs when taken excessively. Refined and hybrid fruit and vegetable sugars slip past the liver like a slipping gear. The liver tries to recognize the sugar, but for the most part, it is unidentifiable and slippage occurs as unprocessed sugar enters the blood rapidly, causing a "high," — or sugar rush — which has been described by many people addicted to refined sugar or even by people hooked on fruit or carrot juice.

Obviously, refined and processed sugars should be released from the diet. But even amongst certain raw foods, there are some sugars that should be avoided. I definitely recommend against the prolonged daily intake of straight carrot or beet juice. Both carrots and beets are extremely hybridized foods. They may heal one to a certain degree (because they are nutrient-rich raw plant foods), but once you reach a certain level of attunement, the body can begin to react to the sugar. I have seen many people on carrot juice cures begin to become unbalanced as they progressed in their cleansing. If used to sweeten juices, consider using no more than one carrot or one beet per 1 quart (1 liter) of juice. You may also choose to use apple or pear to sweeten vegetable juices. Cucumber softens the bitterness of vegetables and is an excellent base for vegetable juices.

I also recommend that we avoid seedless fruits such as: bananas, seedless grapes, seedless oranges, pineapple, seedless watermelon, etc. These foods, are bred for certain genetics and then weakling, sugary plantings and cuttings are spread to gardens and farms everywhere. These weak strains are essentially artificial and loaded with hybrid sugar (however, if these foods have their seeds they are okay). A more detailed discussion of hybrid foods will follow in **Lesson 16: Hybrid Food**.

Hybrid sugar, like refined sugar, can overstimulate the endocrine system, unless it is mitigated with fats, green-leafed vegetables or high-protein foods (such as spirulina, blue-green algae, maca or bee pollen) to "lessen the shock." The glands sense the body is loaded with food, but hybrid foods (especially commercial fruits and sugary root vegetables) are fairly empty of trace nutrients and the body signals more hunger, which leads to an overeating of hybrid sweet fruit (seedless fruit). This overeating can be stopped by eating high-quality green-leafy vegetables, which have the trace elements.

A diet heavy in hybridized sweet fruit can lead to constipation, especially if the individual is not highly active. Because excess sugar spills off into the urine, excessive urination can occur when the sugar is not being immediately utilized (due to a lack of activity). Excessive urination leads to dehydration and a potassium overdose, behind which follows constipation. This process is accelerated if nuts are included in the diet (without greens) as nuts are more difficult to digest and slow the digestive system. If this process continues unabated, a minor diabetic condition will occur as the body is constantly urinating to spill off excess sugar.

Too much sugar in the blood triggers the release of alkaline minerals, such as calcium, from the bones and tissues to buffer sugar's acidifying effects. These minerals are also lost with the urine. So, excessive stimulation of the body by sugars (including hybridized sweet fruit) not only causes constipation, but also leaches minerals from the body in the long term.

This condition is completely reversible through regular exercise, considerably decreasing the intake of sugary fruits, and by adding a large portion of dark green-leafy vegetables and a variety of raw plant fats to the diet (again reference The Sunfood Triangle). The best way to rehydrate the body is with fresh spring water (plus a pinch of full-spectrum salt and a squeeze of lemon) and/or with celery juice. High-sodium foods, such as celery, are excellent to include to rehydrate the body and to relieve constipation as sodium counterbalances a potassium overdose (which could have contributed to the condition).

Refined and hybrid sugars in the form of sucrose ($c_{12}H_{22}O_{11}$) actually take water away from the body. In order to break down sucrose ($c_{12}H_{22}O_{11}$) into two molecules of glucose ($c_6H_{12}O_6$), a molecule of water (H_2O) is required. Thus, drinks or smoothies containing refined or hybrid sugar can actually make one thirstier. This is why I believe it is best to rehydrate the body with fresh green-leafy vegetable juice rather than with fruit juice. Celery/kale/cucumber/lemon juice is another particularly excellent drink we can use to rehydrate.

Excessive intake of refined and even hybridized sugar (those foods listed in the chart below with a typical glycemic index of 70 or above) can cause a hyper-insulinization of the blood. This can lead to drowsiness and fatigue.

The glycemic index is the rate at which sugar is absorbed into the blood. Consider the glycemic index (below) for certain foods (the higher the number, the greater the influx of sugar into the blood).

From this chart we can clearly understand which foods cause sugar problems. Cooked grains and cooked hybrid vegetables (beets, carrots, corn, potatoes) cause a greater sugar rush into the bloodstream than fruit! Sugar imbalances (diabetes, hypoglycemia) are best addressed by removing refined sugars, cooked grains, and cooked or raw hybrid foods from the diet.

The chart makes evident the sugar imbalance that beer can cause. Alcoholics, in general, have a disrupted sugar metabolism, but they can find relief eating moderately sweet fruits (berries) as a replacement for alcohol. Regular fruit meals can keep the blood sugar levels balanced; assorted greens, plant fats, and superfoods (spirulina, blue-green algae, goji berries, maca, bee pollen, etc.) can provide the B vitamins and trace minerals which are usually deficient in the alcohol consumer.

Food Glycemic Index

Maltose (sweetener)	152	Jelly Beans	114
Glucose (pure)	138	Waffle	109
Baked Potato	135	Donut	108
Carrots (cooked)	127	French Fries	107
Honey	126	Commercial Beer	105
Cornflakes Cereal	119	Corn Chips	105
Rice Cakes	117	Mashed Potato	104
Pretzels	116	Cooked Millet	103
White Bagel	103	Baked Yams	74
Dates	103	Frozen Peas	74
Watermelon (seedless)	101	Watermelons	74
Millet (cooked)	101	Orange Juice	74
White Bread	100	All Bran Cereal	73
Melba Toast	100	Pumpernickel Bread	71
Whole–Wheat Bread	99	Baked Sweet Potatoes	70
Shredded Wheat	97	Grapefruit Juice	69
Brown Rice	96	Mangos	69
Croissants	96	Baked Beans	69
Rye Breads	95	Porridge Oats	68
Green Pea Soup	94	Pineapple Juice	66
Pineapple	94	White Spaghetti	66
Seedless Raisins	93	Mixed Grain Bread	64
Cantaloupe	93	Lentil Soup	63
Black Bean Soup	92	Oranges	62
Macaroni & Cheese	92	Grapes	62
Beets (cooked)	88	Wheat Spaghetti	61
Oatmeal	87	Green Peas (dried)	56
Ice Cream	87	Kidney Beans	54
Pizza (cheese)	86	Tomato Soup	54
Split Pea Soup	86	Apples	53
Carrots (juiced)	85	Yogurt	52
White Rice	83	Whole Milk	49
Paw–Paw	83	Chickpeas	49
Apricots	82	Pears	47
White Pita Bread	82	Skim Milk	46
Corn (cooked)	81	Apricots (dried)	44
Pastries	81	Soy Milk	43
Potato (boiled)	81	Lentils (red)	43
Wild Rice (Saskatchewan)	81	Peaches	40
Seedless Bananas	79	Grapefruits	36
Popcorn	79	Plums	34
Sweet Corn	78	Cherries	32
Potato Chips	77	Nuts	16–32
Kiwifruit	75	Soybeans	20

(Chart Sources: Foster Powell K., Brand Miller J. "International Tables of Glycemic Index," **The American Journal Of Clinical Nutrition**," 62:871s, 1995; Jenkins, D.J.A., "The Glycemic Response To Carbohydrate Foods," **Lancet** 2:388, 1981; Jenkins, D.J.A., "Glycemic Index Of Foods: A Physiological Basis For Carbohydrate Exchange," **The American Journal Of Clinical Nutrition**, 34:362-366, March 1981; and various other sources. Overall, these GI values are based on over 80 studies in the peer-reviewed literature.)

On The Sunfood Diet, those with hypoglycemia or diabetes can choose low-sugar fruits initially, then move to high-sugar fruits eventually. However, it is extremely important to mention that those with a sugar metabolism problem still need some sugar and that sugar should come from raw, organic natural fruits (with seeds) and/or unfiltered, wild honey.

Fats

Eat raw plant fats for beauty. They make the skin and hair shine. Natural, raw fatty foods contain oils which lubricate the mucus linings and joints of the body. They help cushion and suspend tissues and organs. Raw plant fats keep everything clean and "well-oiled." Just as sugar is the fuel of the body, raw plant fat is the oil or lubricant of the body.

In this section, we are going to discover why a diet containing a sufficient (and efficient) quantity of raw plant fat is essential for good health.

On the walls of the intestines we find villi. These are small hair-like tissue structures containing capillaries designed to absorb carbohydrates (fruits) and amino acids (green-leafy vegetables, superfoods). The villi of the small intestines contain lacteals (lymph channels), which absorb fats into the lymphatic system after they have been emulsified by bile fluid coming from the gall-bladder and liver into the intestines. The emulsified fat is conducted through the lymphatic vessels to the liver, where the fat is prepared for distribution throughout the body.

All fats are made up of two substances: glycerin and fatty acids. The number and kinds of fatty acids attached to the glycerin molecule determine the fat type.

Some fatty acids are called "essential" because the body is not independently capable of manufacturing these substances at sufficient levels. Nearly all individuals in the Western world are essential-fatty-acid deficient! The essential

fatty acids are linoleic and linolenic fatty acids, both of which are found abundantly in fatty raw plant foods, especially in avocados, nuts, and seeds. The
highly-touted omega 6 and omega 3 fatty-acid groups contain the essential
fatty acids. Omega 6 and omega 3 fatty acids are found in an excellent ratio in
flax seed oil.

Because of their unique biochemical structure, fats "cut" or disguise more
potent substances. This is why milk is used in coffee. It is also why avocados go
well with hot chilies. In Mexico they eat young coconut flesh (high-fat) with
chilies and fresh lime juice. Fats tone down "hot" foods (such as ginger, garlic,
chiles, etc.).

Fatty foods slow the release of sugars already in the digestive track. One can
eat fruit in the morning with an avocado and have a longer time release of sugar,
which allows one to experience a higher energy level longer.

Excellent foods containing raw plant fats and the essential fatty acids include:
avocados, durians, Sun-ripened olives, young coconuts, nuts, seeds, olive oils,
and seed oils.

Plant fats contain no cholesterol. Cholesterol is not found in the plant world.
Every cell in the human body produces the amount of cholesterol that it needs.
Animals and humans produce their own cholesterol. Infants are the only humans
who need dietary cholesterol, which they get from their mother's milk, as they
use it for healthy brain formation. All cholesterol problems are eliminated by
removing animal foods from the diet.

Studies have found that a diet adequate in fat intake is essential for healthy
bone formation and mineralization. Raw plant fats are the "delivery vehicle" for
the minerals in green-leafy vegetables.

Raw plant fats insulate the nerve tissue and protect us from pollution and
from the harshness of present-day civilization. Many raw-foodists I have met
agree that they seem to rarely desire avocados or nuts while living in the woods
far away from the urban centers; however, once they return to the harshness of
cement, cars and big buildings, the desire for avocados and nuts also increases.

Raw plant fats effectively increase the electric tension on cell membranes, making them more permeable to oxygen and nutrients.

All the craze against fats applies mostly to cooked fats. Cooked fats (containing trans-fatty acids) are totally destructive to sound health: they interfere with cell respiration; they are a major source of damaging free radicals; they lack their associated enzyme lipase and thus are difficult to digest. Trans-fatty acids cause the powerhouse of each cell, the mitochondria, to swell and malfunction, becoming less capable of efficiently producing energy. Fats are always incorporated directly into the cell wall; when trans-fatty acids are incorporated into the cell wall, the cell begins to lose control over what substances are entering through the cell membrane. Salt, carcinogens, damaging free radicals and chemicals begin to accumulate inside the cell. The cell becomes susceptible to ultra-violet radiation and cancer.

Cooked fats include any fatty substances that have been heated, hydrogenated, pasteurized or excessively oxidized. To prevent oxidation from light, all oils purchased in stores should be in dark bottles (including coconut oil). All seed oils should be purchased while still refrigerated or else they will oxidize and become rancid.

Cooked fats are thick, heavy, and have a deranged structure. They clog the blood, arteries and the lymphatic system. Because cooked fat is not miscible with water, is clogging and is generally difficult for the body to process, metabolize and eliminate, eating cooked fats causes the body to gain excessive weight.

In contrast, raw plant fats do not cause the body to gain excessive weight unnecessarily (unless one overeats unsoaked nuts). In fact, as one transitions away from cooked food, s/he can actually lose weight eating a significant portion of raw plant fats. Eating fresh coconut flesh, avocados, olives and durian can help a person lose weight because these fats contain lipase enzymes which allow body fat to be burned. Lipase enzymes are typically missing in the excessive fat tissues of the body. Lipase enzymes, from raw plant fats and their oils, help metabolize cooked fat deposits which have stagnated and accumulated throughout the body. Each raw essential fatty acid replaces each cooked trans-fatty acid incorporated into the cell walls. Raw plant fats (in reasonable quantities) are easily recognized by the liver and distributed properly throughout the body.

Raw plant fats do not clog the blood with red blood cell and platelet aggregation like cooked fats do. Long-time raw-food nutritionist, Ross Horne of Australia, tells us in his wonderful book **Improving On Pritikin**: "To prove that the fat of avocados did not cause excessive levels of triglycerides in the blood and did not cause red cell and platelet aggregation and blood viscosity when the avocado was eaten raw, I had blood tests done which clearly demonstrated this..."

Raw plant fats have exactly the opposite effect of cooked fats. Raw plant fats are incredible: they are antioxidants, they insulate the nerves, they protect us from pollution, they moisturize the skin, and they ease digestion by lubricating the delicate mucus lining. I have strong experiential evidence that a high raw-fat diet is the best approach for some, but certainly not all.

Many people who are new to raw diets and vegetarianism think they need protein to fill the empty space left by eliminating animal food; what they need and want much of the time is fat. Most people and nutritionists mistake the desire for fat for the desire for protein as they cannot distinguish the difference between the two. Fats are soft, heavy and full; proteins are dense, abrasive and energetic. Protein alone will not fill the empty space when you stop eating cooked food.

New vegetarians and vegans typically attempt to fill the space for fat with cooked vegetables. Cooking densifies vegetation and gives the body the illusion of "fullness" and satiation that fat provides. Many non-raw-food vegans and vegetarians I have met, to me, look deficient in raw fat and overloaded on cooked vegetable starch. I have observed that a fat-deficient state coupled with sugar imbalances due to cooked starch can lead non-raw vegans and vegetarians back to animal foods to get fat for its own sake, and to get fat to slow the entry of sugar into the blood. For vegans and vegetarians, I recommend replacing cooked starch with cooked non-starchy (mostly cruciferous) vegetables, such as purple cabbage, cauliflower, broccoli, asparagus and artichoke. One can then transition into a raw-food diet, and include more raw plant fat into the diet.

Cooked, densified non-starchy vegetables slow down the absorption of sugar into the blood stream like fats do. I think Arnold Ehret took advantage of this with his low-fat **Mucusless Diet Healing System**. His system of eating raw fruits and non-starchy vegetables cooked or raw with almost no fats is excellent for detoxification, but deficient in fat in the long term.

Fats are the bridge which carry one from a cooked-food diet to raw-food nutrition. Fats fill that empty space perfectly. They are what the body requires to function optimally. They satiate hunger.

The most digestible fats come from the oleaginous fruits (oily fruits) such as avocados, durians and Sun-ripened olives. They have a high-water content and a simple structure, making them easy for the body to identify, metabolize and assimilate.

Those with liver damage, a weak liver or have a slow metabolism for fat digestion may need to moderate their intake of raw plant fats significantly when embarking into Sunfood nutrition. Nuts may have to be bypassed and avocados and/or blended seeds used instead. You will need to tune into your body, to know when you have eaten more fat than your liver can handle (acne or lethargy may result from an excessive fat intake). Usually, when the liver is working hard processing raw plant fats, the appetite will shut down.

Saturated, Monounsaturated, And Polyunsaturated Fats

Research by Dr. Howell in **Enzyme Nutrition** and Udo Erasmus in **Fats That Heal, Fats That Kill** indicates both saturated and unsaturated fats are greatly beneficial as long as they are raw. If the fats are cooked or oxidized, they are altered chemically and may be devoid of lipase (the fat-splitting enzyme) which can lead to health challenges.

There are three major types of fats: saturated, monounsaturated and polyunsaturated fats. Typically all raw plant fats have some of all three; however, the ratio of each to the other differs for each food.

Saturated fats are more stable than unsaturated fats and the most resistant to alterations due to heat. The best saturated fats come from organic, cold-pressed mature coconuts in the form of coconut oil and organic, cold-pressed cacao oil (cocoa butter). With consuming the whole coconut, I have found, because coconut fat is more stable, benefit in drinking the coconut water and leaving the husk at room temperature for one or two days before opening it up and spooning out the white flesh. Leaving the coconut out at room temperature allows the associated fat enzyme, lipase, to begin breaking down the coconut flesh. After a few days of enzymatic breakdown, the coconut flesh generally contains more "energy" and is easier to digest.

Monounsaturated fats are found abundantly in avocados, Sun-ripened olives, durians, olive oil, cacao beans, almonds as well as most nuts and their oils. The slight electrical nature of monounsaturated fats allows them to split and bind with some toxins.

Polyunsaturated fats are dominant in the substance and oil of walnuts, sunflower, flax, hemp, sesame and other seeds. Polyunsaturated fatty acids have a horseshoe shape. Their strong electrical nature allows them to easily split, enabling them to bind with and carry toxins out of the system. Because of their ability to bind with toxins, raw polyunsaturated fats are the most healing fats for the body. Polyunsaturated fats are highly sensitive and are the most subject to structural derangement through heating, hydrogenation and oxidation. Deranged polyunsaturated fats (otherwise known as trans-fatty acids) are the most damaging fats for the body and should be totally avoided.

Because all oils are in some way sensitive to light, oxidation, rancidity and contact with plastic, I recommend only purchasing oils that are packaged in dark glass. Polyunsaturated oils such as flaxseed oil and hempseed oil should be refrigerated.

Fats And Longevity

Living a long and vibrant life is a matter of minimizing free radical damage to the body through a diet rich in antioxidants. A free radical is an electron-deficient oxygen molecule primarily produced when electrons are being stolen from the body by refined and cooked oils (corn oil, safflower oil, etc.), excessive sugar intake and toxins. In seeking to acquire another electron, a free radical is capable of combining with and destroying enzymes, amino acids, collagen and other cellular elements. An antioxidant is not "anti-oxygen" but is in fact an oxygen modulator, that products healthy cells from oxidation.

Raw plant foods, such as citrus fruits, contain the antioxidant bioflavonoids and vitamin C. Deep green leaves contain the powerful antioxidant chlorophyll. Goji berries are loaded with carotene antioxidants, including the richest source of beta-carotene found in any food. The brazil nut is noted for its abundance of the antioxidant mineral selenium. Blue-green algae contains blue-pigment phycocyanin antioxidants. The skin of the great mangosteen fruit contains highly-medicinal xanthone alkaloids. Raw cacao beans, perhaps the most concentrated source of antioxidants found in any food, contain heart-friendly catechin and epicatechin flavonoids.

Up until now, what had been overlooked is that raw plant fat sources are always also powerful antioxidants. Raw plant fats have long-chain fatty acids which help protect cell membranes from oxidation. Raw plant fats deactivate free radicals by giving them electrons. Raw plant fats are loaded with spare electrons and having spare electrons equates into achieving longevity. Essential fatty acids (omega 3 and omega 6) have a particular abundance of electrons. The spare electrons in fats help sweep toxins along to the liver to be eliminated.

Humans should live longer than any other mammal on Earth because humans can consciously control the amount and quality of food material entering the body. If the intake of this food is decreased to a pleasant frugal minimum (but still includes high-quality raw plant fats, which are antioxidants), then the obstructions and free radicals in the system will be decreased to a minimum. In this way, the system becomes abundant in electrons, is more efficient (well-oiled), and operates with less friction, thus maximizing longevity.

Animal Fats

Raw animal fats are typically saturated, so they are not as strong in their cleansing abilities as monounsaturated or polyunsaturated fats, therefore they do not directly help detoxify the body, but certain saturated fats such as lauric acid, found in raw milk and butter are helpful as anti-viral agents.

Animal flesh fats are particularly dangerous today, not only because they bring some form of karmic energy upon the consumer from the animal's death, but primarily because they contain stored toxins collected from the environment. Farmed animals eat pesticide and chemical-sprayed foods which end up stored in their fat cells. This gives the consumer a double dose of negativity. The same holds true for fish liver oil, which can contain all the toxins present in the fish. The liver is the detoxification center of the body, through which all the toxins must pass.

As far as raw milk products go, they are high-fat foods. Generally, raw goat's milk is of a higher quality than raw cow's milk because goats are a cleaner, more discerning animal — if they do not find the food they like, they will go hungry, whereas cows will start chomping anything green, as well as any kind of grain.

Many have lived long lives taking in raw milk, butter, and cheese to fulfill their fat requirements as Professor Hilton Hotema reported in his classic book **Man's Higher Consciousness**, but none I am aware of have ever gone late into life eating large quantities of raw flesh for fat because the negative karma is too great and does come back to entrap the one who ingests too much of such substances.

Raw, organic, dairy products may be used to fulfill the fat category of The Sunfood Triangle for people with weak fat metabolisms or in need of vitamin B12. Raw organic dairy products may also benefit those who have become deficient in alkaline minerals (calcium, magnesium, etc.) from not consuming enough whole green-leafed vegetables and/or who are experiencing a lack of excellent intestinal flora. The karma of raw dairy products is neutral, if the milk is freely given. However, this is rarely the case today, and most dairy animals are enslaved, lead sad lives and are finally killed for their flesh. Also, drinking the milk of another animal, especially after the weaning age, seems unnatural. Raw dairy is mucus-forming and, if taken, should be consumed moderately.

All pasteurized dairy products should be avoided. They contribute greatly to atherosclerosis, encouraging the plaque buildup in arteries that is epidemic throughout the population and cause allergies. The two countries with the highest rate of heart disease, the U.S. and Finland, are also the two countries with the highest consumption of pasteurized dairy products. (For more information on this subject, please read John Robbins' book **Diet For A New America**.)

Tree Nuts

Contrary to popular opinion, nuts are a fat-dominant food, not a protein-dominant food.

Nuts and seeds can comprise part of the daily diet, however, they should be eaten in reasonable quantities (a maximum of 0.33 pounds or 0.15 kg per day). Remember, they are negative karma foods. If overeaten, they should be balanced with green-leafed vegetables and juicy fruits.

It is best to eat nuts moderately — ration them and do not eat more than you set aside for yourself. It is easy to overeat nuts and eat them too fast, especially if you purchase them unshelled. Every couple of months I like to rest my body from nuts for a week or two (sometimes several months).

Because nuts are so concentrated, they should always be eaten with or just before a large meal of green-leafy vegetables.

Some of the best nuts include almonds, brazils, cacao, cashews, hazelnuts, macadamia, pecans, pistachio, walnuts, and pine nuts. Macadamia nuts are the richest nuts of all because they have the most fat and the least protein. However, macadamias can be mucus-forming unless eaten with a significant amount of green-leafed vegetables.

Cashews have a shell filled with a caustic resin that makes cracking the shells, for the most part, difficult. Thus, cashews are often cooked out of their shells. Even if they are labeled "raw," they are usually cooked (I did not like finding this out when I first discovered raw foods, but I eventually got over it!). After many years, I finally tracked down a group that supplies truly raw cashews. Each one is hand-cracked and extracted. I have made these available through links on my website www.davidwolfe.com. What pleasure to eat cashews again!

Tree nuts are also potentially mucous formers. If you eat too many nuts, you may find that clear mucus will flow from your nose. This is because nuts are acid-forming in the body. A mucous discharge is a way for the body to dispel some acid-forming minerals and create a more alkaline internal environment. Eating the alkaline-forming green leaves counterbalances the acid-forming elements in nuts, eliminating mucous discharges.

Quantities should be kept to less than 2.0-2.5 pounds (0.9-1.2 kg) of nuts per week. I recommend seeds over nuts because they seem to be more digestible. If not eaten fresh from below the plant or tree, you might consider soaking nuts and seeds in water and/or sprouting them for 3-12 hours to disarm their enzyme inhibitors. Enzyme inhibitors keep nuts and seeds in their dormant state until conditions are right for growth. If eaten in the dormant state without green leaves to help along digestion, nuts and seeds can burden the pancreas and sit "heavy" in the stomach.

If you eat nuts in moderation and eat nuts with green-leafed vegetables, then you need not worry about soaking or mucus formation. A strong digestive tract, strengthened by months and years of eating quality high-fiber green vegetables, is capable of digesting a small quantity of nuts with little difficulty.

Seeds

My experience and research has revealed that the best seeds are those which contain a reasonable ratio of fat to protein. A good edible seed should contain no more protein than 2 parts fat to 1 part protein (2:1 ratio). These include flax, hemp, pumpkin, sesame (used to make tahini), sunflower and especially young coconut (a coconut is actually a seed).

The seeds that we call "grains" and "legumes" are protein-dominant, not fat-dominant. I recommend against excessive protein-dominant seeds like these.

Raw legume sprouts, such as mung beans, kidney beans, lentils and soy beans, can drain the body of water. If legumes are eaten, the best legumes are chickpeas and peanuts (aflatoxin-free wild Amazonian peanuts are the only peanuts I recommend). Chickpeas should be sprouted. Peanuts may be soaked until plump before eating, although they are nice in their dried state as well. Both chickpeas and peanuts have a higher ratio of fat to protein than other legumes, but chickpeas are still protein-dominant. Soy beans have a high ratio of fat to protein (1:2) so they are one of the better legumes, even if cooked. However, they are such hybridized foods (so far out of the natural wild state) and they are mostly genetically modified that I do not endorse them or products made primarily from them (soy milk, soy cheese, soy burgers, etc). Research is indicating that more than two servings of soy per week can influence hormone metabolism. Soy is known to be thyroid suppressive.

Grains (especially hybridized, weak seeds) do not metabolize cleanly when cooked. Cooked grains, and to some degree sprouted grains, such as oats, rice and wheatberries, may leave a gummy residue behind that will clog up the tiny lymph and blood vessels if overeaten over a long period of time. If one enjoys eating grains, they should be eaten uncooked and unsprouted in their hard, natural state in the way that the Roman soldiers ate them. After a few moments of chewing, they soften and become quite edible. Raw grains mix well with grasses and wild greens. Be careful, as grains eaten in this state contain amylase inhibitors creating digestive distress if any sweet food is eaten within several hours following a raw grain meal.

If one is to sprout or cook grains, the best for this purpose are quinoa and millet. They have a higher ratio of fat to protein than other grains, although they are still protein-dominant. Quinoa and millet are also closer to the wild state.

Protein

Perhaps the biggest misconception in the field of nutrition is the confusion between fat and protein. When someone says, "I need protein," they often need and want fat. Most people and nutritionists cannot distinguish between the desire for fat and the desire for protein. Many raw-food advocates have recommended nuts for protein, when in reality the value of nuts is in their fat. Some people can give up fish much easier than cheese, because fish is mostly protein, whereas cheese is mostly fat.

Protein is what we are; it is the structure of our physical body and each one of our cells. The protein theory essentially states that you need flesh protein to build flesh protein. If that were true, then gorillas should have to eat flesh to develop their incredibly muscular 400+ pound (180 kg) bodies.

Imagine a newborn human baby doubling its body weight in several months on a diet of breast milk. Most breast milk is less than 2% protein and even the heavier "hind-milk" is only about 10% protein. Breast milk itself, is a fat-dominant food.

The construction of proteins actually occurs from the free amino acids available to the body. The body has to break down all protein (if it can) into its constituent parts, the amino acids, before the material can be utilized. Protein is a collection of amino acids. The protein structure consists of amino acids strung together like grapes on a vine.

Protein is important, yet not as important as is being overstated by official ivory-tower-sanctioned sources. Protein, of course, should be of the best plant type. And one should not confuse fat/oil with protein.

Very dense protein-dominant foods (animal muscle), whether raw or cooked, create obstructive residues inside the human body. Plant protein is of a higher and lighter vibration that metabolizes more cleanly.

The best, cleanest sources of protein are green vegetables, seeds (hemp, flax, sesame, poppy, sunflower, chia, etc.) and superfoods.

For clarity, superfoods are plant foods with extraordinary properties. Usually they contain all essential amino acids, high levels of minerals, and a wide array of unique, even rare, nutrients. Some prominent superfoods include:
• Marine phytoplankton (this outstanding superfood forms the basis of the entire food chain for the whole planet. Marine phytoplankton is a source of DHA, EPA, and phospholipids)
• Spirulina (a spiral algae consumed for thousands of years by indigenous people in Mexico and Africa. The highest concentration of protein on Earth)
• Blue-Green Algae (Klamath lake algae has a phenomenal reputation in the health field)
• Chlorella (another high-protein algae that has the special property of detoxifying heavy metals from the brain when used in conjunction with cilantro)
• Bee pollen (wild pollen, not orchard pollen, should be used and should come from ethically harvested sources where bees are treated respectfully. Bee pollen is nature's most complete food)
• Maca (a radish-family root that grows in the high Andes. This root increases the production of progesterone in women and testosterone in men. A warming food, rich in minerals and vigor-increasing properties. Also a powerful aphrodisiac.)
• Cacao beans (this the raw form of chocolate. Cacao is the nut of the cacao fruit. This is likely the most chemically complex food substance in the world. Usually better for weight loss as it inhibits appetite. Please read my book **Naked Chocolate** for more information on cacao, the food of the gods!)
• Goji berries or Wolfberries (this is the most revered food in Tibetan and Chinese herbalism. These closely-related berries look like red raisins and

taste incredible. They contain at least 18 amino acids, are a complete protein and a fantastic source of minerals)
• Hemp seed (the only seed with no enzyme inhibitors. Contains edestin perhaps the most bio-available form of protein. Also contains the youthening sulfur-bearing amino acids and a unique array of minerals)
• Wild young coconuts (not to be confused with white Thai coconuts found in markets, wild coconuts are one of the greatest foods on Earth. The coconut water and soft inner flesh are strength enhancing, electrolyte-rich, mineral-rich, youthening and invigorating. Wild young coconut water is the best base for any smoothie — especially great with other superfoods)

Remember, as with all foods, not all superfoods work for everybody, find the ones that agree with you and enjoy. I usually use them in morning smoothie drinks.

Real strength and building material comes from green-leafed vegetables, seeds and superfoods where the amino acids are found. These are our true "protein foods." They contain all the amino acids we require. We might look at the gorilla, zebra, giraffe, hippo, rhino, or elephant and find they build their enormous musculature on green-leafy vegetation and grass seeds exclusively.

The World Health Organization has established a minimum daily requirement of 32 grams of protein for a 150 pound (68 kg) male. Women require slightly less protein than men, except when pregnant (then they require slightly more than men).

To satisfy the powerful meat and dairy interests in the United States, the U.S. Recommended Daily Allowance (RDA) presents an inflated protein recommendation of 0.8 grams of protein per kilogram of body weight. This is not a minimum daily requirement, but a "recommended" daily requirement that includes an added 30% "safety margin." Under the U.S. RDA, a 150 pound (68 kg) male is recommended to consume 54.4 grams of protein per day.

Interestingly, protein can be adequately supplied by raw plant foods. Animal protein is not necessary to meet protein needs. The consumption of cooked animal protein has been statistically correlated with all the major diseases of civilization. As the cooked animal protein increases in the diet, the rate of disease increases in a one-to-one correlation (for more on this see John Robbins' book **Diet For A New America** and Howard Lyman's book **Mad Cowboy**). Most of the diseases of civilization are actually caused by animal-protein poisoning because protein-dominant animal foods are acid-forming and not natural foods for humans to consume in such large quantities.

Is there enough protein available in the all-raw diet? Consider the following analysis (below) of Day 3, Wednesday, of the All-Raw Menu (**Appendix B: The Sunfood Diet Weekly Guideline And Menu Plan**):

Chart: Protein

Item	Weight(lbs.)	Mass(g)	Protein/100 g	Protein
5 apples	1.8 lbs.	810 g	0.2 g	1.6 g
20 pecans	0.12 lbs.	60 g	7.8 g	4.7 g
25 macadamia nuts	0.18 lbs.	80 g	8.3 g	6.6 g
3 cucumbers	1.2 lbs.	550 g	0.6 g	3.3 g
3 large tomatoes	1.2 lbs.	550 g	0.9 g	5.0 g
1 zucchini	0.35 lbs.	160 g	1.2 g	1.9 g
2 oranges	0.80 lbs.	360 g	1.3 g	4.7 g
Spinach	0.44 lbs.	200 g	2.9 g	5.8 g
Lettuce (romaine)	0.44 lbs.	200 g	1.6 g	3.2 g
Endive	0.44 lbs.	200 g	1.7 g	3.4 g
Kale	0.44 lbs.	200 g	3.3 g	6.6 g
Green cabbage	0.44 lbs.	200 g	1.2 g	2.4 g
			Total Protein:	**49.2 g**

Note: Three tablespoons of spirulina contains about ten grams of protein. Spirulina contains 60 grams of protein per 100 grams of substance and is not even in this list. If it were, it would

I have had individuals walk into my office with severe liver and kidney damage caused by the high-protein diet. Seeing lives trashed by incorrect nutritional advice and fanciful theories sends the message home: Please, stop listening to anyone in any field who is not getting the results you desire.

Consider the words of Morris Krok in his book **Diet, Health, And Living On Air**: "In the metabolism of fats, sugars and starches, the waste which is left behind is carbon dioxide and water. This however is not the case with protein, which leaves as its end-products uric acid and urea, which, if retained in the system, are very harmful. Thus not only is protein not well utilized for bodily heat, but it is also a potential danger to the health of the liver and kidneys, and because of this, is the greatest factor in acidifying the entire membranous tract."

Dr. C. Samuel West describes in his book **The Golden Seven Plus One** that the primary cause of disease is undigested protein trapped in the intercellular fluid between the cells.

Although I am something other than a supporter of them, if acid-forming protein-dominant foods (animal muscle, sprouted grains/legumes) are eaten, they should always be combined with green-leafy vegetables. The alkaline greens neutralize the acidity of the protein food. The fiber in greens helps push everything through the digestive system properly.

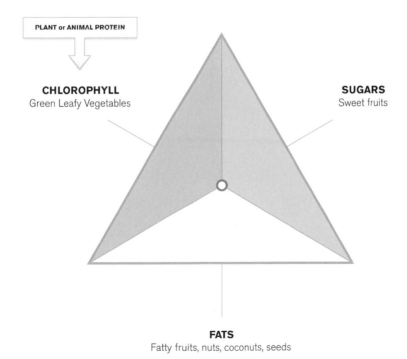

PLANT or ANIMAL PROTEIN

CHLOROPHYLL
Green Leafy Vegetables

SUGARS
Sweet fruits

FATS
Fatty fruits, nuts, coconuts, seeds

The Sunfood Triangle and Protein

For the best health, I recommend that the diet predominantly contain proteins (amino acids) in the form of green vegetables, seeds and superfoods.

The Center Point

Food, first and foremost, is a stimulant. We can do without one of these three classes of foods for a time, if we eat very little and do not stimulate our body too far in one direction. If we go too far in one direction, then the other foods should be brought in to pull us back. For example, if you eat too much sugar, you need fat and chlorophyll to pull you back. If you eat too much chlorophyll, you need fat and sugar to center you.

Many newcomers to raw foods and The Sunfood Diet tend to overeat dried fruit and nuts as a replacement for the heavier cooked foods. They are getting a strong dose of concentrated sugar and nut fat. These foods must be balanced by also overeating green-leafed vegetables, such as kale, or one will eventually be thrown off balance.

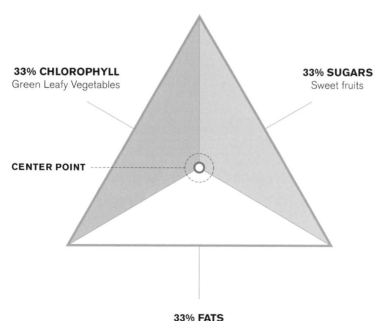

33% CHLOROPHYLL
Green Leafy Vegetables

33% SUGARS
Sweet fruits

CENTER POINT

33% FATS
Fatty Fruits, Nuts, Coconuts, Seeds

The Sunfood Triangle: The Center Point
(Chlorophyll : Sugars : Fat)

The least stimulating food on the human body is a low-sugar, high-water content, low-fat fruit, such as the cucumber. Eating low-sugar, non-fatty fruits keeps us close to the center point. Non-sweet fruits are low stimulation foods. Some low-sugar fruits include:

Food definitely stimulates the body. You can demonstrate this on yourself,

Bell Pepper *(not green)*	Dragon Fruit	Noni	Summer Squashes
Breadfruit *(raw)*	Grapefruit	Okra	Tomatillo
Cranberry	Jalapeno Pepper	Pumpkin	Tomato
Cucumber	Lemon/Lime	Serrano Pepper	Zucchini

when you are tired, perhaps even sleepy, by eating any raw plant food and you will come wide awake. You may eat to stay awake if necessary.

Aside from eating a balance of foods, there are other ways we can become more centered. Deep breathing, exercise, laughter, sex and yoga all help to return us to the center point.

Meditation returns one to the center point. I once spoke with a gentleman who had met and spoken in depth with Fred Hirsch, the publisher of Arnold Ehret's **Mucusless Diet Healing System**. This gentleman described that Arnold Ehret's largely fruit diet was also accompanied by deep meditation, but this was purposely left out of the book, because meditation did not fit the western paradigm of mainstream thought. Meditation is greatly beneficial in centering the mind and body and facilitates the fulfillment of The Sunfood Diet.

Consider that Arnold Ehret's fruitarian diet consisted considerably of apples and raisins with occasional green-leafed vegetables. Back in his time (the beginning of the 20th century), the hybrid foods (such as seedless raisins) available today, did not exist. Arnold Ehret ate apples (sugar) with raisins with seeds (fat) and green-leafed vegetables, which covers the three classes. Real raisins with seeds are a totally different food than most of us know, especially for those living in northerly climates where grapes grow wildly. Raisins can be stored and eaten all throughout the winter.

Fasting also helps return us to the center point. Our spiritual powers are highest when fasting.

Ideal Foods

Good, fresh durian must be one of the most incredible edibles on Earth. Raw-food lore is full of durian stories ranging in content from adventures in southeast Asia to all-night durian-cacao parties in Toronto, Canada.

The durian fruit of southeast Asia contains incredible fat and sugar, putting us right at the midpoint between the two. Added with green-leafy foods, we can live on Durian alone, at least for some time. A raw-foodist once told me he believed durian and raw cannabis constituted humanity's most natural foods. I thought that was interesting. If raw cacao beans and noni were thrown into the mix I would probably say he was right.

We can live for some time on seeded grapes and/or natural seeded raisins. Seeded grapes and natural Sun-dried, vine-ripened raisins with seeds are some of the most incredible foods on Earth. They have the sugar and the fat (the grape seed). Add that to the grape leaves (green-leaves), which come with the grape plant, and we could live on the grape plant alone for quite some time. I did actually eat primarily grape plants (leaf, fruit and seed) for a week once while camping after a horse ate my food.

Watermelon is one of the top foods on the planet. If you chew up some of the seeds for fat (which I have found to be quite an aphrodisiac), and take in the natural melon sugar, you again have a close to balanced picture. Add in the green rind or green-leafy vegetables of some kind and you can go quite some time on those alone.

Apricots are a sweet fruit (sugar) with an edible kernel which tastes like an almond (fat). They also have the sugar and fat wrapped in one package. The Hunzas, one of the longest-lived tribes on Earth, are world-renowned for their diet of apricots. The apricot kernel contains specific compounds that work to repair the prostate. They should be immediately included into the diet of anyone experiencing prostate troubles. I know of several people who have healed themselves of prostate cancer naturally, and who swear by these kernels. (Prostate issues can be helped by releasing pressure in the colon through enemas and colonics and by eating an alkaline diet).

Wild young coconuts are also one of the Earth's most perfect foods. With electrified water and soft, "spoon meat" on the inside, few foods can compare. Again, green leaves are required to make a coconut diet work for you in the long-term. Also, coconuts are a seed and thus they have a negative karma charge, which should be balanced with positive or neutral karma foods (greens).

Fruitarianism

The present-day fruitarian movement finds its philosophical roots in the scriptures (Genesis 1:29), the writings of spiritual masters, such as Sri Yukteswar in his book **The Holy Science**, in the writings of Professor Arnold Ehret, in the fascinating accomplishments and philosophy of Dr. Johnny Lovewisdom, in the writings of Morris Krok in **Fruit The Food And Medicine For Man**, and in the writings of T.C. Fry.

What exactly comprises a fruitarian diet has been the subject of much debate over the years. In this book, I believe I have finally settled the matter. For the record: a fruitarian is an eater of fruits (fatty, sweet, and non-sweet) and green-leafed vegetables.

The fruitarian diet lifestyle is ideally a beautiful way to live, it is in total harmony with the philosophy of Ahimsa (a Sanskrit word that means causing no harm). However, as I have described, raw foods — especially fruits — carry with them a strong karma and energy. For that reason, they must be eaten in a balanced fashion. Too much hybridized sweet fruit will throw the body off balance. The fruitarian diet has to be done correctly (and I would recommend: only for a period of time, not indefinitely). Specifically, green-leafed vegetables must be eaten as they contain heavier minerals, calming properties, fiber and certain intangible items not available in fruits. All frugivorous (fruit-eating) primates include green leaves in their diets; also, fats must be derived from avocados, durians, or olives instead of nuts if one is to remain within the fruitarian Ahimsa paradigm — eating nuts kills the plant embryo.

I do not personally recommend a long-term fruitarian diet, as it brings up the possibility of multiple types of nutritional deficiencies (demineralization and a lack of B vitamins) and potential neurological problems (especially those involving a lack of long-chain omega 3 fatty acids such as DHA and EPA). If one goes too long on a high-fruit diet, the first thing that will happen is that s/he will go deficient in salt (sodium), the next thing that will occur is a deficiency in calcium. However, for those experimenting with a fruitarian diet which is a lot of fun in the short term (a few days or weeks), I recommend the following:

1. Eat no more than 33.3% high-sugar fruits, such as melons, mangos, peaches, etc.

2. Eat plenty of non-sweet fruits, such as cucumbers, tomatoes, nonis, etc.

3. Eat plenty of high calcium, alkaline-forming fruits, especially: figs, olives, oranges, panini (prickly pear), papaya and rambutan.

4. Breathe in pure air.

5. Take in and swim in only pure water (containing no acid-forming minerals, such as chlorine).

6. Avoid stress-inducing and acid-forming environments (e.g. cities).

7. Eat plenty of silicon-based foods: peppers, chilies, okra, etc. Silicon can be biologically transmuted into calcium by the liver (see **Biological Transmutations** by Kervran).

8. Avoid all nuts! (They are too acid-forming. One will be thrown off center by eating them if no greens are in the diet. Nuts must be balanced with greens).

9. Eat a sufficient quantity of olives. Olives have a naturally high sodium content (even when unsalted).

Keys to a high-fruit diet:

1. You must be active to burn up all the sugar (fuel) you are putting into your body.

2. You must be mentally positive.

3. You must be emotionally stable.

4. You must have the right metabolism for this kind of diet.

The Ideal Spiritual Diet Of Humankind

"AND BY THE RIVER UPON THE BANK THEREOF, ON THIS SIDE AND ON THAT SIDE, SHALL GROW ALL TREES FOR MEAT, WHOSE LEAF SHALL NOT FADE, NEITHER SHALL THE FRUIT THEREOF BE CONSUMED: IT SHALL BRING FORTH NEW FRUIT ACCORDING TO HIS MONTHS, BECAUSE THEIR WATERS THEY ISSUED OUT OF THE SANCTUARY: AND THE FRUIT THEREOF SHALL BE FOR MEAT, AND THE LEAF THEREOF FOR MEDICINE." — *Ezekiel 47:12*

To elevate the spiritual powers, consider eating a mineral-rich, Live-Alkaline Fruit (LAF) Diet of green leaves and fruits for a few days. Increase your positive karma by consuming avocados for fat, wild green-leafed vegetables and non-hybridized sweet fruits of a high alkaline content (i.e. blackberries, cherries, currants, figs, grapes, kumquats, lemons, limes, loganberries, mameys, mulberries, oranges, papayas, prickly pears, raspberries, sapodillas and tangerines).

The Ancients, Longevity and The Secret

The longevity of the biblical patriarchs is legendary.

One of the most startling discoveries I came across by suggestion of my friend Steve Adler was the "Bible Code" concept. It has been discovered that the first five books of **The Bible**, commonly known as the Torah, are encoded. What is interesting for us is the dietary law laid down in Genesis 1:29 — herbs and fruits. By analyzing Genesis 1:29 after understanding the Bible Code it was discovered that it contains, in code, the seed-bearing plants which existed in the Garden of Eden. The seven seed-bearing plants embedded in this verse are: barley (grass), wheat (grass), vine (grapes), dates, olives, figs and pomegranates. The three food classes are there. For more on this fascinating subject, please see **Cracking The Bible Code** by Dr. Jeffrey Satinover.

Consider how the Bible Code discovery mirrors the 8 most important bio—active fruits of the ancient Essenes: grapes (vine), dates, olives, figs, pomegranates, apricots, carob and small yellow apples. The Essenes are a religious group originally based in the Dead Sea region of Israel. They are historically known for their raw-vegetarian dietary philosophy, well-developed wisdom and remarkable longevity. The Essenes are still around today. In fact, your author has been involved with the Essene church since 1996.

The ancient Britons, according to Plutarch, only began to grow old at 210. Their food consisted almost exclusively of acorns, berries and water. The ancient Greeks of the pre-heroic age lived on oranges and olives. We know from our understanding of The Sunfood Triangle that it is highly likely that wild green-leafy foods were included as well. The fat is there, as well as the fruit, and the green leaves. They all must be there.

Again we see such longevity in the Bulgarians, who are the longest-lived people in present-day Europe. They often reach ages exceeding 105 and even up to 125. Their simple diet consists of fruits (sugar), vegetables (chlorophyll) and sour milk or buttermilk (fat). They are a thin people typically weighing between 122 and 130 pounds (56 and 59 kilograms). This again goes to show the truth that the less weight you carry the longer you live — we have yet to discover an obese centenarian.

THE SECRET REVEALED

1 Decide today to include significant portions of green-leafy vegetables, sweet fruits (with seeds) and raw plant fats/oils in your diet. These food classes could constitute 75%+ of the diet.

2 Balance the three food classes against each other to achieve exceptional health!

3 Begin experimenting with different superfoods and determine which ones agree with you.

Three Food Classes and their Benefits

THE BENEFITS OF CHLOROPHYLL (RAW):
- Insure good, daily elimination.
- Chlorophyll: Nature's medicine.
- Counteract acid-forming foods such as nuts, seeds, durians, cooked foods, apple cider vinegar, proteins, animal products.
- Counteract acid-forming air toxins such as carbon dioxide, carbon monoxide, sulfuric acid, nitrous oxide, chlorine, etc.
- Greens are the lung cleansers.
- Deactivate, combine with, and help wash out heavy metals.
- Alkaline-forming foods. Greens make the body alkaline.
- Best source of alkaline minerals (calcium, sodium, magnesium, iron and trace minerals).
- Balance the endocrine system (*especially if wild greens are eaten*).
- Green-leaves naturally brush and clean the teeth.
- Green-leaves naturally broom out the entire digestive tract as they pass through the body.
- They ground the mind.
- They calm the system.
- They are karmically neutral.
- Antioxidants.

Three Food Classes and their Benefits

THE BENEFITS OF SWEET FRUITS (RAW):
- Glucose/Fructose/Sugar: Immediate energy.
- Karma: A positive role in spreading fruiting plants and trees about brings us good luck.
- Pleasure.
- Captured nutrients from the Sun — Sunfood!
- Cleansing food: Fruits are relentless cleansers and mucus dissolvers.
- Vitamin C.
- Antioxidants.

THE BENEFITS OF FATTY FOODS AND OILS (RAW):
- Builds better brain tissue.
- Insulates the nerves; protects the body against pollution.
- Helps reverse heart disease and atherosclerosis because the lipase enzyme present in raw plant fats (except nuts) helps metabolize the cooked fat clogging the arteries and lymph system.
- Replace trans-fatty acids which have hindered the respiration of each cell.
- They are a stabilizing factor in raw diets.
- They ground the body.
- Long-term fuel.
- They deliver minerals to the bones; they help with the assimilation of minerals, including calcium.
- They help transport vitamins A, D, E, and K, along with other nutrients, to the tissues.
- Antioxidants.

Three Food Classes and the Effects of Overdose

SYMPTOMS OF A CHLOROPHYLL OVERDOSE
- Spaciness.
- Laziness.
- The feeling of being too passive.
- Feelings of being too cold *(with the exception
  of wheatgrass juice which can make one feel too hot.)*

SYMPTOMS OF A SUGAR OVERDOSE
- Excessive urination.
- Light-headedness.
- Tooth sensitivity.
- Edginess. Anxiety.
- Constipation.
- Sores in the mouth
  *(this can be caused by a potassium overdose:
  eat sodium-residue foods, such as celery or kale,
  to help relieve this condition).*
- Black circles under the eyes *(adrenal exhaustion)*.
- Grogginess.

SYMPTOMS OF A FAT/OIL OVERDOSE
- Mucus elimination.
- Liver stagnation.
- Edginess.
- Sluggishness.
- Oily pores.
- Pimples.
- Constipation.
- Feelings of being too hot.
- Feelings of being *"hung over."*
- Strong body odor.

The Best Sugary Fruits include:

Apples

Apricots

Berries of all types

Black Sapotes

Blackberries

Blueberries

Cacao fruit *(chocolate fruit)*

Cherimoya

Cherries *(wild are best!)*

Crab Apples

Dates of all exotic types

Figs of all types *(wild are best!)*

Goji Berries

Grapes with seeds

Incan Berries

Jackfruit

Loquat *(they are close to the wild state)*

Lychee

Mango

Mangosteen

Melons with seeds

Mulberries

Oranges with seeds

Papaya *(must be organic, all conventional are now genetically modified)*

Passion Fruit

Paw-Paws

Pears *(the wilder, the better)*

Persimmons with seeds

Plums

Pomegranate *(extremely strong fruit, resists hybridization)*

Raspberries

Sapodilla

White Sapote

All wild sweet fruits and berries

The Best Fatty-Foods include:

Akee *(a relative of the durian fruit that grows in West Africa and the West Indies)*

Avocados

Borage seed oil

Cacao beans *(chocolate nuts)*

Coconut oil/butter

Durians

Flax seed and its oil *(cold pressed)*

Grape seeds

Hemp seed and its oil *(cold pressed)*

Nuts of all types *(cashews must be soft to be truly "raw")*

Nut butters *(almond butter is excellent)*

Olives and their oil *(stone pressed if possible, cold pressed is also good)*

Peanuts *(must be certified aflatoxin free)*

Pili nut *(a tasty, oily tropical nut originating in the Philippines)*

Poppy seeds

Pumpkin seeds and their oil *(cold pressed)*

Sesame seeds

Sunflower seeds

Tahini *(sesame butter)*

Unhulled tahini *(an alkaline fat, high in calcium)*

Young coconuts *(young Thai coconuts are available in the US at Asian markets)*

The Best Green–Leafed Vegetables include:

Arugula

Bok choy

Celery *(very important; an excellent source of sodium)*

Cilantro

Crane's bill

Collards

Dandelion

Dark green cabbage

Endive

Fennel *(wild)*

Kale *(especially dinosaur kale)*

Lamb's quarters *(goosefoot)*

Lettuce *(all types)*

Malva

Mustard *(wild)*

Parsley

Purslane

Spinach

Spring onions *(green)*

Sunflower greens

Wild radish

All green herbs

All wild edible greens

Algae *(blue-green, chlorella, spirulina, and marine phytoplankton; these are alkaline-green protein superfoods, they are not true leafy-vegetables; nevertheless they can be used in this category)*

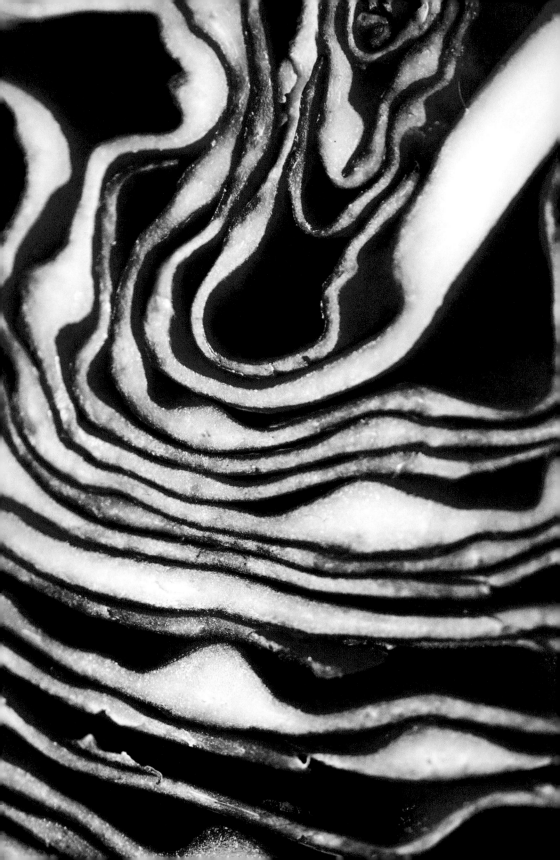

12

THE TRANSITION DIET

"...FOR THE TEMPLE OF GOD IS HOLY, WHICH TEMPLE YE ARE."
— *I Corinthians 3:17*

"YOU DON'T BECOME A RAW-FOODIST, YOU ALREADY ARE ONE.
YOUR BODY IS DESIGNED TO PROCESS RAW MATERIALS."
— *Raw Aphorism*

First, we understand that The Sunfood Diet transforms you in three specific stages, all of which will elevate you to a new understanding of your inner potential:

1. DETOXIFICATION
2. REJUVENATION
3. REFINEMENT

Second, we understand every life process is reversible. It might take from a few months to many years to make the transition back to the most fitting diet for your body, but once we embark on the path, the benefits will be worth the effort.

Third, we must know that we are always in control. Success philosopher Napoleon Hill was well known for his belief that the power of thought is the only thing over which any person has complete, unquestionable control.

Napoleon Hill was wrong. The power of thought is not the only thing which any person has complete, unquestionable control. Any individual has complete and unquestionable control also over their food choices. No one has ever accidentally eaten a meal in their whole life. Now that fact is truly astounding. It means, unequivocally, you may choose to give your body the very highest-quality foods and it will, in turn, give you the very highest-quality performance. Eat the best food ever and experience the best day ever!

What To Eat

The Sunfood Diet is not about restriction, it is about abundance. Eat any kind of raw plant food you like in the quantities you like, keeping in mind the balance outlined in The Sunfood Triangle. Try adding new raw foods into your diet and allow them to crowd out the old food choices naturally. Don't try — "try" is a lie. Avoid guilt. Allow and flow with what is happening.

The Sunfood Diet requires green-leafed vegetables, sweet fruits and fatty plant foods. But it can contain all kinds of raw plant foods: all fruits, herbs, vegetables of all types, sea vegetables, nuts and seeds, as well as superfoods (cacao beans, goji berries, wolfberries, spirulina, blue-green algae, maca, etc.), all preferentially in their wild state, and secondarily grown at home or organically from heirloom, non-hybrid strains. As a transitional stage The Sunfood Diet incorporates cooked vegetables with a preference for more natural plant varieties. For example, choosing baked sweet potato or yam preferentially over the standard hybrid potato. This program is to be coupled by individually advised short and long fasts on vegetable juices and or water.

Organic Food

Let's begin the transition with organic food. Organic foods are not sprayed, grown with pesticides or fungicides, or genetically modified. Pesticides and fungicides are chemicals specifically designed to kill living organisms. They should not be used on our pristine lands, put on our foods or fed to our children.

Spend the extra money for organic food, you are worth it. That investment will come back to you multiplied a hundredfold. You will also be supporting the organic farmers and organic food distributors who need our financial assistance.

The famous 12-year Schuphan study tested the nutritional superiority of organically grown foods. Among other things, Schuphan found:

1. Organic foods have far higher mineral and trace mineral contents, with the exception of sodium. Organic produce contains far more iron, potassium, magnesium and calcium than conventional crops. (Most studies of this type demonstrate that organic foods have 2 to 10 times the mineral content of conventional foods — you really do get more value for the money).

2. Organic spinach contained 64-78% more vitamin C.

3. Organic Savoy cabbage contained 76-91% more vitamin C.

4. Organic crops had a dry weight (after dehydration) of 69-96% more than conventional crops, demonstrating a higher food-value content.

In 1993, Bob Smith, a trace minerals laboratory analyst, began a small experiment. For two years he visited stores in Chicago and purchased 4 to 15 samples of both organic and commercial produce. He brought these samples back to his laboratory and tested them for trace elements. His conclusions were as follows:

1. Organically grown wheat had twice the calcium, four times more magnesium, five times more manganese, and thirteen times more selenium than the commercial wheat.

2. Organically grown corn had twenty times more calcium and manganese, and two to five times more copper, magnesium, molybdenum, selenium and zinc.

3. Organically grown potatoes had two or more times the boron, selenium, silicon, strontium and sulfur, and 60% more zinc.

4. Organically grown pears had two to nearly three times more chromium, iodine, manganese, molybdenum, silicon and zinc.

Overall, organically-grown food exceeded commercial-grown crops significantly for twenty of the twenty-two beneficial trace minerals. Organic foods also had lower quantities of toxic trace elements, such as aluminum, lead, and mercury.

Pesticides are poison. According to data gathered from the Internet, the top 10 worst commercial fruits and vegetables based on pounds per acre (lbs./acre) or kilograms per hectare (kg/hectare) of pesticides used are:

Chart: Pesticides		
	lbs./acre	*kg/hectare*
Strawberries	302 lbs	340 kg
Dates	140 lbs	158 kg
Carrots	119 lbs	134 kg
Pears	112 lbs	126 kg
Cabbage	102 lbs	115 kg
Lemons	93 lbs	105 kg
Grapes	91 lbs	102 kg
Sweet Potatoes	88 lbs	99 kg
Peaches	71 lbs	80 kg
Nectarines	70 lbs	79 kg

The lowest pesticide use was in the following:

	lbs./acre	*kg/hectare*
Figs	2 lbs	2 kg
Avocados	2 lbs	2 kg
Pecan	3 lbs	3 kg
Garlic	3 lbs	3 kg

Increasing Digestive Strength

The digestive organs act as one big muscle. If you have weak digestion, you can strengthen your digestive capacity by slowly increasing the raw green vegetable juices in your diet over time. If no juicer is available, one may help their digestion along by soaking green-leaves in olive oil for two to three hours before eating them. Chew your food well. One will automatically increase their digestive strength by introducing more and more fresh juices and raw foods at an appropriate pace, allowing the body to adjust.

After about 6 months on raw foods, once the eating disciplines are in place, it is a great idea to do a raw herbal cleanse. These cleanses typically last 2-4 weeks and consist of taking various combinations of healing herbs, clays, and

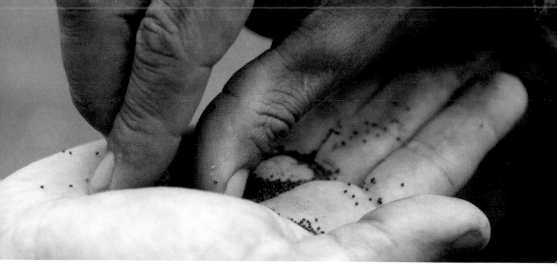

Poppy seeds are nature's primary plant source of zinc. Zinc is a critical mineral for detoxification, transition and maintenance.

probiotics. A cleanse will help strip out impacted mucus in the digestive tract, thus increasing digestive strength.

In my experience, I have found that drinking freshly-made green vegetable juice increases digestive strength. It supplies the minerals needed to digest the whole food.

Chinese oriental medicine claims that some people do not have enough "fire" in their constitution to thrive on raw foods. Anyone, however, can increase their fire to help digest raw foods — especially easy-to-digest blended foods. The best way to increase the fire in one's constitution is to Sunbathe. It is my experience that the more direct Sun energy the body receives, the greater is the digestive strength. Other ways to increase the fire in one's constitution is to practice vigorous exercise, deep breathing and astanga yoga. In yoga we find the "breath of fire," which entails inhaling passively, exhaling in bursts through the nose as you pull the lower belly in, drawing up from the perineum.

Eating Healthy In Social Situations

What do you do when you go out to eat? Visit family? What about business lunches? Plan ahead. Bring one or two avocados and/or one or two apples with you. Order a salad, and mix the avocados and/or apples in with it. Generally, restaurants do not serve organic food, but we have to do the best we can in each circumstance. I have found that the best approach is to intelligently avoid the situation altogether. Do something different. Business people are tired of doing the "standard business lunch." Take them to a juice bar or, where possible, a raw-food restaurant. Take them to a park. Without food in the way, you can conduct business quickly and efficiently — this will save you the expense and time in your day. Another idea is to hire a raw-food chef to cater business meetings. Check with your local raw-food restaurants to locate a raw-food chef in your area.

You have the most sophisticated computer in the world between your ears — use it! Leverage your mind to figure out a way to redirect family events and business lunches to fit your dietary health habits.

My experience as a raw-foodist has taught me a wonderful lesson: The way people react to you and your diet has nothing to do with the diet itself, with other people, or with anything else; the way people react has everything to do with what is going on in your own mind! Once your mind is set right, everything else will set right.

People have thousands of preconceived notions about vegetarian diets, but no preconceived ideas about eating raw foods. So you can say it is anything you want. Eating raw fruits and vegetables makes sense to most people, but eating tofu, seitan, or millet does sound strange to the average person.

When your attitude is positive and supportive towards other people and their food choices, they will not feel threatened by you, but will feel uplifted by you. Once we change, everything else changes around us.

Peer Pressure

Imagine if everybody smoked cigarettes and one day someone decided to stop. Imagine also, that as soon as the withdrawal symptoms began all the cigarette experts would get together and accost and attack anyone who did not smoke cigarettes for being nicotine deficient.

You are going to face peer pressure; it is part of the process. All great endeavors have their challenges, or they wouldn't be great.

When people offer you toxic food, they may be projecting upon you their own lack of information or fears. Let them know why you are making other choices.

If they persist with negative behaviors towards you, and make you feel uncomfortable, then you should minimize or eliminate spending time with those people. Use these incidents of negativity to drive you to stay resolute with your own diet and spiritual path.

Eating While Traveling

Cucumbers, nuts, seeds for eating and sprouting, dried fruit, sea salt, spirulina, blue-green algae, cacao beans, goji berries, grass powders for chlorophyll and minerals, as well as all-raw organic superfood powders that combine many of these ingredients, are beneficial to take with you while traveling. You may find that it is easy to be a Sunfoodist while traveling, especially in Europe and Mexico during the summer, because fresh fruit stands are abundant. In tropical countries fresh coconuts become a staple while traveling.

Water is another factor while traveling. Airplane travel dehydrates the body as cabin air is extremely dry. Be sure to bring quality water with you while flying.

I once spoke to a Mormon missionary on the phone who had befriended a raw-foodist as they were both working to spread their message in a third-world country. On the phone, the missionary told me that the raw-foodist was known for cooking his water, instead of his food! The lesson I picked up from this conversation was valuable: if you are in a less-developed country with a questionable water supply, boil your water to kill any parasites, then recharge it by placing pink salt or sea salt, MSM powder, large quartz crystals and fresh lemon juice in the water before drinking it. Water-borne parasites are a primary source of illness in less-developed countries.

Consider packing powdered cayenne with you on your travels. Powdered cayenne has been shown to protect against water-borne amoebic dysentery, a common ailment afflicting travelers in less-developed nations. Powdered cinnamon has also been shown to be very effective.

Eating while traveling requires planning ahead. Leverage your mind. You have built within you the intuitive ability to intelligently set goals and think ahead.

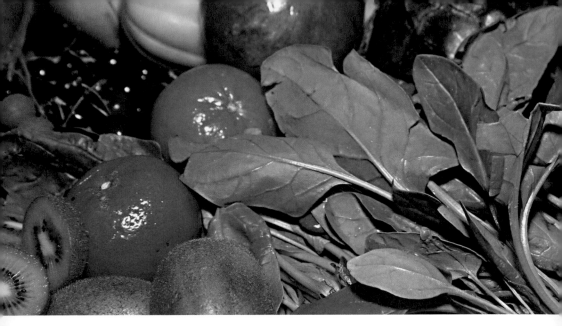

**Fresh produce is available just about anywhere on the planet.
If unavailable, one has the opportunity to explore wild food options.**

How To Eat Raw In The City

Cities typically abound with chemicals and toxins. Because of all the toxicity in the air and water, we need to protect ourselves. I have found that densifying the body with more young coconuts and nuts protects the body from pollution. If we are totally purified on a raw-food diet containing little or no fats, pollution can filter into us (things move from areas of greater concentration to areas of lesser concentration). By eating nuts we provide a dense fat substance which moves into the lymph and thickens our tissues — this protects us. Nut fats (especially from cacao nuts) also provide us with more antioxidants to protect against free radicals formed from city toxins.

I have also found protection in the city by eating significantly more ripe hot peppers. Every city contains ill people who are carrying within them large amounts of toxicity that may be breeding virulent bacteria. City life often brings us into direct physical contact with these people. Hot peppers contain phyto-antibiotics that wipe out harmful bacteria, thus aiding our immune system. Hot peppers may be eaten with avocados or nuts to "cut" their heat. If hot peppers are too strong for you, you might want to add other antibiotic foods, such as garlic, onions or ginger to your diet while in the city.

Of course, Nature's lung cleansers, the green vegetables should be increased when breathing polluted air. I generally achieve this by drinking more green vegetable juice while staying in big cities such as New York, Los Angeles, Toronto or London.

Eating Food Naturally

Food tastes better when you eat it naturally. The taste is altered when utensils are used. Have you ever eaten juicy, ripe, organic watermelon without a knife, just with your hands? One time my cousin and I decided to eat a ripe organic watermelon (I had grown in my backyard) without using a knife. We waited until it was ripe and soft enough for us to punch into the shell with our fists. Then, under a shiny afternoon Sun, we broke into the melon and began scooping out handful after handful of luscious melon. It was one of the most incredible eating experiences I have ever had. The melon tasted better. The seeds never got in the way, because when a watermelon is eaten naturally, the seeds slip through your fingers. Watermelon seeds only get in the way when the melon is eaten unnaturally with a knife! Those types of insights make life new and wonderful. Try eating a watermelon with your bare hands and see what happens.

Superior Food Combining

Natural hygiene is a philosophy that promotes entirely natural means to heal the body by using properly combined whole plant foods, exercise, Sunshine, and rest. The principles of food combining espoused by natural hygiene in books such as the Diamond's **Fit For Life**, and Herbert Shelton's **Food Combining Made Easy** work extremely well for the average individual who is new to this diet information. They worked for me when I first applied them. These principles essentially demonstrate that cooked proteins (fish, tofu, etc.) and cooked carbohydrates (potatoes, rice, etc.) should not be eaten together, and that all cooked foods should be eaten with a salad. They also demonstrate the vital point that only one type of concentrated (cooked) food should be eaten at a meal. Also, they suggest fruits should be eaten alone on an empty stomach.

The challenge with the old food combining principles is that they are outdated and much has been learned since they were formulated decades ago. My new

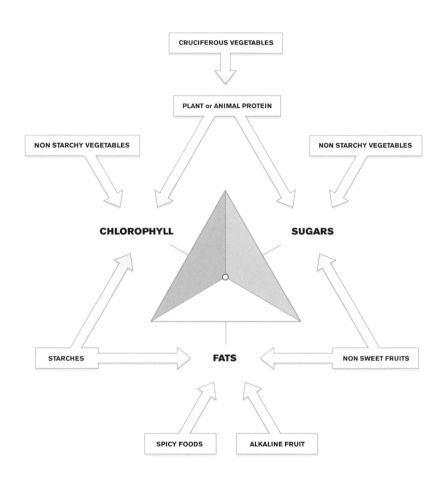

Food Combining Chart	CHLOROPHYLL	SUGARS	FATS
Plant or Animal Protein	YES	Sometimes	Sometimes
Cruciferous Vegetables (Broccoli, etc.)	YES	NO	Sometimes
Non Starchy Vegetables (Greens, etc.)	YES	YES	YES
Starches (Baked potato, etc.)	YES	NO	Sometimes
Non Sweet Fruits (Cucumber, etc.)	YES	YES	YES
Alkaline Fruit (Citrus, Figs, etc.)	YES	YES	YES
Spicy Foods (Garlic, Cayenne, etc.)	YES	Sometimes	YES

guidelines are not strict (but helpful!) — eating should be fun. Below, I have listed my suggestions for superior food combining:

1. If cooked or dehydrated foods are eaten, try to eat only one type per meal and eat them with green vegetables.

2. For beginners, fruit digests best on an empty stomach. One may try eating sweet fruits with green vegetables and/or fats/oils; this is fine as long as no gas/flatulence is created. Sweet fruits may be eaten with light green-leafy vegetables such as lettuce or mint leaves.

3. The following fruits combine well with fat-dominant foods: bananas, apples, dried fruits and alkaline fruits (citrus, figs, papaya, berries). Fat-dominant foods include: avocados, olives or olive oils, nuts, seeds or seed oils, coconuts, durian and raw dairy. Combining sweet fruits and fats will allow the sugar from the sweet fruit to be time-released, providing more long-term energy.

4. If sweet fruits are eaten with cooked or steamed non-starchy vegetables (asparagus, cauliflower, broccoli), the fruit should be eaten first. Combining sweet fruits and non-starchy cooked vegetables may allow the sugar from the sweet fruit to be time-released, again providing more long-term energy; this does not work for everybody. Sweet fruits should otherwise not be mixed with cooked or dehydrated foods due to the potential for fermentation and gas.

5. Initially, if you are very sensitive, stay with one type of sweet fruit at a time. One may eat multiple types of sweet fruit together as the digestive strength increases over weeks, months and years of eating raw plant foods.

6. Green-leafy vegetables of different varieties may be eaten together.

7. Green-leafed vegetables should always be eaten with any cooked starches (bread, pasta, rice, cakes), except for crispy or crunchy starches (corn chips, potato chips, toast, popcorn), which should be eaten with fats (avocados, olives or their oil, young coconut, seed oils, etc.). Crispy or crunchy starch is very coarse and harsh on the soft tissues of the body. Fats soften the abrasive quality of these foods.

8. Foods dehydrated below 120° Fahrenheit are great for transition diets and

as raw treats because the enzymes are intact and they provide a bridge away from cooked food. Typical dehydrated foods should be eaten with green-leafy vegetables. Crispy dehydrated foods should be eaten with plant fats. When transitioning onto raw foods, I found benefit in squeezing lemon or lime juice on cooked foods and dehydrated foods. This adds flavor, enzymes, and alkalinity without contributing to fermentation of the food in digestion.

9. Cooked foods and dehydrated foods should not be mixed together as it may cause a clash, fermentation and overall poor digestion. Again, only one concentrated food should be eaten per meal.

10. Plant protein (superfoods) such as hemp protein, goji berries, algae, bee pollen, etc. may be eaten with light green vegetables such as lettuce and celery. They also may combine well with oils and sweet fruits in smoothies. This works as long as they do not produce gas/flatulence. The fiber-bound plant proteins, such as sprouted grain and sprouted legumes, should be eaten with alkaline green vegetables to balance out their acids. These fiber-bound plant proteins typically do not mix well with fats/oils or sweet fruits. Animal proteins (except dairy protein such as whey) also do not mix well with fats/oils or sweet fruits. Animal proteins are recommended to be eaten with green-leafy salads for additional fiber and alkalinity.

11. Initially, stay with one type of fat per meal. Eventually, one may eat multiple types of raw fats together (e.g. avocados with nuts in a salad) as the digestive strength increases over weeks, months and years of eating raw plant foods.

12. Spicy foods, such as hot peppers, garlic, onions, ginger, etc., are not toxic if they are amenable to you. Eat them with fats and/or green vegetables. I can eat ripe red jalapeno peppers one after the other while feeling only a slight heat. (And that is an important point, peppers must be ripe, not green, or they may be allergenic or toxic.)

13. Low-sugar fruits and raw cruciferous vegetables may be eaten together (e.g. okra and cauliflower). Different types of low-sugar fruits may be mixed together (e.g. cucumbers and tomatoes). Different types of cruciferous vegetables (e.g. broccoli and cauliflower) may be mixed together.

14. Low-sugar fruits may be eaten with greens or fats. Low-sugar fruits can

be juiced with green vegetables.

15. For purposes of food combining, seaweeds (dulse, nori, kelp) may be treated as green-leafy vegetables; however, they are not a replacement for green-leafy vegetables.

16. Raw fermented foods (e.g. seed cheeses, kim-chi, sauerkraut, etc.), which often appear in accelerated healing diets due to their high enzyme activity, may be eaten with green-leafy vegetables to calm their digestion. Raw fermented foods can combine well with cooked and/or dehydrated crackers.

17. Raw cruciferous vegetables and sprouts are typically more bound up in fiber than other vegetables and may be difficult for some people to digest. For this reason, when eaten with fruit, gas/flatulence commonly arises due to incomplete digestion of both foods. Raw cruciferous vegetables and sprouts may be eaten with green-leafy vegetables and oils. In some people they mix well with avocados and olives.

18. After some time of eating all raw plant foods you may find your digestion will have strengthened to the point where you can combine almost any raw foods together without any adverse reactions. I have even combined water-melon, macadamia nuts, avocados, cucumbers, kale, and tomatoes at the same time without an adverse reaction.

Transition Guidelines

1. Control and direct your thoughts. The more you think about yourself as you could be, rather than as you perceive you are, the more excited you will become about increasing your health. You will begin to see yourself as a radiant being. You will be convinced you can do it. One day you will succeed in performing something you previously thought of as quite impossible to accomplish. You may not even notice this extraordinary deed. But as you keep on performing impossible acts, or as impossible things keep on happening, you become aware that a sort of power is emerging.

2. What you do must be the product of your own conclusions. At some point on this dietary journey, you are going to have to have faith: faith in the restoring power of natural foods; faith in yourself and your own good judgment. No degree of

success is possible without some degree of trust in our intuition and the unknown. This is laid out in nearly every spiritual book, including Napoleon Hill's master-piece **Think And Grow Rich**. In fact, he dedicated a whole chapter to faith, and I present you a lesson on this subject as well.

3. Guard your mind against the negative influences of other people. Critically think through free advice. Anything acquired without effort and without cost is generally not helpful. Seek out and listen to those who are getting the results you desire.

4. Transition smoothly away from the meat-based diet as calmly and as quickly as possible. People often first let go of red meat, then pork, then chicken and then fish. This pattern works extremely well. Replace meat with avocados, young coconuts, olives, nuts and seeds. By transitioning from a cooked-meat diet to a vegetarian diet, happier feelings, more vigorous health experiences and positive emotions will arise more often.

5. Transition smoothly away from dairy foods by first letting go of eggs, milk and then cheese. Move to raw organic milk or cheese if you feel it is necessary. One may replace dairy foods with green-leafed vegetables for calcium and avocados, young coconuts, olives, nuts and/or seeds for their excellent raw plant-fat content.

6. Continue to eat a large percentage of raw plant foods throughout your transition. Once you have let go of animal foods and have adopted a vegan diet, then you may find the transition to more and more raw foods easier.

7. The body feels a shake up and discomfort with a sudden change in diet. Counselors who have worked with drug addicts know that it can be dangerous to stop a drug habit too abruptly. The body can be shocked by being deprived of a certain poison, such as cocaine, especially when this drug's constant use has forced the body to adapt itself to the poison. A drug can actually become a physiological necessity one must wean away from. This same principle holds true with many addictive cooked foods. Transition at your own pace, but continue moving forward. To be successful in anything, you must be willing to step outside of your comfort zone. Push the bounds of your potential. All successful people have this in common. You may realize your comfort zone was

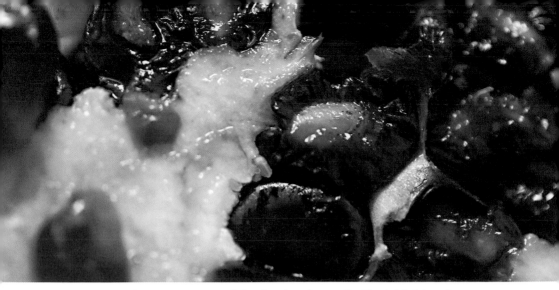

**If you have never enjoyed the ripe, bursting, antioxidant-rich juice of
the pomegranate then certainly one of life's great pleasures has escaped you.**

never really comfortable! Stabilize at 70% raw, then 80%, then 90%. Try eating
a 100% raw plant-food diet if that is possible for you.

8. The ultimate diet, weight loss success formula: "Increase raw, decrease
cooked." It works every time.

9. Take massive raw-foods action. Start consistently putting significant
amounts of high-quality raw plant foods into your body instead of cooked food.
Just get the raw food into your body and everything else follows. Get the old
juicer out of the cupboard or invest in a new juicer. Drinking fresh vegetable
juice daily (about 1/2 liter or more) is extremely important in the transition
process and beyond. Drink slowly; mix the juice well with your saliva before
swallowing. Drinking fresh vegetable juice allows minerals to reach the blood
and tissues quickly.

10. Eat wild, home-grown and/or organic food. Organic food is grown without
pesticides and other dangerous chemicals, such as chemical fertilizers (see the
section on Organic Food above). Organic food also is free of genetic modifica-
tion. Eating pesticide-free and non-genetically-modified foods are extremely
important for all healthy populations to observe into the future.

11. For the ideal digestion and assimilation of fruits, maintain a mono-diet
(one fruit at a time) whenever comfortable. If you do eat more than one type of

fruit, try to give yourself 30 to 60 minutes between fruit types. Fruits may be combined, but the mono-diet is simplest for digestion. The mono-diet is based on the realization that when you eat any fruit in its original state, its taste changes at some point from pleasant to unpleasant. This means that when the organism has filled its need for that particular food, it no longer wants any more and the taste of the food changes. Pineapple, for example, gives a very strong taste change and can actually burn the mouth if one continues to eat past the signal. This is called an aliesthetic taste change.

12. For ideal digestion and assimilation, eat green-leafy vegetables with raw plant fats and eat raw plant fats with green-leafy vegetables.

13. Chew your food well (50 to 100 chews per mouthful). This is going to take some concentration. An East Indian proverb states: "Chew your food well for the stomach has no teeth." Another proverb states: "Drink your food, chew your juice." Remember, the entire premise behind digestion is to turn the food into a liquid so it may be absorbed.

14. Eating seasonal fruits and green-leafed vegetables is Nature's way of telling you what to eat and when.

15. Eat fruits which contain good, strong, viable seeds. Eat fruits in their perfectly ripe stage. A perfectly ripe jalapeno pepper is red. A perfectly ripe lime is yellow. A perfectly ripe eggplant is yellow.

16. Eat more sweet fruit and/or seeds if you are active. Eat more green-leafy vegetables and/or non-sweet fruits if you are sedentary.

17. Be aware that certain cooked-food cravings present themselves when you are tired (at the end of a long day). Be prepared. Go to sleep early if necessary. Drink a glass of pure water with a twist of fresh lemon. Persist, break the old cycles and soon the desire disappears. Cravings are always temporary.

18. For ideal food use and assimilation: eat only when actual hunger exists. Avoid "emotional" or "boredom" eating.

19. Exercise is the key to metabolizing food. Food is best metabolized when the desire is created for it through movement. Exercise creates a "draw" for nutrients within the blood and lymph systems. *To thrive on a raw-food diet, exercise is essential.*

20. Digestion is an art. Try eating while standing. When you are sitting, your internal organs are compressed and digestion is hindered. Also, try fully squatting, instead of sitting, during a bowel movement-elimination.

21. Make a practice of eating the foods that agree with you.

22. Food itself is an anchor that accesses different emotional states. To break food addictions, identify which emotional state you are trying to reach and then discover a way to get there without food. Periods of food obsession will pass, just stay the course. Work through emotional addictions to food. You can do it. Ask for help.

23. Have a relative, friend, spouse or lover do The Sunfood Diet with you. Support each other.

24. Get a job, career, or simply volunteer in either the diet, exercise, health or success field! This will challenge you to walk your talk and keep pushing beyond former boundaries. It will bring you in contact with positive, supportive people. Introduce this book to new, positive acquaintances to help them along.

25. Consider donating all the cooked foods, pots, and pans in your home to charity. When you decide to make the "jump," go to local organic food stores, farmer's markets, or farms and purchase a massive amount of raw plant food — get a good variety — and let the fun begin.

26. If interested in eating an all-raw diet, I recommend initially experimenting with it on a small scale. First go 100% raw for a day. Then extend that to a week, or a month. Set in advance a specific date and mark each successful day on a calendar. Understand that after you go 100% raw for five to seven months straight, your body will not readily accommodate a return to a previous cooked-food diet because you will be too cleansed, sensitized and purified for your body to handle other foods.

27. What is the method by which your body returns to its natural diet? It is the pain/pleasure principle. As your body becomes more and more in tune with itself, the pain/pleasure principle takes over. Raw plant foods are so pleasurable that other choices disappear!

28. Meet other people excited about eating a raw plant-food diet. Hold regular raw-food potlucks. Place a raw-food potluck notice on the bulletin board of your local natural-foods markets.

29. This book has been designed as a constant source of motivation. My desire is that the intensity of the emotion and the inspiration with which I live my life and which I have put into this book are passed along to you consistently. This book was created for you. Refer to it often. For support, reference my Internet websites (www.thebestdayever.com, www.davidwolfe.com). If you do not have a computer, Internet access is available at any public library.

30. Educate yourself. Saturate your mind (see **Lesson 25: Saturation Point**). Read, listen to audio recordings, watch DVDs and videos about natural, raw plant-food nutrition. Discuss the idea with others. What you think about comes about.

Cooked Starches

Cooked starches (breads, pastas, cakes, rice, corn chips, potato chips, baked potatoes, popcorn, crackers and cookies) are typically the last cooked foods to go for most people as they transition into raw foods. This is because cooked starch is the most addictive and the most blood-sugar-altering food. LifeFood nutritionist Dr. David Jubb has pointed out that starch does not appear in foods growing wildly, starch develops as foods are domesticated, genetically cross-bred and hybridized (see **Lesson 16: Hybrid Food**).

A diet heavy in cooked starch over many decades can cause arteriosclerosis (hardening of the blood vessels), ossification of the tissues and joints, skin thickening, and premature aging. As Professor Arnold Ehret pointed out, the reason a cooked-meat eater might live longer than a starch-eating vegetarian is because the first produces less obstructions than the starchy overeater; but the meat-eater's later diseases are always more dangerous because of the accumulated poisons, pus and uric acid found in the meats.

To help overcome addictions to cooked starch, one can switch to dehydrated starchy foods. Every little discipline adds upon every other. Another useful tool to stay off starches is to combine sweet fruits and fats together in a meal. For example, oranges can be eaten with avocado or apples with nuts. This simulates the gradual sugar release from the breakdown of complex carbohydrates (cooked starch) in digestion.

Dehydrated Food

Dehydrated foods (foods heated below 118° Fahrenheit) are an excellent tool to help succeed with the raw-food approach. Dehydrated foods still have the enzymes intact and my experience has been that they do not dampen the raw-food "high." However, I rarely eat dehydrated foods (except dehydrated flax crackers) and I imagine they could alter the raw-food "high" if overeaten regularly. Many raw-food recipe books describe how to make dehydrated foods. I recommend **Raw Transformation, Rawvolution, I Am Grateful, Raw Food Real World**, and **RAW: The Uncook Book**. There are many other great recipe books on the subject.

Frozen Food

Generally, freezing food destroys anywhere from 30% to 66% of the enzymes in the food. Freezing is not as damaging as cooking. My own experiences and experiments have demonstrated that freezing alters the water and fiber in food and causes slow or constipated digestion if frozen food (even if defrosted) is eaten in excessive quantities. Water expands when frozen. The delicate fibrous structures inside all fruits and vegetables are damaged as water expands during the freezing process.

Some raw plant foods are more tolerant of freezing than others. Durians, for example, tolerate freezing well. Berries are tolerant of the freezing process. Nuts and seeds are also tolerant of freezing temperatures as they possess a rich content of fats and oils and a low content of water.

Overeating

Every Sunfoodist grows through periods of eating large quantities of raw plant foods, especially during the transition and beyond. This is part of overcoming food cravings and releasing emotions. I recommend that you tune in to the aliesthetic taste change, progressively simplify your diet (by living mostly on liquids), face sunken emotions when they come up, and enjoy the process of becoming healthier, happier and more joyful.

My personal feeling is that occasionally overeating raw plant foods is okay. You still get the results and the spiritual connection. A gorilla might eat 60 pounds (27 kilograms) of fruits and vegetables a day! Considering that a gorilla weighs three times as much as the average person, we may deduce that eating 1/3 of a gorilla's fare would not be overeating. 1/3 of 60 pounds is 20 pounds of fruits and vegetables! Nobody can eat 20 pounds (9 kilograms) of raw fruits and vegetables every single day.

If you overeat one type of food, such as sweet fruit, remember The Sunfood Triangle: balance by eating more fats and green-leafed vegetables. Many new Sunfoodists overeat dried fruit and nuts; this is okay, as long as this behavior is balanced by green-leafed vegetables (see The Sunfood Triangle). Also, it is better to overeat avocados and olives than nuts, as avocados and olives are more digestible.

Something to keep in mind: a raw-foodist once shared a great piece of knowledge when he told me that, "Any food is addictive, if you eat too much of it." Switch your common foods around occasionally. Also, sometimes skip a meal and just drink water. Drinking water helps to alleviate hunger.

Eating more high-quality mineral-rich food stops us from overeating. This demonstrates that overeating is often caused more by a desire for minerals, and less by the desire for calories.

The best way to overcome the desire for eating is to be so busy striving for and achieving goals that no time is left to eat!

Enjoy your new diet. Once you feel capable, begin experimenting with eating less until you feel comfortable with less food. Refine your diet with time — be patient. The saying goes: "Eat a little, that way, you'll be around long enough to eat a lot." Systematic undereating slows the aging process.

Flatulence

When one begins The Sunfood Diet, fermentations may occur which form gas and flatulence in the intestinal tract. This may have several causes which are listed below:

1. When Sunfoods reach plaque encrusted intestines (impacted with mucus and hardened fecal matter), they will not digest properly and fermentation may occur. To alleviate this situation, one should have a series of 5 to 8 colonics conducted by a registered colon hydrotherapist and also undertake an herbal cleanse.

2. Foods are being combined haphazardly in less than ideal combinations. It is best to eat one type of food at a time, and then wait twenty minutes to an hour to consume the next item.

3. Foods that are difficult to digest, such as bean sprouts, wheatberry sprouts, or soaked oats, are eaten in large quantities without being mixed with a sufficiently large quantity of green-leafed vegetables.

4. Overeating apples and pears (or their juices). These foods contain large quantities of pectin and other bowel cleansing compounds that can increase flatulence.

5. Undereating full-spectrum salts (sea salt , rock salt) and/or sodium-residue foods — especially greens (kale, celery, dandelion, spinach). These foods cool the intestines. When the intestines are heated by too much potassium or sulfur-residue foods, flatulence results.

6. A candida overgrowth or another microbial/fungal imbalance of the digestive tract is occurring. This can be overcome by an organic no-sugar, no-starch diet, probiotics containing: acidophilus, bifidus and bulgaricus, supplemental enzymes, more dietary greens, green juices, seeds, seaweeds, superfoods, grapefruit seed extract, olive leaf extract, vitamin C (from powdered berries), MSM powder (1-2 tablespoons per liter of water) and garlic.

If one repeatedly experiences gas and fermentation from eating sweet fruit as a mono-diet, this could be a sign of a candida overgrowth. If this is your situation, please review **Lesson 13: How To Use The Sunfood Triangle** under the section **Eating To Overcome Candida**.

Natural healers know that snakebites are dangerous, not only because of the venom, but also due to the fermentation they cause in the tissues. Ice on a

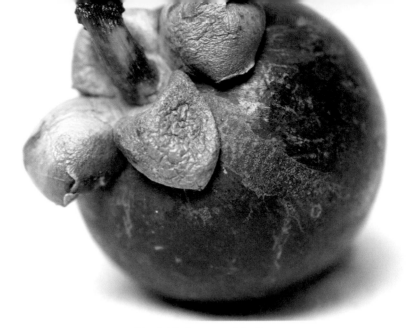

The fabled queen of fruits —
The Mangosteen

snakebite will halt fermentation (and also decrease circulation to slow the spread of the venom). To stop digestive fermentation, place a cool object or ice-pack on the diaphragm, or get into cold water. Sucking on ice cubes for 15 minutes may also be helpful.

Better Choices

Choose positive friends over negative relatives.

Choose wine over beer. Most wine is raw. Wine is simply the product of grape fermentation. Beer is brewed (cooked)! An occasional glass of wine does not break or hinder the Sunfood "high." Beer, however, always snapped the spell for me and I gave that up years ago. Choose organic wine containing no added sulfites. I personally do not consume alcohol anymore.

Choose dandelion over iceberg lettuce. Commercial iceberg lettuce contains relatively little nutrition. Dandelion is a wild food and it contains a full complement of minerals and vitamin C.

Choose yams over potatoes. Potatoes are genetically weak, hybridized foods. Yams are closer to the wild state; they contain far better nutrition.

Choose raw corn over corn chips. Have you ever eaten raw corn? We call it the "raw corn revelation." Even though it is a hybrid food, a little white sweet corn in the summer time is a beautiful thing. Watch out for genetically modified strains. Even better is to grow sacred, heirloom purple corn at home.

Choose ocean water, seaweed, Himalayan pink salt, or celtic sea salt over table salt. Discover the taste sensation of ocean water or dulse seaweed with lime, tomato and avocado! If any sprinkled salt is to be used, use highly-mineralized pink salt or celtic sea salt.

Choose dried fruit over candy. Dried fruit is filled with natural sugar which the body can recognize. Candy contains refined sugar that the body does not recognize and which acts as a powerful behavioral drug. Eat green-leafy vegetables with or following dried fruit to clean the teeth.

Choose cruelty-free, organic, raw wild honey over conventional orchard honey. Because most farm bees are cruelly treated and have their honey (food) taken away and replaced with sugar-water and antibiotics, I do not recommend conventional orchard honey. I recommend cruelty free, organic, raw wild honey. Problems with bread addiction may find relief by spreading a high quality honey on their bread. The enzymes (amylase in honey) will begin to predigest the bread starch.

Choose raw cacao beans (and raw honey) over cooked chocolate. To conquer addictions to cooked chocolate, replace cooked chocolate with the real thing that all chocolate is made from — cacao beans! I had an encounter once at one of my seminars with a group of women who cheered when they found out they could eat raw chocolate without guilt, fear or anxiety! (More information on chocolate is found at www.sacredchocolate.com and in my book **Naked Chocolate**.)

Choose dried prunes over dates. If you feel dates are too sugary or too strong, switch to dried prunes. If dates are eaten, they should be eaten in the fall and winter when they are in season. As far as dried fruit is concerned (while you are in the transition stage), prunes are a better choice than dates.

Choose dried figs over raisins. Raisins are great, if they have seeds. Without seeds they are hybrids (seedless). Dried figs are full of crunchy little seeds that compliment the taste and encourage thorough chewing.

THE TRANSITION DIET

1 Enjoy your food without fear or anxiety. Eat 100% love. As long as you are eating the food and it is entering your body, allow it to be fully enjoyed and metabolized! Eat your food naturally — relax. How relaxed are your face, stomach and hands while you eat?

2 Immediately act upon the transition guidelines outlined in this lesson. How can you adopt the transition principles into your lifestyle today and enjoy the process?

3 Use the Superior Food Combining table from this lesson daily until it becomes embedded in your consciousness. Photocopy the table and post it in your kitchen or dining area.

4 If you are not able to get organic fruits and vegetables, what do you do?
   a Ask for organic food at your local store.
   b Order organic foods to be delivered by mail to your home (see the **Resources** section at the end of this book).
   c Start your own garden. If you do not have a yard, ask a friend if you can grow a garden in her/his yard.
   d Search for local organic growers. Perhaps you can volunteer your services in exchange for food?
   e Start your own organic farm!
   f Write a letter to your local politicians, newspapers and other media outlets, telling them how you feel about the difficulties of finding non-poisoned food in your area.
   g Eat wild foods.
   h Plant fruiting plants and trees wherever you legally can and enjoy the harvest each year.
   i Consider moving to a better location where higher-quality foods are available.
   j Contact the gardening advocacy group: Food Not Lawns.

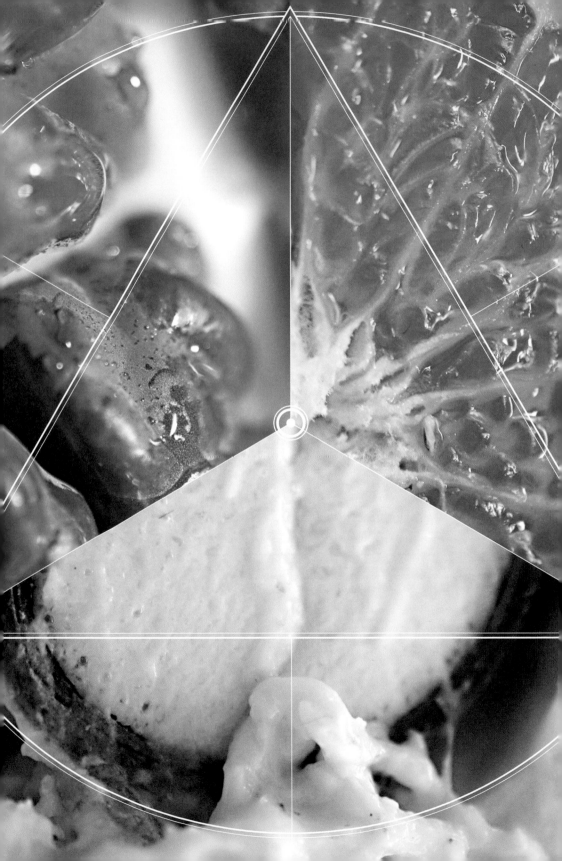

13

HOW TO USE THE SUNFOOD TRIANGLE

The charts provided in this lesson become applicable when 70-100% of your food intake consists of raw food. By balancing the three food classes: green-leafy vegetables, sweet fruits and fatty foods against each other in different ratios, we can feel different effects. If we eat more greens, and less sweet fruits and fats, we will be calmed and mellowed out. If we eat more sweet fruits, and fewer greens and fats, we will achieve more instantaneous energy. Basically, we can move the center of The Sunfood Triangle around to experience different results.

Many of the suggestions provided in this lesson are temporary measures. We do need a good, healthy amount of all three food classes in our diet. In some sections below, I recommend a certain food class may be limited, or totally elim-inated, from the diet. This is a temporary measure only! For example, if we are "Eating For Spirituality" we would remove fat from the diet. We will eventually need fat in the diet; however, this is a temporary suggestion to achieve a specific result.

The diagrams in this lesson are keyed to following dry weight ratio of the three food classes — chlorophyll:sugar:fat.

Eating For Weight Loss

A diet of raw plant food easily takes off those unwanted pounds. Any cooked foods eaten should be properly combined. This means that cooked starch (complex carbohydrates) should not be combined with cooked protein (fish, meat), and any cooked foods should be eaten with a large green-leafy salad.

Specifically target and minimize cooked fats (heated oils, pasteurized milk and cheese, cooked eggs, as well as fat-dominant meats, such as bacon) and cooked starch (bread, pasta, cakes, cookies) in the diet as they both put on the extra pounds. Pizza and cooked ice cream both contain a high dosage of cooked starch and cooked fat, and are both particularly fattening. Cooked fats, devoid of lipase (the fat-splitting enzyme), accumulate in the body as they are difficult to metabolize and this results in weight gain (raw fats, such as

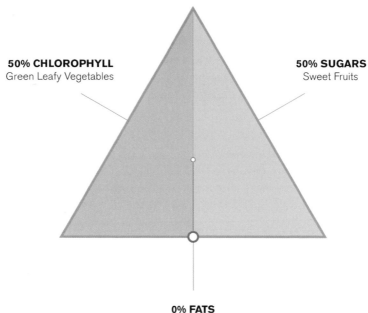

50% CHLOROPHYLL
Green Leafy Vegetables

50% SUGARS
Sweet Fruits

0% FATS
Fatty Fruits, Nuts, Coconuts, Seeds

To Lose Weight center at 50:50:0
(Chlorophyll : Sugars : Fat)

avocados, can actually help one lose weight as they contain lipase — which the body can use to help metabolize stores of cooked fats). Cooked starch is essentially sugar, and if this sugar is not used as fuel, or urinated away by the body, it is converted to fat. This is also true of all processed sugars including barley malt, corn syrup, rice syrup and brown or white sugar which should also be avoided.

The best strategy is to eat the raw fruits and vegetables that you like the best. As you progress, you will gradually decrease the amount of cooked food that you are eating, and you will develop a taste for different raw, healthy fruits and vegetables. I know at least a dozen individuals whom I have met over the years who have lost 150 pounds (67 kg) eating raw plant foods. I have seen individuals over 3 years drop from 300 lbs. to 150 lbs. (135 kg to 67 kg). This kind of weight loss dramatically effects a life transformation. Weight loss is easy when it is done intelligently and naturally with raw, organic plant foods.

If one simply remains within The Sunfood Triangle regime at a high-raw level, the body will take off the necessary weight over time. However, if one is looking to accelerate weight loss, then one should cut fats out of the diet (or at least minimize them) until you have reached your desired weight. Nuts, in particular, should be eliminated from the diet for weight loss.

The best snack foods for those in search of weight loss are cacao beans (raw chocolate), cucumbers, tomatoes, bell peppers, raw okra, bok choy and celery because they contain very few (if any) calories and are satisfying. Cacao beans make a fantastic addition to smoothies and raw desserts because they are a natural appetite suppressant.

Eating For Weight Gain

How many obese animals do we see in Nature? Animals carry exactly the weight they need and no more. Every animal in Nature is at a perfect weight without exception. What is considered a normal weight by civilization's standards is actually an artificial weight created by a demineralized cooked-food diet. Your natural weight might be five to ten pounds (2.3 to 4.5 kg) lighter than what is recommended in the common body weight charts. However, these charts are not always accurate as people differ in bone size, bone and tissue density, musculature, etc.

Initially, when you adopt The Sunfood Diet, you will most likely lose weight as your body detoxifies wastes it has accumulated over a lifetime. This is a necessary process. Don't worry about it, embrace it. First and foremost, allow your body to detoxify.

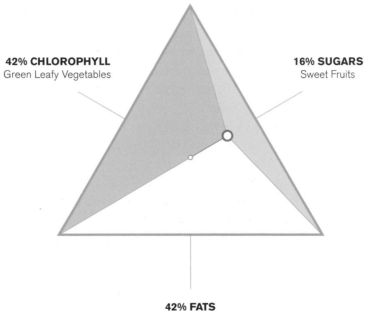

42% CHLOROPHYLL
Green Leafy Vegetables

16% SUGARS
Sweet Fruits

42% FATS
Fatty Fruits, Nuts, Coconuts, Seeds

To Gain Weight center at 42:16:42
(Chlorophyll : Sugars : Fat)

The inability to gain weight when eating raw plant foods may in some cases actually be caused by eating cooked-food. Eating cooked starch (bread, cookies, pasta, rice, etc.) with certain metabolisms actually promotes weight loss when one is significantly purified and has been eating 95%+ raw food for more than 6 months. In some cases, when the body is at that level of purification, digesting cooked starch drains living water and vital energy, leaving one sallow.

The inability to gain weight when eating raw plant foods may also be due to an encrusted intestinal tract, which hinders food absorption and causes emaciation. Encrusted mucus on the intestinal wall may eventually be dislodged over time if one eats raw foods, small green salads, juices, blended soups, as well as supplemental enzymes and incorporates yoga exercises to condition and strengthen the abdominal area. And, the process may be accelerated by a series of 6-10 colon irrigations (colonics), incorporating probiotics (friendly intestinal bacteria) into the diet (acidophilus, bifidus, L. salivarius, etc.) and an herbal cleanse program.

The inability to gain weight when eating raw plant foods may also be due to parasitic infections which may cause emaciation. If you suspect that you have a parasitic infection, I recommend that you "burn" them out with daily meals containing one or more of the following: garlic, onions, hot peppers, ginger, papaya seeds and spicy wild greens (wild mustard is excellent). High-quality herbal remedies can be effective against parasites. Oxygen therapies are also effective (read Ed McCabe's book **Flood Your Body With Oxygen**)

Once the body is significantly detoxified, which may take anywhere from four months to two years, depending on the toxicity of the body beforehand, then you can gain all the healthy weight you desire. I recommend you do so in the method shown in the previous diagram.

The secret to gaining strength and weight by eating a raw plant-food diet is to eat green-leafed vegetables and plant fats together — and fewer sweet fruits — as well as by adding superfoods (spirulina, raw hemp protein, maca, etc.) into one's diet. More non-sweet fruits may be included as well. Consuming these foods in a blended state is recommended. My own experience proved this true. I found it worked for thousands of others. Test for yourself and see.

Think of the gorilla: pound per pound the strongest land mammal. The gorilla possesses a fantastic musculature and is capable of bench pressing 4,000 pounds (more than 1800 kg). In his wonderful book, **L'Homme, Le Singe, Et Le Paradis (Humans, Primates, and Paradise)**, Albert Mosseri describes:

(Translation) "The gorilla is not interested in eating so-called protein foods. How can they develop all that muscle mass, weighing many hundreds of pounds, eating only green vegetables and fruits? This fact is of great importance."

Since gorillas eat nearly 80% green-leafed vegetation and have a similar digestive physiology to the human body, the lesson here is that eating plenty of green-leafed vegetation increases strength and muscle mass.

All the building blocks necessary to construct and energize your body are present in plants. Out of the 22 amino acids found in the body, 8 must be derived from food. The body is capable of recycling and manufacturing the other 14 amino acids. All 8 essential amino acids are packaged in abundance in raw plant foods, especially in green leaves and superfoods (spirulina, blue-green algae, bee pollen, maca, goji berries, wolfberries and hempseeds).

Raw plant fats are "fatty." They are heavy and of course help with weight gain. They will put just the right amount of fat on your body to give you excellent proportions and a good shape. They also add weight indirectly by providing fuel for working the muscles to build muscle mass. However, eating more fats alone will not cause weight gain, greens must be added. Fats help the body assimilate the amino acids and minerals from greens.

My personal salad formula for gaining weight consists of the following 3 foods:
> a) Tomatoes (Non-sweet fruits with a high water-content)
> b) Macadamia nuts (High-fat nuts)
> c) Kale leaves (Dense in minerals, amino acids, and protein)

I have eaten this mixture for lunch and dinner on many occasions. After several years of following a raw-food diet, my weight stabilized at 150 pounds (68 kg). This type of salad combination and eating style, in conjunction with vigorous exercise, helped me gain 18 pounds (8.2 kg) and reach 168 pounds (76 kg) in a span of two years while maintaining my all-raw diet and a body-fat level of 9.4%. I am 6 feet tall (190 cm).

Another good weight gain combination I have enjoyed is eating avocados with olives and chasing them with green juice.

The heaviest tissues in your body are muscle, fat and bone in that order. It has been estimated that 40% to 50% of our body weight is muscle! Muscle is best constructed out of green vegetables and superfoods.

Consistent exercise is also important for gaining weight. Engage in rigorous exercise; work and enlarge your muscles; increase your muscle mass by doing more resistant, anaerobic exercise.

Also, consider the wise words of the Greek historian Herodotus: "Exposure to the Sun is highly necessary in persons whose health needs restoring and who have need of putting on weight." The ancient Greeks and Romans knew the Sun feeds the muscles. For males, the Sun's rays on the skin and the genital organs stimulate the production of testosterone which increases muscle size and sexual potency. The muscles receive an increased amount of blood flow when they are exposed to Sunlight. This helps to provide nutrients to build strength. Vitamin D (which is actually a hormone not a vitamin) strengthens bones and helps to increase bone mass and mineralization. Vitamin D is formed internally by exposure of the skin to the Sun.

Slowing the metabolism will allow one to increase their weight. There is great value in avoiding frequent snacks. The way to gain weight on The Sunfood Diet is to eat more food, less often. The more often you eat, the quicker your metabolism runs, and the more weight you will lose. The less often you eat, the slower will be your metabolism, and the more weight you will gain or retain. Also and again, to gain weight one must eat more green-leafy foods, fats and superfoods and eat less sweet fruits, as described above.

People who are of an ayurvedic vata constitution (typically a person who tends to be thin already) will find great weight gain value in blending smoothies and salads to create soups (see Sequoia's Calcium Soup in **Appendix C: Sunfood Recipes** of this book for more information on blended raw soups). Blending food adds more caloric value and increases the mineral density of foods, both of which have a balancing effect for a vata constitution.

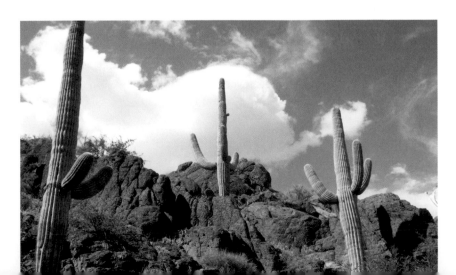

Feeding Healthy Children

The most beautiful children I have met or seen have been children raised on raw plant foods. They are alert, content, happy and eager to explore life. In the final (seventh) edition of his famous book, **Baby And Child Care**, the world's most famous childcare specialist, Dr. Benjamin Spock, recommends breast-feeding until solid foods are introduced. He specifically recommends a vegetarian diet at that point and, beyond age two, a vegan diet with an emphasis on raw plant foods. Dr. Spock's own vegetarian diet had given him "a new lease on life." He wanted the seventh edition of his book to be in the forefront of linking the consumption of meat and dairy with disease.

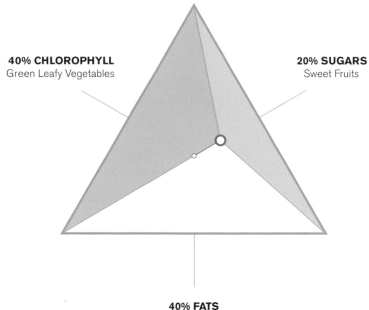

40% CHLOROPHYLL
Green Leafy Vegetables

20% SUGARS
Sweet Fruits

40% FATS
Fatty Fruits, Nuts, Coconuts, Seeds

To Feed Children center at 40:20:40
(Chlorophyll : Sugars : Fat)

Children naturally gravitate towards sweet, bright-colored fruits. Parents must keep in mind that children also need fat, chlorophyll-rich foods and superfoods. Calcium and magnesium are extremely important for growing children, and if not coming from the mother's breast milk, it must be in the diet in the form of green-leaves and/or green juices in sufficient quantities.

If your children have trouble eating green-leafed vegetables, try mixing apples or pears with green-vegetable juice — all freshly made. Try feeding your children Sequoia's Calcium Soup found in **Appendix C: Sunfood Recipes** at the back of this book. Because some children resist bitter compounds in vegetables, you may also use dried, powdered grasses (mixtures of powdered barleygrass, wheatgrass, etc.) in fruit or coconut water smoothies. These powders will allow you to get the minerals in without the child resisting based on taste. Very young children sometime prefer the taste of grass to typical green vegetables. Also, lead by example. Children do what you do, not what you say (as I am sure you have already discovered!).

Pregnant mothers should also balance their Sunfood Diet with more greens and fats with lots of variety to feed the growing baby. Foods with plenty of trace minerals (edible wild plants, organic seaweeds, wild bee pollens, seeds, superfoods, etc.) should be included in the diet of children and pregnant mothers. A very important addition for mothers and young children is the raw, vegetarian form of "fish oil" that is actually algae oil or DHA. This oil helps to promote: proper brain formation, increased intelligence, excellent eyesight, strong nerves and the alleviation of depression. An ample supply of vitamin B12 is also vital for the nerve health of breast-feeding mothers and growing children.

For more information on breastfeeding, natural childbirth, mother-child bonding and raw-food parenting, please read **Conscious Eating** and **Rainbow Green Live-Food Cuisine** by Dr. Gabriel Cousens. Also, **The Continuum Concept** is a classic book on natural childcare.

Eating For The Elderly

Imagine that the entire digestive tract from the mouth all the way through the body is one big muscle. Over a lifetime of eating processed, microwaved, pasteurized and/or cooked foods lacking in fiber, vitamins, minerals, amino acids, various nutrients and enzymes, the digestive "muscle" becomes weakened. A weak "muscle" may not be able to handle a large quantity of nutrient-rich, fiber-rich fresh fruits and green leaves immediately. Therefore, it is best to ease a more mature digestive system on to raw plant foods in a manner which allows strengthening and progress without shocking the system. I have found this principle of comfortable transition particular applicable to those over the age of 40 on macrobiotic diets who are switching over to raw foods.

By consistently drinking fresh vegetable juices, eating a small, though increasing, amounts of fiber-rich foods (such as non-sweet fruits and green-leafed vegetables) and chewing them very well before swallowing, the digestive "muscle" will be strengthened and cleaned over time.

Elderly people are typically not as active as the younger generation; therefore I recommend less sweet fruit in their diet. The soft, comforting fruit fats (especially avocado) help soothe the more mature digestive system and are an appropriate balancing food for menopause.

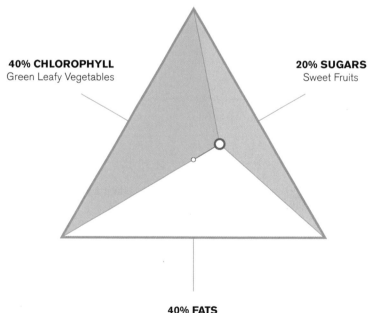

40% CHLOROPHYLL
Green Leafy Vegetables

20% SUGARS
Sweet Fruits

40% FATS
Fatty Fruits, Nuts, Coconuts, Seeds

The Elderly can center at 40:20:40
(Chlorophyll : Sugars : Fat)

Additionally, elderly people require more amino acids in their diet as the liver's amino acid pool (amino acid reserves) decreases with age. Therefore amino acid rich seeds (hemp, flax, pumpkin) and superfoods (spirulina, bee pollen, propolis) become more important in the diet with age.

Of special note, the two raw foods known to have superior longevity properties are royal jelly and wolfberries or goji berries. These should be eaten daily as part of a youthening program.

Eating For Detoxification

By eating a diet of 100% raw plant foods, you will automatically begin to detoxify and heal poor health and disease conditions.

To accelerate detoxification and healing, we remove fat from the diet. Juicing and blending foods saves the body digestive energy channeling more energy for healing and detoxification. Dr. Norman Walker recommended a sugar-rich food (carrot, beet, apples) and green-leafed vegetables in nearly all his curative juice recipes. He did not quite understand the problems with hybrid, over-sugary, foods (foods were not as hybridized in his day as they are now), but he did understand the power of juice fasting. He understood the detoxification power of chlorophyll foods and natural sugar foods with no fatty foods included.

If you are doing an extended juice fast (15 days +), you may want to include small portions of cold-pressed olive, hemp or flax oil in with your drinks to provide the body with necessary fat to maintain some equilibrium.

In reality, eating for detoxification is more about not eating for detoxification. Generally, the less you eat, the longer you live (so the more you get to eat!). Eating less has thus far been the only scientifically proven method to extend the lifespan of humans, animals, birds and worms. Simple reasoning would suggest that eating less exposes the organism to less foreign materials, less toxins and less energy-draining foods.

It seems that as soon as one stops eating, all the toxins forced in through mucus pressure due to eating, especially toxic food, begin to flow out. A coating on the tongue will form, one may feel unwell, weakness can set in, hypoglycemia (low blood sugar) will make its appearance and other symptoms will arise.

The power of fasting in healing is formidable. Generally, however, the average individual living on chemicalized, antibioticized, pesticide-sprayed, genetically-modified, sugarized, microwaved, processed, pasteurized and/or cooked food is too toxic to fast. Fasting can draw out too many toxins at once and drain vital mineral reserves.

A better, safer idea would be to fast short periods on fresh vegetable juice (containing lemon), plenty of high-quality water and superfoods (spirulina, bee pollen, powdered grasses, blue-green algae, etc.) so that enough minerals are present to help escort toxins out of the body.

One interesting working theory that I agree with is that (when an individual

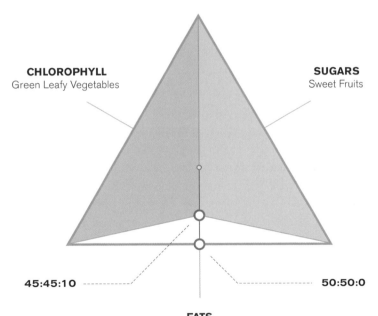

CHLOROPHYLL
Green Leafy Vegetables

SUGARS
Sweet Fruits

45:45:10

50:50:0

FATS
Fatty Fruits, Nuts, Coconuts, Seeds

For Detoxification center at 50:50:0 to 45:45:10
(Chlorophyll : Sugars : Fat)

is ready) one should continue on a juice fast cleansing program until all excessive body fat is eliminated. Body fat is where most of the body's poisons are stored.

Eating To Overcome Hypoglycemia And Diabetes

Eating animal foods typically aggravate the system to the point where hypo-glycemia (moodiness) and diabetes manifest, but (aside from the obviously dangerous white sugar and high fructose corn syrup) cooked hybridized plant starch is the real culprit. Hypoglycemia and diabetes are caused by eating cooked hybrid starchy foods — the worst of which includes white or wheat breads, beer, cooked corn of all types, stewed carrots, refined (beet) sugar, baked potatoes, white rice, french fries, cookies, potato chips, seedless fruit, etc. All these food types contain hybrid sugars the liver does not fully recognize and cannot regulate. These sugars send the glycemic index of the blood shooting sky-high causing either too much or too little insulin to be secreted by the pancreas (reference the Glycemic Index Chart in **Lesson 11: The Secret Revealed**).

Hypoglycemia is a condition where too much insulin is secreted into the blood by the pancreas to control blood sugar. Too much insulin in the blood causes blood sugar to drop too rapidly causing mood swings and erratic behavior. Avocados contain a seven-carbon sugar that depresses insulin production, which make them an excellent choice for people with hypoglycemia. Prickly pear cactus fruit juice (panini juice), mesquite beans (mesquite powder), and many seaweeds are raw food choices with some satisfying sweetness that also help control hypoglycemia.

Diabetes (type II) is one-step beyond hypoglycemia, when too little insulin is secreted into the blood. This is an eliminatory process of unused and/or unas-similable sugars, with the pancreas for a time stopping its secretions of insulin so the cells can unload their stocks of undesirable sugars into the bloodstream, and from there send the sugars into the urine to be eliminated. By stepping in at the critical moment and blocking this purge, injected chemical insulin forces the body to live with unacceptable sugars it can hardly tolerate, without being able to dismiss them.

To restore a healthy pancreatic condition, find the center in The Sunfood Triangle. Use good sweet fruits (with seeds) to boost the blood sugar when you feel it is dropping. Fats or protein (green vegetables, spirulina, hemp protein) can be used to thicken the blood if blood sugars rise too quickly. Green leaves (especially fresh green vegetable juice) and superfoods eventually provide the body with the alkaline protein and minerals it needs to restore itself to a healthy metabolism.

Beneficial supplements that I have noted over years to be helpful with pancreatic conditions include: supplemental enzymes and MSM (methyl-sulfonyl-methane) powder.

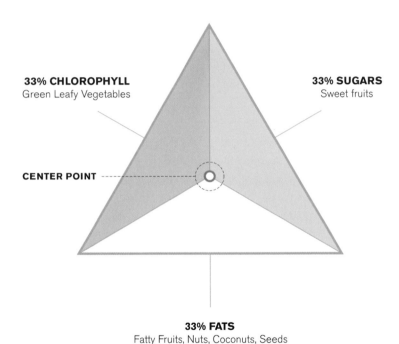

33% CHLOROPHYLL
Green Leafy Vegetables

33% SUGARS
Sweet fruits

CENTER POINT

33% FATS
Fatty Fruits, Nuts, Coconuts, Seeds

The Sunfood Triangle: The Center Point
(Chlorophyll : Sugars : Fat)

If you are on insulin injections, please contact a naturopathic doctor to devise a plan to wean yourself down or completely off from insulin.

It takes years to heal a diabetic condition, but it can be healed by staying the path. Many years ago, through a series of synchronous events, I ended up on **The Dating Game**. I met one of the show producers backstage. We started talking about raw foods. She told me her roommate had diabetes and was just beginning to get interested in raw-food nutrition. I called her roommate and we became fast friends. After about eight months of detoxification and natural foods, she was able to stop taking insulin for the first time in eight years.

My friend Sergei Boutenko was diagnosed with juvenile onset diabetes at age nine. This was after he collapsed into a near coma from bingeing on Halloween candy. The doctors said he would have to go on insulin for the rest of his life. His mother, Victoria, became determined and set out to find a better way. She asked everybody. Finally, in line one day (two weeks after Sergei's collapse) at the local natural food store, she randomly asked the woman in front of her if she knew anything about helping a child with juvenile onset diabetes. The woman told Victoria she had to get the child on the raw-food diet immediately, and recommended some books by Dr. Ann Wigmore. Sergei went raw immediately, his whole family (all of whom were suffering from a variety of illnesses) soon followed suit. Within two months he was completely back to normal. The entire family was also healed of their various conditions.

Sergei first visited me in January 1998. He spent a week at my house helping me with business and just having fun. Sergei, his sister, and parents travel around the United States and Canada catering raw-foods events and teaching people the incredible benefits of raw-food nutrition. Sergei has his own book out now called **Eating Without Heating**.

Eating To Overcome Candida

Candida is a type of fungi that excretes toxic waste that can get into the bloodstream and cause symptoms of bloating, clouded thinking, depression, diarrhea, exhaustion, halitosis (bad breath), menstrual pains, thrush (pasty saliva), unclear memory recall, yeast vaginitis and fungal nail conditions.

Conventional diets high in cooked-starches (bread, baked potato, cakes, cookies, pasta) and diets loaded with refined or hybridized (seedless) fruit sugars both feed candida. When all this sugar is added into a body whose levels of good intestinal bacteria (probiotics) are low and whose tissues have become acidic due to a prolonged lack of alkaline mineral salts (which come from vegetables and superfoods) in the diet, then candida proliferates.

Those suffering from candida typically have had a history of antibiotic use. This eliminates much of the good intestinal bacteria and also allows candida to spread.

Systemic yeast infections (candidiasis) find growth potential in a damp, musty condition in the body. Candida is a yeast and then a fungus when its rhizoids (long roots) penetrate the tissue mucosa and bridge the boundary between the internal body and digestive tract.

Candida can thrive only in a dark, moldy, oxygen-deprived environment. The very first recommendation I give to those with candida is to get more direct Sunlight on the skin. Yeasts and fungi are destroyed by direct Sunlight. Those

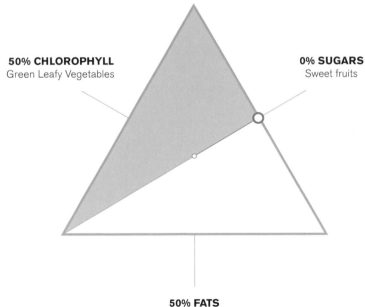

50% CHLOROPHYLL
Green Leafy Vegetables

0% SUGARS
Sweet fruits

50% FATS
Fatty fruits, nuts, coconuts, seeds

To Overcome Candida center at 50:0:50
(Chlorophyll : Sugars : Fat)

Excellent Low–Sugar Fruits include:
Avocado *(fatty fruit, excellent)*   Bell Pepper *(not green; green peppers are harsh and unripe)*   Bitter Melon   Breadfruit *(raw)*   Cranberry   Cucumber *(very healing)*   Grapefruit   Lemon *(may irritate the candida sufferer)*   Lime *(may irritate the candida sufferer)*   Noni   Okra *(very healing)*   Olives *(not from a can)*   Pumpkin   Sour apples   Squash   Tomatillo   Tomato   Zucchini

with candida must get their naked body into the Sun as much as they can. Oxygen is another key factor. Increasing oxygenation through oxygen therapies is a valuable aid in healing candida (please read **Flood Your Body With Oxygen** by Ed McCabe for more information on oxygen healing).

An anti-candida diet can include raw vegetables (mostly greens or non-sweet vegetables such as nopales or jicama...no potatoes or beet/carrot juices), green juices, occasional soaked nuts and seeds, seaweeds, superfoods (powdered grasses, chlorella, and green formulas), superherbs (reishi, horsetail, pau d'arco), young wild coconuts (not sugary Thai coconuts), raw coconut oil butter, raw cacao butter, a wide variety of low-sugar fruits and (only if necessary, but not recommended) one mildly medium-sized sweet fruit or small fruit serving per day (berries are best).

A food that provides particularly excellent benefits is raw coconut oil butter. Coconut oil butter is easily digested and is excellent for people who have trouble digesting fats. It consists of 48% lauric acid, a substance that exhibits anti-microbial, anti-bacterial and anti-fungal properties. All of these characteristics help to combat a candida overgrowth.

High doses of healthy intestinal probiotics (acidophilus, bifidus infantis, L. salivarius, L. plantarum, L. bulgaricus, etc.) that will colonize in the intestines are required to overcome candida.

Prebiotics are also valuable. These are foods that nourish probiotics (healthy bacterial flora). Prebiotics include foods such as chicory root, dandelion root, and yacon root.

One can find great benefit sugar fasting (eating no sweet fruit for several weeks or months and simultaneously dosing up on probiotics). For more detailed information on low-sugar, raw, anti-candida diets please read Dr. Gabriel Cousens' book **Rainbow Green Live-Food Cuisine**.

Sprouted grain can yield a slight quantity of usable sugar. When fasting from sugar for long periods, the little bit of sugar from sprouted grain can be beneficial and will not foster candida growth. Sprouted grains must be clean of fungus and of a high-quality or heirloom seed stock.

In the long term, when the desire for real sugar appears it must be addressed with high-quality, seeded sweet fruit, and not with cooked starch. Some sweet food must be eaten or the body will eventually go off balance. One to two pieces of non-hybridized fruit (0.4 pound or 0.2 kg) each day should be fine. Fermentation of the fruit from too many combinations must be avoided. If cooked foods are eaten, they should be non-starchy vegetables (such as broccoli, cauliflower, asparagus, artichoke, etc.).

Supplements that can be helpful with candida include: olive leaf extract, grapefruit seed extract, supplemental enzymes, MSM (methyl-sulfonyl-methane) powder, small amounts of fully-mineralized sea salt or rock salt, edible clays and powdered vitamin C-rich berries such as camu camu berry powder. MSM detoxifies mercury. Mercury poisoning seems to be a common underlying factor in candida.

Herbs that are great allies against candida include: oregano, garlic, pau d'arco tea, and cat's claw tea.

One may cautiously return to eating more sugary fruits in the diet once the body is cleansed and the candida symptoms have disappeared.

Anti–Candida Salad

Cilantro	Avocado
Lettuce	Flax Oil
Parsley	Sprouted Wild Rice or Barley or Sprouted Rye

I recommend following a cleansing and intestinal rebuilding program either before or after a sugar fast. Important guidelines for herbal cleansing while overcoming candida:

1. Do not have fruit juice if you have candida, especially while on an herbal cleanse. Use only vegetable juice or water for the psyllium shakes.

2. Take a high-quality probiotic formula containing at least acidophilus, bifidus and L. bulgaricus, at least 1 hour before bedtime throughout all the cleansing steps, 1/2 hour after each set of herbs, and 1/2 hour after each meal.

3. Take ample amounts of the probiotic bifidobacterium infantis through rectal implants (either through enemas or have your colon hydrotherapist do the implant). Bifidobacterium infantis is found in breast-fed infants, and is probably the most basic of all intestinal bacteria in the human species. Be sure to have your colon hydrotherapist provide you with an implant of bifidus bacteria following each session.

There is a psychology necessary to heal chronic candida. Candida is associated with subconscious self-destructive feelings of rejection and a lack of self-worth. Negative, self-destructive thoughts destroy good bacteria in the intestinal tract and allow candida to proliferate. Positive, self-confident thoughts help good bacteria proliferate in the intestines.

An emotional cleansing is required to overcome chronic candida. Be aware that unresolved issues usually involve parents or past lovers. While healing

candida (and while moving into raw foods in general) one should seek out counselors, friends, books, DVD's and/or audiotapes that can assist with emotional
releases.

In review, a candida condition can be remedied by the elimination of cooked
starch and antibiotics, lots of Sunshine on the skin, an increase of oxygen,
wholesome raw nutrition, fasting from sugar, adequate dosages of coconut oil,
superfoods, probiotics, prebiotics, specific supplements, superherbs and a
rebuilding program with colon cleansing as well as emotional cleansing.

Some additional recommendations: Those with candida should keep a clean
house; musty, moldy homes are bad for the candida sufferer. Panty hose should
not be worn; they trap moisture and lead to yeast vaginitis. All body orifices
should be allowed to breathe oxygen.

Eating For Mental Clarity

To achieve the maximum clarity of mind, fast or eat only one type of juicy,
sweet fruit for several days.

Two or three days of only sweet fruit (not overdone) will heighten your mental
clarity. Your brain runs primarily on glucose, which is best derived from sweet
fruit. In fact, several parts of this book were written while I was on a six-day
watermelon fast.

Once one is cleansed and remineralized, fasting on water places one right at
the center of The Sunfood Triangle — perfect balance. After your body is purified and you fast on water for several days, your mind will become so clear it will
astonish you. Fasting intensifies thoughts and wishes. Fasting and prayer are
mentioned 66 times together in the **Bible**. Remember, one should only undertake a water fast when the body is in balance and the blood is clean.

While fasting, stored glycogen (super-densified glucose) is released from the
liver and from within the cells to fuel the body. As one purifies their diet over a
long period of time, the cells and liver will accumulate stores of glycogen,
allowing one to fast longer and longer without a major blood sugar drop. In his
book **The Golden Seven Plus One**, Dr. C. Samuel West reports that each unit of

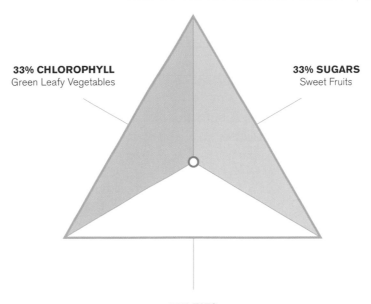

33% CHLOROPHYLL
Green Leafy Vegetables

33% SUGARS
Sweet Fruits

33% FATS
Fatty Fruits, Nuts, Coconuts, Seeds

For Mental Clarity center at 33:33:33
(Chlorophyll : Sugars : Fat)

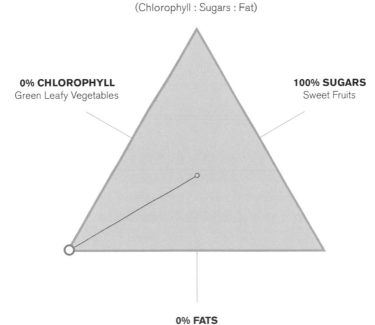

0% CHLOROPHYLL
Green Leafy Vegetables

100% SUGARS
Sweet Fruits

0% FATS
Fatty Fruits, Nuts, Coconuts, Seeds

For Mental Clarity center at 0:100:0
(Chlorophyll : Sugars : Fat)

glycogen contains 27,000 units of glucose — all of which can be released at once.

Eating For Athletics And Endurance

I advise athletes to stay right in the center of the triangle by increasing all three food classes equally. This provides more calories to burn for endurance. More sweet fruit, more fat, more green-leafed vegetables. Instead of "carbo-loading" (loading up on cooked starch, such as pasta, bread, and baked potatoes), the athlete should be loading up on a wide variety of agreeable, nutrient-rich raw foods and superfoods for several days leading up to the event. From my experience with surfing, I have noted that pumpkin seeds, in particular, provide excellent endurance fuel for me. Sweet fruits should be eaten regularly throughout competition to keep the blood sugar up. If the blood sugar bottoms out, the athlete can lose mental poise and quickly experience fatigue. Chewing green-leafed vegetables can be time consuming for an athlete; so green juices may be substituted for salad for athletes during peak training periods. Superfoods (spirulina, hemp protein, blue-green algae, maca, bee pollen, wolfberries and goji berries) are also valuable for their extraordinary protein and nutrient content.

I have worked with several world-class athletes and they have found great benefit from my green drink formulation. It consists of: kale, celery and cucumber put through a juicer. The kale provides the heavy minerals necessary to nourish the muscles (its alkaline elements neutralize lactic acid build-up); celery replaces the sodium lost through perspiration; and cucumber provides excellent fluids and soluble fiber.

Another excellent drink for athletes is coconut water, which is the highest source of electrolytes found in Nature. Electrolytes are electrically-conductive, charged minerals in solution that, once in the digestive system, directly nourish the tissues. Adding powdered superfoods to coconut water is a great idea.

Eating To Warm The Body

"Nevertheless, the calorific value of foods definitely exists. A number of years ago when I swam during the winter, I found that on a diet consisting mainly of salads and fruits, the body would take a minute or more to warm up and withstand the cold water. However, the reaction would be almost instantaneous when nuts, dried fruits and cereals were added

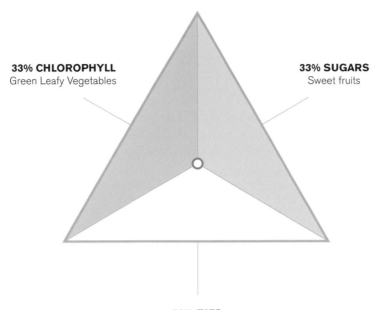

33% CHLOROPHYLL
Green Leafy Vegetables

33% SUGARS
Sweet fruits

33% FATS
Fatty Fruits, Nuts, Coconuts, Seeds

For Athletics and Endurance center at 33:33:33
(Chlorophyll : Sugars : Fat)

TO THE DIET. ADDING THESE FOODS ENABLED ME TO STAY LONGER
IN THE COLD WATER." — *Morris Krok, Fruit The Food And Medicine For Man*

The feeling of coldness when one begins a Sunfood Diet is typically caused by a thickening of the blood during detoxification episodes; this decreases circulation. It is also caused by an increased blood flow to the internal organs — which are finally given a chance to heal — and a corresponding decreased blood flow to the extremities.

As was demonstrated earlier in **Lesson 1: The Principle Of Life Transformation**, life change comes from the inside out. This is also true with the internal structure of the body. The most vital, central organs heal and transform first (the blood focuses there first). The musculature and the outer perimeter of the body are the last to heal.

After you persist through the transition and detoxification — through the feeling of coldness — you will discover that your resistance to both cold and hot weather will increase by eating raw foods.

A doe in the forest survives the harshest winters on a diet of simple grass. She has no cooking pot or stove.

Eating hot food can actually decrease your resistance to cold weather in the same way that a hot shower decreases your resistance to the cold. Just as a cold shower increases your resistance to cold weather, "cold" raw food also increases your resistance to cold weather.

To keep the body warm, consider eating food that is at room temperature. Cold refrigerated food will cool the body. Perhaps you can adjust your refrigerator to the warmest temperature it will allow.

Serving raw soups in warmed ceramic bowls may be helpful in cold winters. Warm water with a twist of lemon juice or herbal and medicinal teas are also wonderful. Paul Kouchakoff, the Swiss scientist who discovered that eating cooked food causes a white blood cell immune system reaction in the blood also discovered that water "corrupts" due to heat somewhere around 159° Fahrenheit (61° Celsius). This is valuable information for tea makers!

We can eat certain types of food to warm the system.

Fats warm the system. Fats contain the same elements as the carbohydrates, but the hydrogen is present in a much larger quantity, and this results in more heat being produced by its breakdown and digestion. Maca is a "fatty" vegetable superfood (usually powdered) that has incredible warming properties.

Potassium-rich foods are warming foods. Some nuts, such as macadamias, have a high level of potassium, as do seeds, such as sunflower seeds. Most fruits are rich in potassium. Some of the most warming, highest-potassium fruits are: avocados, dates, durians, persimmons (with seeds), prunes, pumpkin, raisins (with seeds), and sun-dried apricots. You will also notice that these fruits correspond to what is available in the fall and winter.

Sulfur-residue foods warm the body. Sulfur-residue foods include: cruciferous vegetables, garlic, and onions. Durian has a high sulfur and potassium-yield. In Asia, one who overeats durian is often said to have "hot eyes."

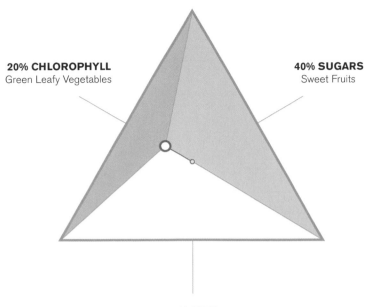

20% CHLOROPHYLL
Green Leafy Vegetables

40% SUGARS
Sweet Fruits

40% FATS
Fatty Fruits, Nuts, Coconuts, Seeds

To Warm the Body center at 20:40:40
(Chlorophyll : Sugars : Fat)

Eat a meal that is high in fats, potassium, and/or sulfur and you will notice a heating reaction within 45 minutes as the food begins to digest. This reaction will become more pronounced over time as one becomes more purified by eating a raw-food diet.

Eating To Cool The Body

"THE LIFE FORCE FLOWS THROUGH THE BODY, AND BY ACTING ON THE RESISTANCE OFFERED BY FOOD, GENERATES HEAT AND ENERGY AS A BY-PRODUCT." — *Dugald Semple, The Sunfood Way To Health*

We can do five things to cool the body nutritionally:
1. Fast. When you fast, your body temperature lowers.
2. Eat cold, refrigerated, frozen food or ice.
3. Eat only green-leafy vegetables. Green-leafy vegetables do not produce

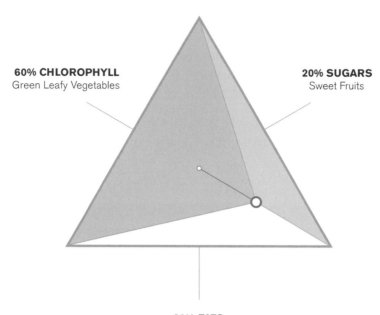

60% CHLOROPHYLL
Green Leafy Vegetables

20% SUGARS
Sweet Fruits

20% FATS
Fatty Fruits, Nuts, Coconuts, Seeds

To Cool the Body center at 60:20:20
(Chlorophyll : Sugars : Fat)

much heat as they pass through the human digestive system. They lack calories.

4. Eat sea or rock salt or high-sodium foods. Sodium-rich foods are cooling foods. Dark green-leafy vegetables, such as kale, dandelion, and spinach, are cooling. Celery is an excellent summer-time cooling food. Seaweeds are also cooling, unless the salt is washed off. Wild coconut water has a sodium yield and is a great cooling cocktail on hot, humid days.

5. Eat special cooling foods such as cucumbers, melons and cacao fruits.

Eating To Ground The Body

When one becomes ungrounded, a mineral deficiency is the primary cause. Vegetarians, vegans and raw-foodists who become ungrounded typically are eating weak, mineral deficient food. Animal foods — especially fish — due to its concentration of minerals, tends to bring people back to earth who have become ungrounded. There are other ways to ground oneself with plant foods.

Grounding occurs due to increasing the mineral-content of foods in one's diet. The more minerals in the food, the more grounded you feel...the more minerals, the more "ground" — literally. Generally, organically-grown, fatty foods (especially nuts and seeds) and green leaves are good sources of minerals. So, to ground the body, one would balance there and avoid commonly-found, mineral-deficient fruit.

Superfoods and seaweeds play an important role with keeping individuals grounded as well. Superfoods and seaweeds are generally dramatically more mineral- and protein-rich than everyday organic produce.

Edible clays and sea or rock salts, because they are earth, are also grounding.

Eating For Spirituality

"ALL PHILOSOPHY IN TWO WORDS — SUSTAIN BUT ABSTAIN."— *Epictetus*

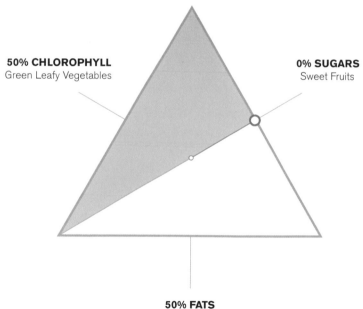

50% CHLOROPHYLL
Green Leafy Vegetables

0% SUGARS
Sweet Fruits

50% FATS
Fatty Fruits, Nuts, Coconuts, Seeds

To Ground The Body center at 50:0:50
(Chlorophyll : Sugars : Fat)

Dr. Johnny Lovewisdom taught me the spiritual value of avoiding fats for a selected period of time with his Vitarian Diet. Lovewisdom himself attempted to completely eliminate fats from his diet by swearing off all avocados, nuts and seeds (see his book **Spiritualizing Dietetics: Vitarianism**). He eventually introduced goat's milk (pure fat) into his diet (see Viktoras Kulvinskas' book **Life In The 21st Century**) – which justifies the conclusion that fats are essential.

We have already seen the value of a momentary period of a fatless diet for detoxification. When you strip away all the internal insulation created by fats, after all improper foods have been removed, then you tune directly into the cosmic spiritual energy that pervades all things. This is the Vitarian Diet, which contains few fats, and only fruits and vegetables of a high-water content.

This kind of fat-free diet can allow one to reach a tremendous, though passing, high. Years ago, my friend Joshua Rainbow told me that he became so sensitive on the Vitarian Diet that simply turning into the wind became an ecstatic experience. One must be careful with such lean diets in the long term as pollution in food, air and water makes the nerves more susceptible to damage when fat is absent in the diet. Also, mineral deficiencies, omega 3 fatty acid problems, and vitamin B12 issues may, over time, make their appearance with such nutritional approaches.

Because the desire for fat (and its insulation) increases the closer one is to civilization (pollution), this type of spiritual diet is heightened when one is living in Nature – far away from toxicity.

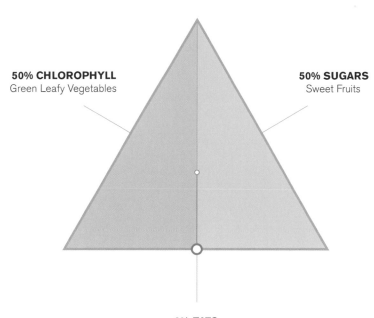

50% CHLOROPHYLL
Green Leafy Vegetables

50% SUGARS
Sweet Fruits

0% FATS
Fatty Fruits, Nuts, Coconuts, Seeds

For Spiritual Clarity center at 50:0:50
(Chlorophyll : Sugars : Fat)

A magnificent Kirlian photograph
of an organic jujube (sometimes called a Chinese date).
The jujube is generally considered a low-sugar fruit and
has been used for thousands of years in
Chinese medicine as a counterpoint to ginseng.

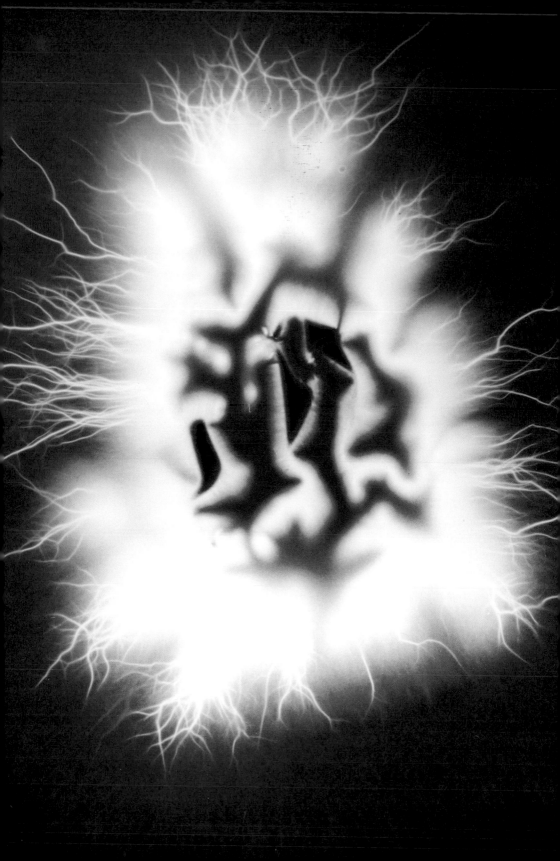

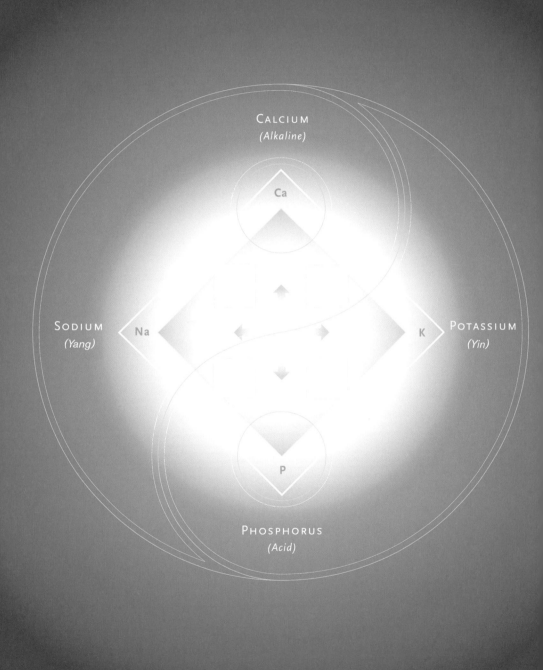

14

ALKALINE AND ACID

There are many different meanings to the terms "alkaline" and "acid" as they relate to human health. General lore on the subject proclaims that we should become alkaline and ingest alkaline substances. This may or may not be true depending on the individual context of what is meant by alkalinity and acidity. These meanings fall into three different categories: electrical charge, hydrogen content of water, and the dominant minerals in food.

Alkalinity and Electricity

The electrical meaning of "alkaline" is a highly negatively charged electrical potential. This is similar to a common battery, where one side is negative (alkaline) and the other is positive (acid). As long as the battery has a high negative electrical potential it is an "alkaline" battery.

Clint Ober, in his book **Earthing** and also in his subsequent research, has demonstrated that we are electrical beings long before we are chemical beings. Electrical energies have instant effects upon us. It has been shown for over one hundred years that the Earth itself is negatively charged and the atmosphere is positively charged. The two opposite charges dance in dynamic disequilibrium creating weather, and when highly polarized, also create thunder and lightning.

Some negative charge bleeds over into the atmosphere near waterfalls, breaking ocean waves, small campfires, or even the burning of beeswax candles

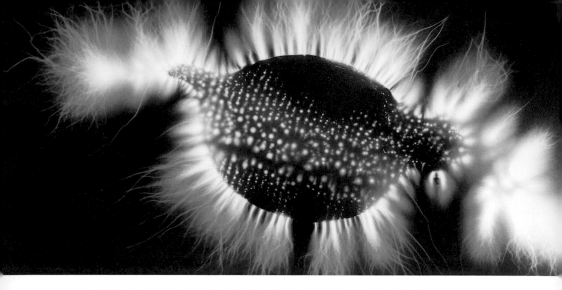

A Kirlian image of a radish. Radish juice is a great aid against kidney stones. Based on the minerals they contain, radishes are neutral (not too alkaline or too acidic).

producing negatively-charged ions. And some positive charge bleeds over into the Earth such as in radioactive materials (e.g. uranium) naturally found in the Earth. Nevertheless, the electrically negative alkaline charge of the Earth and the electrically positive acid charge in the atmosphere dominate.

We may have heard that we are suffering from "acidity," "acidosis," or an acid condition in the body. What we may not yet have heard is that we are suffering from excess acidity, in large part, due to our separation from the Earth's alkaline negatively-charged electromagnetic field. The implications of this discovery indicates that we must connect with the Earth directly as party of our holistic health regime. Our plastic sandals, rubber-soled shoes, wooden floors, asphalt (bitumen) roads, bicycles, automobiles, airplanes, carpets, high-rise buildings, etc., separate us from a direct skin-to-skin contact with the Earth — they block our electrical connection to the Earth with electrically insulating materials. Getting grounded again as our ancestors did when they walked barefoot upon the Earth is important to our overall health. When we are walking barefoot the Earth itself supplies a natural negative electrical charge to our body that is typically absorbed through the "kidney 1 meridian point" (also known as the "bubbling spring" point) on the ball of the foot. This natural electricity can also be absorbed by any other part of our skin that is actually touching the Earth or a body of water upon the Earth such as the ocean or a lake, creek, river, stream, etc.

Our electrical skin-to-skin reconnection to the Earth and its waters has been shown to: accelerate healing, play a role in improving auto-immune disease, decrease susceptibility to oxidation damage (slow aging), cause our red blood cells to become electromagnetically charged (thus increasing oxygen delivery and decreasing platelet aggregation), raise our energy, improve alkalinity, help reverse adrenal fatigue, improve thyroid function, increase bone density, improve our body's natural electrical meridian system, fortify our resistance to corrosive damage by the electromagnetic fields produced by electronic devices (such as computers, kitchen appliances, radios, televisions, mobile phones, live wires, etc.), and much more. Basically, by reconnecting to the Earth's electrical field, we become healthier.

Devices have now been developed by Clint Ober that assist us in being "Earthed" (grounded) by connecting us to the negative alkaline charge of the Earth even in our ungrounded homes and workspaces. These devices are known as grounding technologies and include computer mouse pads, desk pads, sleeping systems, grounded shoe wear and more. A revolution in grounded shoeware is imminent (and is especially important) in cities and in places where parasites and contamination due to the excrement from dogs and other animals preclude barefoot safety.

In the context of electricity and alkalinity, we should avail ourselves of as much of the negative, alkaline, electrical charge of the Earth as possible.

In situations where it is impossible to be properly grounded (such as while being transported in an automobile, bus, or airplane) it is recommended that one use a Longevity Zapper (www.longevitywarehouse.com) to at least approximate the natural healing energies that come from the Earth.

Alkalinity and Water

One meaning of alkalinity is in regards to the hydrogen content of water. This is associated with a predominance in the water of free radical hydroxyl groups (OH^- molecules). This is undesirable for drinking and causes free radical damage (aging). Natural, cold spring, drinking water typically comes out of the Earth at acidic pH values ranging from 5.6 to 6.8 this means that the water is rich in hydrogen in the form of hydronium (H_3O^+). Hydrogen is what creates hydration. Hydrogen in its root derivation means "generator of water."

Sometimes acidic, toxic sulfur compounds are present in well water (or bore hole water). In those cases, the water may have long-range toxic effects on the body. This type of water, even though acidic, is unfavorable for drinking.

Alkalinity in regards to water may also reference the predominant major minerals present in the water. Water rich in calcium and/or magnesium is considered alkaline. Drinking alkaline, calcium-rich water exposes the body to excess inorganic calcium that can lead to the formation of calcification diseases such as heart disease, arthritis, kidney stones, cataracts, etc. Calcium-rich water is associated with the troublesome formation of scale (lime build-up) in pipes, bathing tubs, and sinks. On the other hand, water rich in magnesium (in the form of magnesium bicarbonate) is alkaline, yet has healing effects on the body and tends to have a healing effect on arthritis and other calcification conditions. The same could be said for spring waters rich in the alkaline mineral lithium – the effects are positive.

As we have seen, depending on the context, both alkaline and acidic waters may be beneficial or harmful to consume.

Alkalinity and Food

An additional (yet probably the most widely used) meaning of alkalinity is in regards to food and nutrition.

In this context, the major mineral content of foods and herbs is considered. The mineral content of edible substances helps us scientifically decide which foods are acid-forming (phosphorus dominant) and alkaline-forming (calcium and magnesium dominant). By "dominant" I mean, the ratio of these minerals will favor alkalinity (calcium and magnesium are greater than phosphorus content) or will favor acidity (calcium and magnesium content is less than phosphorus content).

Another consideration is which foods are potassium dominant and which are sodium dominant, based on their minerals. Potassium and sodium are not directly associated with alkalinity or acidity. Because potassium ash is considered alkaline in most nutrition books on the subject of acidity and alkalinity, a mistake becomes evident, because all high-potassium foods (nearly all raw foods are rich in potassium) are considered alkaline – even if their phosphorus levels are high (as in nuts and seeds). This creates the false impression that nuts and seeds such as almonds, walnuts, and pumpkin seeds are alkaline. They may be more alkaline than fried chicken, but based on their mineral content, nuts and seeds are acid-forming foods. Sprouting or soaking nuts and seeds in water will lower their phytic acid content and enzyme inhibitors, however, based on their major minerals, the nuts and seeds will still be acidic.

In the realm of food and nutrition, we require a healthy balance of alkalinity and acidity. We also require a healthy balance of potassium and sodium. In the beginning stages of cleansing and detoxification more alkalinity and potassium are required in the form of non-sweet fruits, green-leafy vegetables, vegetable juice, grass juice, green sprouts, edible flowers, herbs, certain superfoods (aloe vera, noni, bee pollen, royal jelly, chlorella, blue-green algae, marine phyto-plankton, and acai) and superherbs (these include the most powerful herbs from great dynamic herbal systems, such as reishi mushroom, chaga mushroom, ginseng, schizandra berry, tulsi, ashwaganda, shatavari, pau d'arco, cat's claw, nettle, passionflower, etc.). This type of cleansing diet should be low in sweet fruit and low in fat-dominant foods. In general, this cornucopia of cleansing foods, superfoods, herbs, and superherbs not only contain alkalinity in the form of minerals, they also contain subtle alkaline-forming compounds. On top of this, potassium draws out old, stale dietary salt deposits from the tissues that hold in toxicity.

Eventually, once one has brought their alkalinity up to achieve an acid-alkaline balance, and the old toxic salt residues are drawn out, a new dietary balance must be found. This new Sunfood Diet should contain a balance of alkaline foods (vegetables, vegetable juices, sprouts, seaweeds, green super-foods, herbs, and superherbs as mentioned above) and acid-forming foods (nuts, seeds, sweet fruit, fatty foods).

Let's look at some examples of how balance may be achieved by under-standing the influence of the major dietary minerals. For instance, if you eat foods high in sodium and phosphorus (cooked animal foods), you need to balance that stimulation out with foods high in calcium and potassium (green vegetables) — this is right in line with the food combining principles that have been taught for decades. If you eat foods high in potassium and phosphorus (nuts and seeds), you tend to crave foods high in calcium and sodium (spinach and kale).

For clarity, based on their dominant minerals, most fruits are slightly acid forming, not alkaline-forming. Almonds, we see, are phosphorus-dominant foods, and are not an excellent source of alkalinity. Carrot juice, long recommended for its alkalinity, is also found to be phosphorus dominant and thus acid-forming to a certain degree (although in the context of all beverages, more alkaline than soda pop).

Understanding the dominant minerals in foods helps us to understand cravings. I have known many new raw-food enthusiasts who eat too many potassium-rich foods without balancing with sodium-rich foods, such as kale or seaweed. They typically end up craving and eating salty cooked foods, such as corn chips or potato chips. Cravings for cooked foods may actually be cravings for minerals.

The importance of organic sodium is important for long-term vitality and energy. I have worked with many people who have spent years eating a low-sodium raw-food diet; they have found that their digestion improved and endurance increased when they added more sea salt and sodium-residue foods (kale, celery, dulse) into their diet.

Calcium, magnesium, phosphorus, sodium and potassium are not the only minerals in foods. Other alkalizing minerals include iron and silica. Other acid-forming minerals include chlorine and sulfur. These are usually secondary and tertiary minerals in foods. Generally, foods high in magnesium (such as olives) are usually high in calcium; foods high in chlorine (such as avocados) are also usually high in phosphorus. Some exceptions exist: cacao (raw chocolate) is extraordinarily high in magnesium, though low in calcium; because cacao is high enough in phosphorus to balance out the magnesium, it is generally considered slightly acidic.

To clear any confusion: Many alkaline fruits contain citric and other acids; thus, they will have an acid pH reaction in digestion, but because of their high content of alkaline-forming minerals (calcium, magnesium), their reactions can be alkaline in the body tissues. Thus, they usually alkalize the body and neutralize the acid-forming mineral residues. However, if one is already deficient in alkaline minerals, citric acid will not be broken down properly and thus citrus fruits will be acidic because the alkaline minerals within the food cannot be accessed properly. In addition, some people simply do not metabolize citric-acid-containing foods; so these food choices should be avoided.

The major groups of alkaline foods based on their minerals and subtle properties include:

Green-leafy vegetables
Grasses: wheatgrass, barleygrass, etc. (any grass that has sprouted a green blade)
Alkaline superfoods: aloe vera, noni, bee pollen, royal jelly, chlorella, blue-green algae, and marine phytoplankton, acai, etc.
Sea vegetables: dulse, nori, kelp, sea palm, sea lettuce, hijiki, wakame, arame, etc.
Herbs: oregano, thyme, marjoram, rosemary, etc.
Superherbs: reishi mushroom, chaga mushroom, ginseng, schizandra berry, tulsi, ashwaganda, shatavari, pau d'arco, cat's claw, nettle, passionflower, etc.
Alkaline fruits (if you can digest them properly): citrus fruits, olives, figs, ripe peppers, okra
*In animals, the alkaline minerals are found primarily in bone marrow.

The major groups of neutral plant-based foods (some slight alkaline and others slightly acidic) based on their minerals and subtle properties include:

Root vegetables
Fruits: cucumbers (all types), melons (all types), cherries, berries (except strawberries), papaya, avocados, apricot
Flowers (edible)

The major groups of acidic foods based on their minerals and subtle properties include:

Nuts
Seeds
Fruits: most sweet fruits are on the acidic side, including banana, mango, apples, pear, plum, peach, plum, fruits, strawberries, cacao fruit pulp, durian, mangosteen fruit (not the alkaline rind), cherimoya, soursop, etc.
*In animals, the acidic minerals are found primarily in the muscles (meat).

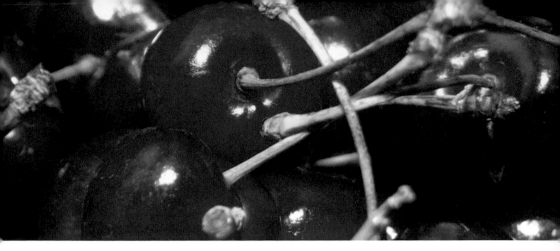

Cherries are the richest natural source of melatonin, which helps remove bad estrogen accumulation and assists with sleep. Based on the minerals they contain, cherries are neutral (not too alkaline or too acidic).

The philosopher Herbert Spencer wrote that perfect correspondence always prevails in Nature — one thing is always balanced by another. You will find by incorporating The Sunfood Triangle in conjunction with a balancing of the major minerals found in foods (alkaline calcium and magnesium versus acidic phosphorus) and (potassium versus sodium) that a great balancing occurs and an incredible health arises.

ALKALINE AND ACID

1   Every day, be sure to ground (or Earth) yourself for as many hours as possible by using one or more of the following strategies:

    • Walking barefoot (walking on beach sand is ideal for new barefooters)
    • Getting your hands in the soil via gardening or playing
    • Swimming in a natural body of water
    • Using a grounded mouse pad
    • Sleeping using a grounded sheet system
    • Using a grounded desk pad
    • Wearing grounded flip flops or other innovative, grounded footwear

    Twelve or more hours grounded each day is ideal for healing, yet even 1 minute grounded is better than zero minutes.

    Note: You may obtain grounded mouse pads, sheets, desk pads, and more as well as a Longevity Zapper (to use when you are not grounded) from www.longevitywarehouse.com

2   Journey to a local cold spring in your area where people have been drinking the water for centuries. Test the pH of the water using a pH meter or pH strips (these are available at any pool supply shop). You will find that most cold springs range from 5.6 to 7.2 pH. Any reading under 7.0 is considered acidic. Acidic spring water at the source means that the water is high in hydrogen and therefore increases hydration.

3   Every day that you eat, be sure to eat green leafy vegetables, green superfoods, herbs, sea vegetables, and superherbs to improve your alkalinity.

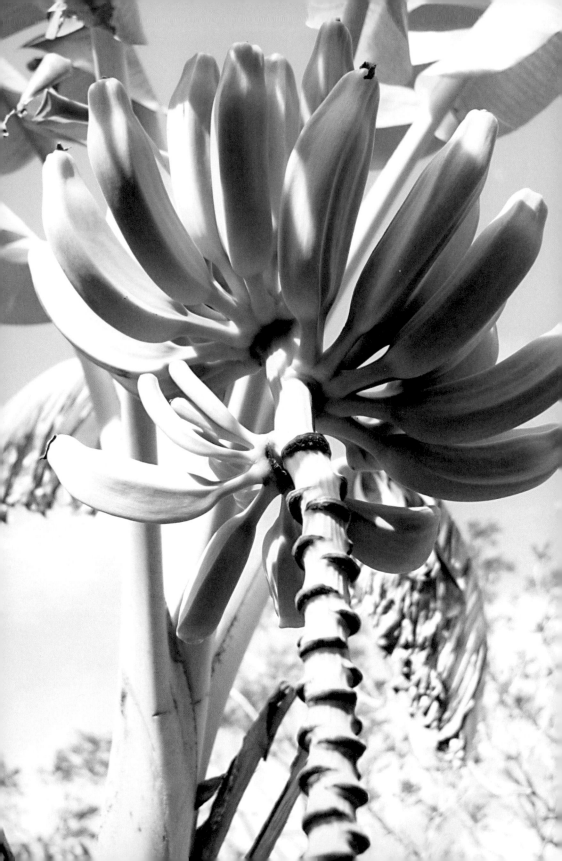

15

HYBRID FOOD

Some philosophers, such as the great writer, translator, and thinker Edmond Bordeaux Szekely, believed humans were once a frugivorous creature, but have been altered due to centuries of unnatural feeding. However, it is not humanity's biological form which has changed, it is the food itself, which has been altered and hybridized.

When the earliest humans first began cultivating crops and fruit trees, they unwittingly also began to protect these crops and fruit trees from natural selection (which, as we have seen in **Lesson 9: Origins**, does occur within a species, but cannot create a species). The cultivated crops were cross-bred for better taste, longer durability, stronger skins, etc., yet at the same time were growing genetically weaker as the unfittest strains were allowed to survive as long as they "tasted better" or "lasted longer." Eventually, certain crops and fruit trees were grown for so long in protective environments (away from wild Nature) that they no longer had sufficient "genetic energy" to survive in wild Nature untended. These foods I have termed "hybrid foods."

Hybrid foods are foods that will not grow in Nature. My colleague, Dr. David Jubb, tells us that hybrid foods are "missing vital electrics." They are foods, which must be nurtured and protected by humans, or else they will be overcome by birds, insects, worms, fungi and bacteria.

Most fruits sold in large supermarkets are cross-bred and hybridized to some degree, but are still excellent foods; often they are still capable of reverting back to a wild or semi-wild state. Fruits, such as avocados, cherimoyas, jalapeno peppers and tomatoes are great examples of these. As a general guideline, fruits which have been hybridized too far include all seedless fruits or fruits with non-viable seeds. These fruits should be avoided, because they are genetically altered and weak.

Also, grafted trees produce awkward fruit, often without seeds. Grafting is a process apparently developed by the Chinese, whereby one variety of fruit tree is united to another variety of the same fruit tree. Many varieties of orange trees are actually two trees in one. The root stock is of a totally different variety than the stem and branches. Again, focus on the seeds; if they do not exist, or are not viable, then avoid those foods.

The biblical verse Genesis 1:29 actually warns of the danger of hybrid foods. The verse advises us to eat only herbs *bearing seed* and fruits *bearing seed*.

Seedless foods are so hybridized they can no longer reproduce. The inability of hybrids to reproduce stems from a deficiency in the procreative cells. Hybrids can lack a double set of chromosomes in their reproductive cells, and this leads to the inability to produce viable seeds.

Common hybrid fruits, grafted fruits or fruits grown from cuttings include: seedless apples, bananas, most common date varieties, kiwis (their black seeds are not viable), seedless pineapples, seedless citrus fruits, seedless grapes (raisins), seedless persimmons and seedless watermelons.

The standard bananas we all know are excessively hybridized foods. I was raised on bananas and this was difficult for me to accept. The black "seeds" found in the common banana are not seeds at all, but are non-viable remnants of what should be semi-hard, pellet-sized, walnut-tasting seeds. I transitioned away from bananas by eating fewer and fewer until I finally let them go.

Hybrid fruit is not only unnaturally high in sugar, but is also low in minerals. I have noticed that I can eat super-sweet wild berries in massive abundance and get no unusual reaction or high at all. I have also noticed that if I eat a mildly sweet hybrid fruit I get a "weird" reaction from just a small amount — seedless

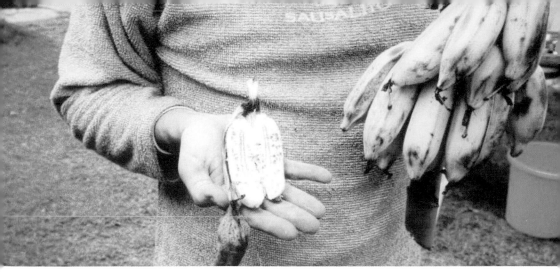

**A real non-hybrid banana with seeds that I found while in Bali, Indonesia.
This type of banana is so filling that it is difficult to eat more than one.**

grapes send me into "la-la" land (sugar high).

Hybrid foods are devoid of the proper mineral balance all wild foods contain. Excessive hybrid fruit consumption leads to mineral deficiencies. It is not only that hybrid fruits and sweet/starchy vegetables (carrots, beets, potatoes) themselves are unbalanced in minerals, it is that an overconsumption of hybrid sweet fruit and sweet/starchy vegetables causes the body to bring heavy minerals from the bones into the blood to buffer the hybrid sugar, which is not completely recognized and dealt with by the liver and pancreas. The minerals and the sugar are then spilled off into the urine. So, in the long-term, hybrid sweet fruit and sweet/starchy vegetables can actually overstimulate you, causing you to lose minerals.

Common hybrid vegetables include: beets, carrots, corn and potatoes.

Most of the vegetation people eat is not found growing wildly in Nature. The fields in which they grow are protected from natural forces. The natural insects are poisoned with pesticides, the soil microbes are poisoned with fertilizers. Crops grown chemically are artificial — their cultivation is unnatural.

Common brown and white rice varieties are hybrids. Commercial oats, barley and wheat are hybrid plants.

Common, controversial alfalfa sprouts (often criticized for containing toxins) are hybrid foods. Clover sprouts are a better, more natural choice and should be chosen over alfalfa.

Most commercially available legumes are hybrids. I once grew lentils from seeds in wild "survival of the fittest" fashion. Only one out of hundreds grew to fruition. When I harvested the lentils from that one plant, each lentil displayed an amazingly beautiful design on the seed surface — totally unlike the dull orange/brown lentils available from the store. Amazingly, the lentil plant had reverted back to its natural, wild state!

Many primitive peoples, and all wild primates, eat foods from at least 100 varieties of plants. The majority of the world's population now, on civilization's various diets, consume only 13 varieties of plants: bananas, beans, beets (beet-derived sugar), corn, oranges, potatoes, rice, wheat, soy beans, sugar cane, sweet potato, cassava and coconut. The first 9 of these 13 listed are such hybridized foods (or genetically modified) that they are either seedless or produce seeds incapable of surviving independently in Nature. Due to the deficiencies of nutrients in hybrid foods, this situation presents an enormous health challenge for the world; and yet, it also presents a tremendous opportunity to improve the health of the world.

People become addicted to bread, corn chips, french fries, baked potatoes, and even carrot juice, because these foods come from hybridized plants that contain an addictive quantity of sugar and a low-level of minerals.

I have noticed that hybrid foods are attacked by different forms of fungi than wild food. Hybrid foods are much more susceptible to early decay. For example, I can have extremely hybridized yellow seedless grapefruits outside in my back patio in the Sun alongside seeded ruby red grapefruits. The ruby reds (though not a wild strain) will last months out there as they ripen to perfection (citrus ripens best in the sun, on the ground), however, the yellow seedless grapefruits will be overcome by bright to dark green mold outlined by white. You will never see this type of mold attack a wild fruit.

From these types of observations, it is clear how hybrid fruit can feed fungal conditions in the body, such as candida. Whereas non-hybrid or wild fruit does not trigger such a condition.

How To Make Hybrids Work For You

Hybrid foods are everywhere and most of us still need to eat something! It is possible for you to make hybrid foods work for you. The effects of hybrid foods on the body are usually not felt physically or consciously until one is significantly purified after many months and years on a pure diet.

Remember: start where you are now. When I started on raw foods I was probably eating 90% hybridized food. My health dramatically improved when I shifted my choices. I realized that I could not thrive on hybridized foods, grafted foods and foods grown from cuttings. Over time I learned to fine tune my diet and body to achieve an extraordinary level of health.

Hybrid fruits and vegetables may be eaten in small amounts. Mixing bananas with fat (avocados, nuts, olives) lessens the sugar effect of that fruit on the system. Eating more green-leafed vegetables and avocados, nuts, or olives with hybrid sweet fruits or vegetables will decrease their effect on the blood sugar and increase the utility of elements in the food. Hybrid grains may be eaten straight or sprouted.

Even if hybridized, whenever possible eat food grown locally, indigenously under the Sun, under truly organic conditions.

Eat food that is in season. I have noticed that I can eat dates in abundance (up to 30 in a day if I am extremely active) when they are in season (fall and winter). But when I eat dates out of season, they give me a strange reaction similar to the feeling of eating too much hybrid fruit and I cannot even eat two or three dates.

Importantly, non-hybridized wild foods are available when you look closely. These valuable foods include: all seaweeds, blue-green algae, wild bee pollen, wild honey, and, of course, all food substances found growing wildly in nature.

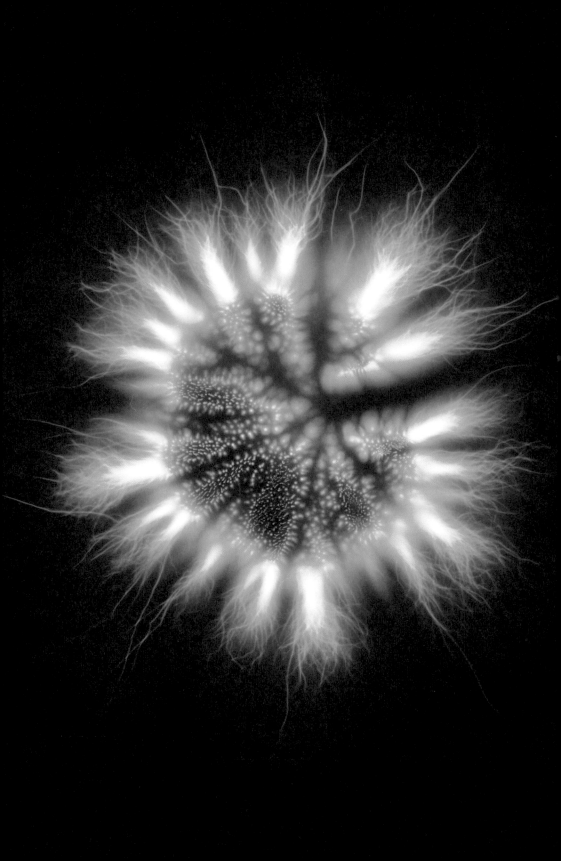

HYBRID FOOD

1 Identify the hybridized foods (raw or cooked) in your diet. Decide to replace these foods with more natural foods as soon, and as often, as possible. Particularly watch out for foods high in sugar and low in minerals.

2 The solution to hybridized food? Grow your own food from heirloom seeds (contact heirloom seed banks through the Internet). Also, whenever possible, eat wild plants and fruits.

3 Participate in a hands-on class — in the field — with a local herbalist.

A magnificent Kirlian photograph of a wild malva leaf. Malva leaves are one of Nature's great delicacies.

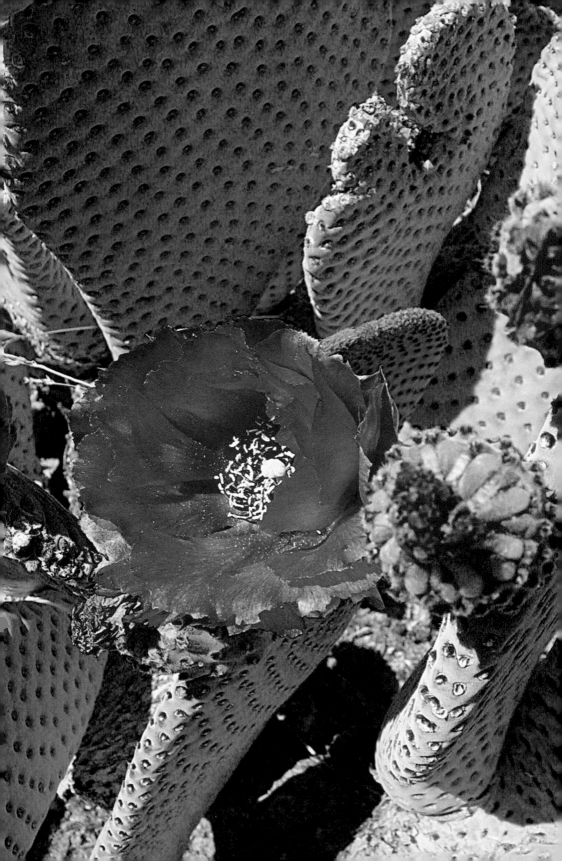

16

WILD FOOD

"IN THE FIRST AGE FOOD CAME BY WISHING AND GREW FROM EARTH WITHOUT TENDING." — *Ramayana*

"IN THE FIRST AGE FOOD CAME BY WISHING AND GREW FROM EARTH WITHOUT TENDING." — *Ramayana*

"ELECTRIC FOODS ARE THE MOST IMPORTANT COMPONENT OF HEALING. THEY MAKE THE BODY ALKALINE. THESE ARE ALL FOODS THAT ARE ABLE TO GROW IN THE WILD."
— *Annie & Dr. David Jubb, Colloidal Biology & Secrets Of An Alkaline Body*

The basis of natural nutrition is wild, raw plant food. The Germans call this "original food." It has been the original food here since the beginning of time.

Wild food connects you immediately to the land. Eating wild food growing in your area acclimates you to the environment. I used to suffer from all kinds of allergies: hay fever, pollen, feline, etc. I completely conquered my allergies by undertaking The Sunfood Diet, by eating wild indigenous food, using MSM powder in my drinking water and through homeopathy. People who are allergic to the pollens of local plants can eliminate these allergies by eating local wild leaves, flowers, fruits, honeys and acclimating themselves to the environment. Many people never eat anything growing locally or wildly in their life! This is not the lifestyle for which we were designed.

Wild food is a revelation. When you eat wild food you will discover how domesticated standard food really is. As long as one is eating a wide variety of mineral-rich, wild, raw plant food, one stands ready to experience outstanding levels of clarity, compassion, vitality, health and connection with nature.

Brian Clement, director of Hippocrates Health Institute in West Palm Beach, Florida, has reported that, based on his research, wild greens have the highest energy frequency of any food. I have experienced their energy first-hand by eating plenty of wild green salads. They send me into a new plane of thought. Evenings after eating such meals are filled with incredible clarity of thought and electricity.

Seaweeds and sea vegetables of all kinds have never been cultivated. They are still in their wild unaltered form. They fit within the wild raw plant-food category, and are high in trace minerals. This is an important factor in a world where many are suffering from endemic mineral deficiencies brought about by consuming pharmaceuticals, chemicals, pesticides and cooked conventional foods that drain the vital energy.

Wild Fruit

Wild food is Sunfood — food grown in abundance under the Sun (and moon!), not under artificial conditions of any type. It is food as the Earth has given it to us in its normal state. Wild food is true to our Creator's original intent.

Store-bought fruitarianism is not workable in the long-term. Fruit enthusiasts should seek out perfectly ripe fruit. Perfectly ripe fruit picked fresh, "from the tree right to me," is an unmatched experience.

Wild fruit is high in minerals, and always lower in sugar than commercial fruit. It is less stimulating and thus is closer to the center point of The Sunfood Triangle.

Wild fruits are the sustenance of the immortals. Fruit has tremendous spiritual power. The more natural (nonhybridized) the fruit is, the greater its spiritual value.

Common fruits which are close to the wild state and/or are extremely viable when grown from seed include: avocados, cherimoyas, crab apples, guavas, heavily-seeded citrus fruits, jackfruits, mangos, most melons, most peppers or

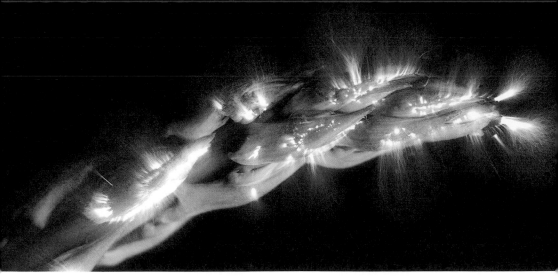

A Kirlian image of the developing head of asparagus.

chilies, papayas, peaches, tomatoes, tomatilloes, olives, white sapotes and others.

A good quality citrus fruit should contain 14-15 seeds, even if the fruit is small in size. The more seeds in citrus, the better. The less seeds in citrus, the more hybridized or grafted is the strain. After you purchase or pick them, keep citrus fruits in Sunlight or on the windowsill so they remain at their maximum nutritive value and quality. The more ripe and Sun-exposed the citrus fruits, the sweeter and less acidic are its contents.

Common vegetables which are close to the wild state and/or are extremely viable when grown from seed include: dandelion, garlic, kale, lamb's quarters, malva, mint, mustard, onions, watercress, wintercress and others.

One of my favorite wild foods is malva (mallow). Malva seems to love growing on the outskirts of civilization — in canyons, back alleys and back yards. Malva is one of those phenomenal greens that tastes incredible when eaten alone. In the winter I typically start off the morning with fruit blended with superfoods, then eat malva for lunch and have a salad with some raw plant fats for dinner along with vegetable juice.

Common nuts and seeds which are close to the wild state and/or are extremely viable when grown from seed include: coconut, macadamia, quinoa and sunflower.

Every locale you find yourself in possesses wild foods with which to eat and live. Get out and explore your local canyons, fields, forests, hills, valleys and mountains. A great reference book is **Edible Wild Plants: A North American Field Guide** by Elias & Dykeman. Take it with you on your hikes and identify your local edible greenery.

In his writings, the herbalist Earl Mindell has confirmed my experience. He has described that less than 1% of all plants are poisonous to eat.

The power of wild foods cannot be underestimated. Eating wild plant foods reconnects you with Nature in a most profound way. One time I was out hiking in a canyon near my home. On the way, I encountered several children ranging in age from seven to ten. We started talking and soon agreed that I would show them all the edible, interesting and poisonous plants growing in the area. We had an extraordinary time together. After several hours, all the children had gone home except one. The two of us were hiking up a hill through brush on our way to a field of young dandelion when we almost walked into a coyote. The coyote looked at us and bolted away. The young child's eyes were wide open. Although earlier he had told me he had seen coyotes, I knew after that incident he had not — at least not like this. These moments are priceless, and this moment all came about in the fun of foraging for wild food.

The goal is to eat the highest quality food possible — the best food ever! The more mineralized and natural your food, the more mineralized and natural you will become. Wild plant foods make you strong and robust and put you "in tune" with your local natural environment.

If you cannot get wild food, or it is impractical, please eat organic. You deserve it. You are worth it! You and your family are worth more than anything on Earth; give your family the best fuel possible. The organic farmers also deserve your support for not spraying pesticides (poisons) on the Earth. If you have to pay twice as much or more for organic food, do it. It is an investment in yourself (which always comes back multiplied). Organic food has more vitality, minerals and value than commercial food. In my experience it is totally worth paying even three to four times as much money for organic food.

Vitamin B12

Although animal and dairy products are a source of vitamin B12, the natural soil microbes, insects and bacteria found on wild food, unwashed garden plants, in earthy soil and also those supplied by plant fermentation, are typically adequate to supply some vitamin B12 needs. The natural microbes and bacteria in the soil need to be duplicated and colonize in our intestinal tract for optimal absorption of nutrients and elimination of waste without excessive fermentation or internal putrefaction. Vitamin B12 is produced by these natural microbes and bacteria as they colonize the intestines. The best source of these organisms is wild, unwashed food.

Vitamin B12 (cobalamin) represents a family of compounds that are one hundred times the molecular size of any other vitamin and contain the mineral cobalt. Vitamin B12 helps maintain the myelin sheaths that insulate the nerve fibers. Problems with vitamin B12 absorption and assimilation can result in nerve degeneration. A vitamin B12 deficiency, when in conjunction with a folate deficiency (due to a lack of green-leafy vegetables), can also cause pernicious anemia.

A problem with the formation of vitamin B12 occurs when there is a sterilization that happens between the picking of the fruit or vegetable and the moment it reaches one's mouth. Sterile environments are unnatural. The soil microbes and bacteria that grow on raw fruits and vegetables need to be duplicated in the intestinal tract for the proper assimilation of vitamin B12 to take place. Dr. Victor Herbert described in the **American Journal of Clinical Nutrition** (1988, vol.48, p. 852-858) the experiences of Dr. James Halsted who traveled to Persia to study a colony of Iranian vegans who did not experience any vitamin B12 deficiencies. He found that their naturally fertilized vegetables were eaten without being carefully washed. He discovered that strict vegetarians who do not practice thorough hand washing or vegetable cleaning may be untroubled by a vitamin B12 deficiency.

Studies have shown that those eating a typical diet of animal products actually require more vitamin B12 than those who do not eat animal products. This is because the typical diet leads to digestive atrophy. Because vitamin B12 is peptide bound in animal products and must be enzymatically cleaved from the peptide bonds to be absorbed, a weakening of all gastric enzyme secretions (due to poor nutrition) causes an inability to efficiently extract vitamin B12 from external food. Raw-food vegans with powerful digestion, actually get more vitamin B12 by reabsorption from the bile (liver secretions into the duodenum) than they do from external food.

The vitamin B12 standards recommended based on studies of the average cooked-food consumer are 0.0000001 ounces (3-4 micrograms) per day. Studies by Dr. Victor Herbert reported in the **American Journal Of Clinical Nutrition** (1988, vol.48, p. 852-858) demonstrate that only 0.000000035 ounces (1 microgram) of vitamin B12 are required per day. This is enough to produce a "beautiful hematologic response." These minimum vitamin B12 requirements are inadequate to explain the needs of well nourished individuals with strong digestion who require even less vitamin B12 due to excellent gastric strength, enzymatic activity and a high ability to recycle vitamin B12.

Dr. Gabriel Cousens, a long-term raw-food vegetarian, has included an excellent discussion of vitamin B12 in his book **Conscious Eating** and on the Internet. Dr. Cousens feels that a vitamin B12 deficiency, which is rare, is typically caused by a lack of absorption in the intestinal tract or a dietary lack of the vitamin. He states that vegetarian and meat-eating pregnant and lactating women alike seem to be susceptible to a vitamin B12 deficiency. He states that macrobioticists and fruitarians may also be susceptible. I have found that individuals who have damaged their digestive system with a high-protein diet are susceptible as well. A link seems to be present between weak digestion and vitamin B12 assimilation.

My own experience working with people who I have discovered were vitamin B12 deficient corroborates Dr. Cousens' hypothesis, but I have narrowed it down to a more specific cause: poor hydrochloric acid production and/or low levels of intestinal flora.

Sugar, as I have mentioned, is an antibiotic. So a long-term high-sugar diet, whether the sugar is coming from refined sources or hybridized fruit, can damage or wipe out the intestinal flora.

Cooking also destroys microbes. A highly-sterilized, cooked-vegan diet (macrobiotics) may not provide the intestines with enough excellent flora.

To insure an excellent quality of vitamin B12, be sure to regularly eat unwashed garden plants. Leave foods unwashed that were grown wildly, home-

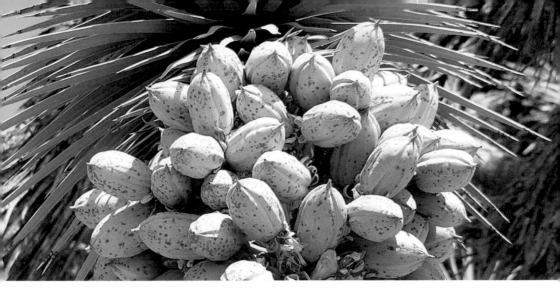

**The sacred Joshua Tree (a member of the Agavaceae family)
produces an edible wild fruit.**

grown, or picked by you from an organic farm. Store-bought food is much different, it should be washed because it can be layered with mold, pollution and toxins.

Getting some soil microbes into your body is very important. Consider the words of Annie & Dr. David Jubb in **Secrets Of An Alkaline Body**: "You can receive help virtually overnight for: seizures, diabetes, arthritis, pneumonia, Parkinson's disease and immune challenges by simply ingesting some soil-born organisms. People have lived in such a sterile antiseptic environment that these necessary symbiotic organisms have been less than present in their diet... By ingesting soil-born organisms, you maintain an enormous reservoir of un-coded antibodies ready to transform specific pathogens... Iron metabolic challenges are solved by living the way Nature intended, occasionally eating a little dirt..."

I eat plenty of unwashed wild food to supply good bacteria for my intestinal flora. However, I have met many long-term raw-foodists (20+ years all-raw) who do not eat unwashed food and who are very healthy. They do eat seaweed and sometimes include spirulina, chlorella, and/or AFA blue-green algae (two to three teaspoons a day). These aquatic plants contain vitamin B12 analogues and perhaps human-active vitamin B12 (more research is required). Also, healthy raw-foodists regularly eat fermented foods, such as raw sauerkraut, which supplies the digestive system with good intestinal flora to manufacture B12. Instructions for creating fermented live-food dishes may be found in nearly all of the raw-food recipe books available, including the books by Dr. Ann Wigmore.

Many nutritionists feel that a vegan diet does not supply enough vitamin B12 for the body. This may or may not be true. My experience of meeting vegans and raw-food vegans who have been following those diets for 20+ years indicates that vitamin B12 deficiencies can arise in certain cases. It seems that if one is clever with their diet or occasionally uses vitamin B12 supplements and follows a healthy lifestyle, there is little chance of a vitamin B12 deficiency. A vitamin B12 deficiency is usually (but not always) symptomatic of a larger problem (high sugar diet, poor absorption, poor or absent flora, also a lack of Sunlight) manifested in weak digestion, pale skin, emaciation and extreme fatigue.

When I lived in Santa Barbara my friends and I would surf the beaches there. Since those beaches are loaded with pockets of tar and oil, lots of tar would bubble up into the ocean water and get on our wetsuits and surfboards. It was such a hassle to clean and worry about that one day I said, "I've had it, I'm through. I am no longer going to even worry about this anymore." And you know what? It was never a problem again. It is my opinion, that the vitamin B12 hype is used most often to scare people away from wonderful vegetarian and vegan diets. If you were to put the vitamin B12 issue out of your mind, and follow the action steps below, you might be surprised to find that it disappears from your consciousness. Vitamin B12 is important, should be addressed and then put away so as to avoid excessive focus on the issue.

WILD FOOD

1   Read and study books and media on edible wild plants. Take a plant book with you on hikes through Nature. Begin identifying the wild edible plants growing in your area. Begin experimenting with eating some of the wild foods you identify.

2   For excellent intestinal flora and vitamin B12 assimilation, include one or more of the following in your daily diet:
a. Unwashed garden plants.
b. Wild plants.
c. Seaweeds (e.g. dulse, nori, etc.).
d. Roots, such as burdock root, have been shown to contain levels of B12 absorbed from soil organisms up to 0.5 mm into the outer skin.
e. Spirulina or blue-green algae (three tablespoons per day). Spirulina may contain a great ratio of human-active vitamin B12 as compared to B12 analogues. More research needs to be conducted in this area.
f. Occasional fermented foods (e.g. raw sauerkraut) when appropriate.

3   If the options in (2) are not available at the moment or are not strong enough to do the job, taking a vegan-quality vitamin B12 supplement (methyl-cobalamin form) daily is appropriate, especially when one is under stress, at risk of a heart attack or stroke, pregnant, nursing and/or culti-vating increased neurological health. Also, including some raw, organic cultured dairy products (e.g. kefir, raw cheese, etc.) may be required to improve B12 levels and also raise the level of the important, bone-mineralizing vitamin K2 for a successful pregnancy and for complete chil-dren's nutrition.

4   If you feel your intestinal flora and food absorption are not excellent, consider regularly including supplemental enzymes and probiotics in your diet. Supplemental enzymes increase digestive efficiency. Probiotic colonies help synthesize nutrients, they counteract pathogenic microbes, and they improve the overall internal environment. These recommendations are especially important for those with a history of prolonged antibiotic, or other drug use, as well as for those who have a history of sugar addictions.

5   To learn more, read Dr. Gabriel Cousens' writings on vitamin B12 including those in his book **Conscious Eating**.

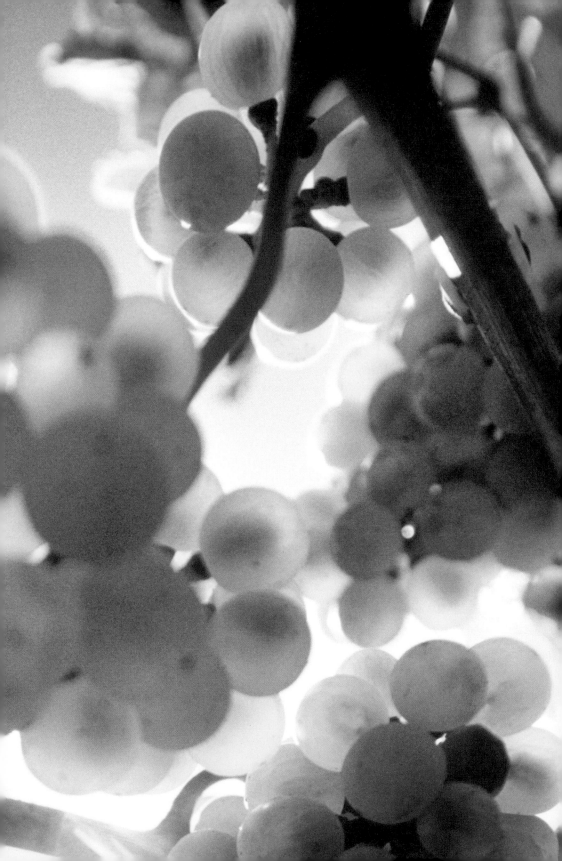

17

MY PERSONAL DIET

Words alone cannot describe the level of health I have been privileged to attain over all these years of exploring The Sunfood Diet. All that comes to mind is that I feel an immense gratitude. I feel incredibly fortunate to have even found or discovered the type of health information I have included in this book. I feel honored to be able to share this information with others.

When I went raw, I began to study the simple things, like my fingers and toes. I marveled at their dexterity and the functions they served. I became very aware of all my bodily systems: respiratory, circulatory, cardiac, glandular, reproductive, neurological and digestive. I was awestruck at the efficiency of our human organs. How could I ever have taken my body for granted? How could anyone? It was like being a billionaire and not realizing that you are rich. I thought about the less tangible things like sleep cycles, dreams, synchronicity and the true nature of Life. I was filled with a new-found reverence for all living and "non-living" things.

I think about things differently now. My outlook on life is something I would describe as glorious. Life is so grand, so incredible, so full of amazement! What can match the grasp of a child's hand in your own, the crisp flavor of a fresh-picked apple, the kiss of a friend or lover, the smell of a spring breeze, the Sunlight penetrating your naked body, the inspiration of highly-emotional music, the feel of sand beneath bare feet, the flow of ocean water through your hair in the mid-summer?

When I initially embarked on the raw path, I was faced with overcoming addictions to bread and corn chips. I was losing a lot of weight. My face was changing and I did not look my best. In the midst of this, a wave of peer pressure from friends, family and relatives descended upon me. But I persevered. Throughout the process two thoughts were dominant in my mind: Jim Rohn's saying, "For every disciplined effort there is a multiple reward," and Andrew Carnegie's saying, "Anything worth having is worth working for."

I kept pushing forward, reading and learning. I began to find that I was transforming in a most profound way and other people were noticing it. I found that many would take the time to listen to what I had to say. I found I was attracting certain people who were acting upon the raw-food information. I stopped trying to convince doubting friends and family and started teaching this diet system to people with dreams.

I found I had to walk my talk. To really inspire others to become healthy I had to become incredibly healthy myself. Many of the spiritual books I have read advise that addictions should not be fought, that they dissolve away when the mind is right. This may be good advice for some, but it did not work for me. I had to fight and conquer processed-food addictions. And I succeeded, and so can you.

I feel incredibly fortunate for having created the opportunity to communicate the raw nutrition message through mass media (radio, television, magazines, newspapers and the Internet). Over the years, I have had the incredible privilege of meeting and communicating with thousands of raw-foodists the world over. The Internet and e-mail have allowed communication and networking on this subject to reach a remarkable level. The time for this information to reach a worldwide audience has come.

Through my seminars, retreats, books, websites, exotic raw foods, video recordings and audio recordings I am helping, along with all other raw-foodists, to chart uncharted territory. I believe I am helping to do for nutrition what Roger Bannister did for running when he broke the four-minute mile barrier. Bannister overcame all the doubters and pessimists. What was once considered impossible became possible. The year after Bannister broke the four-minute mile, 37 other runners broke the four-minute mile. And many thousands have done it since. Did human physiology change? No. What changed were the beliefs about human physiology.

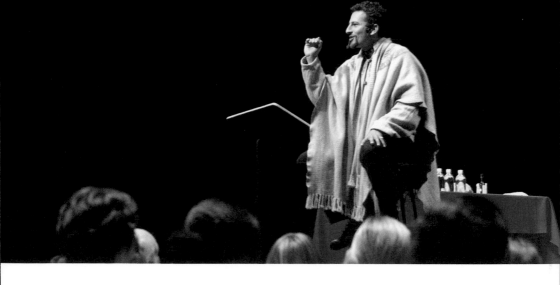

A scene from a lecture I gave to nearly a thousand people in New York City. What an incredible afternoon: The Best Day Ever!

Remember: if one person can achieve the unachievable, then what is possible forever changes.

The Sunfood Diet, when balanced correctly with The Sunfood Triangle and other tools, creates a path to achieve eternal, resonating beauty. This is such an incredible secret. I feel The Sunfood Diet turned me into a lovely being, alive in each recess, capable of understanding every feeling, soothed and healed of past injuries. It taught me that excellent health is essential to truly enjoying every moment of life.

Perhaps I was predestined to be a raw-foodist. My ethnic heritage comes from Persia where there is a long history of raw-foodism and veganism. In fact, in the Persian language (Farsi) there is a specific term for a raw-foodist: Khom Gia Khori (raw plant eater). This term is about as popular in Persia as the word "vegan" in the United States.

My diet may at first seem limited compared to the standard fast-food diet called "moderation," but the way I eat is actually filled with great pleasure, because I have developed the capacity to enjoy the simplest foods and so can you.

In my personal life, the longer I have eaten raw, the more I find I prefer to eat alone, standing up, in a meditational state, listening to success tapes or reading

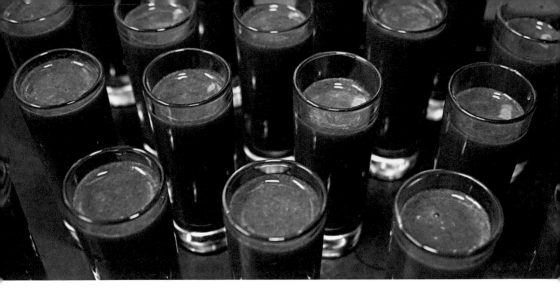

The liquid diet makes everything so much easier!
One day I hope to be a liquidarian 100% of the time.

books. I love eating the best food ever!

I am often asked what I eat. I usually drink a lot more than I eat. I might consume the following in a typical day:

1. One or two avocados, 5-10 ripe olives and/or 35-45 pumpkin seeds.
2. One to two pounds of celery, lettuce, kale and/or wild green food picked or harvested from my gardens or foraged from the canyons near my house consumed mostly as a green juice.
3. Two to three handfuls of citrus fruit, apples, berries or another juicy fruit in season (peaches, plums, nectarines, mangos, etc.). Sometimes I will add these to a smoothie.
4. One or two ripe hot peppers (usually jalapeno or habanero).
5. Two to four strips of nori or dulse seaweed.
6. Three to four tablespoons of spirulina, bee pollen, maca, goji berries and other superfoods. Often these are blended into a morning smoothie with some of the fruits mentioned above.
7. 15-20 cacao beans (raw chocolate nuts). These may also be blended into an evening smoothie with aloe vera, superfoods and water.

I typically eat two large meals a day: one at 11:00 am (usually a superfood smoothie), the other at 7:00 pm (usually a salad). This works wonderfully for me. I may snack between these meals on fruits, seeds or juices.

I love to eat green-leafy vegetables (I chew them like gum sometimes if I am bored!). I have found that bitter green foods are very healing. When you cultivate a taste for bitter food, you will see a marked improvement in your health.

Ripe hot peppers are one of my favorite foods. For centuries, herbalists have told us of the beneficial effects of hot "cayenne" peppers in healing heart conditions. Hot peppers are also great for stimulating the digestive tract and for "burning" out parasites in the intestines. These foods are natural antibiotics and they contain an excellent quantity of liver-supporting sulfur. (The type of sulfur needed to produce glowing skin, hair and nails, is of another type found in aloe vera, spirulina, hempseed and MSM powder).

From both my experience and the experience of other long-time raw-foodists, I definitely disagree with the natural hygiene philosophy of including no hot peppers and other spicy raw foods (onions, garlic, ginger) in the diet. These foods play important roles for some body types (for example, Ayurvedic kapha body types are balanced by these foods) even though they may unbalance other body types (such as Ayurvedic pitta body types being aggravated by hot chilies).

I do not eat complex raw-food recipe dishes often — in the beginning, when I had weaker digestion, a recipe for me was usually for disaster. Now, I love the experience of raw-food restaurants. Raw restaurants and raw recipe books are excellent dietary tools and fun for family, friends and parties. There are dozens of raw-food recipe books available. There are more and more raw-food restaurants opening up all around the world. There are also many fantastic chefs who specialize in "uncooking."

Many commercial supplements are lifeless and overwhelm and confuse the body with too many concentrated synthetic elements (petrochemical vitamin pills, non-soluble mineral tablets, heavy colloidal mineral tinctures, animal protein powders, etc.). I only consume the highest-quality, naturally-derived supplements. I particularly enjoy MegaHydrate, Crystal Energy, my liquid David Wolfe's Ormus Gold, fully mineralized sea salts, and others. In my opinion, high quality organic foods and superfoods are the best sources of nutrients and supplements there are to enhance specific needs, requirements and/or desired nutritional goals. My thoughts have changed on supplements over the years. I began years ago with the opinion that they are unnecessary. Through experience I now feel that high-quality supplements can be quite helpful.

If you feel too restricted eating exactly what I recommend, you can always take up the fall-back position: eat a wider variety of raw plant foods including fruits, vegetables, herbs, nuts, seeds, sprouts, sea vegetables, raw plant-food recipes, etc. Remember, the initial goal here is to eat as much raw plant food as we can adjust into our diet. Make your nutrition fun.

Water

I am often asked what I do for water. The best book I have found on the subject of water is **Living Energies** by Callum Coats. **Living Energies** is essentially a compendium of the greatest pieces of research done by Austrian water wizard Viktor Schauberger. I have always felt a close affinity with the Greek philosopher Thales who believed that everything on Earth consists of various quantities of water and that water is the basic substance of all matter. Later, by studying the writings of Viktor Schauberger, I found Thales philosophy detailed scientifically. Hydrogen apparently cannot be completely disassociated from oxygen (water cannot be destroyed) that is why a catalyst is always required to conduct electrolysis in pure water. Because the catalyst is changed due to electrolysis, it is then not a true catalyst and indicates some deeper scientific truth underlies the reaction.

Viktor Schauberger's philosophy focuses on the ennoblement of water: life is about ennobling water in a dynamic interaction between the Heavens and the Earth. Essentially, Viktor Schauberger and many spiritual adepts throughout history have understood that water responds to our thoughts and intentions. Water is a living, conscious entity. Dr. Masaru Emoto has demonstrated this fact in his books **The Messages of Water** (volumes 1, 2 and 3).

Viktor Schauberger states emphatically that the best water to drink is fresh, spring water coming forth from the earth at cold temperatures (preferably 39.2 degrees Fahrenheit or 4 degrees Celsius). I personally drink fresh spring water and glacial run-off water in copious amounts whenever possible. However, when living in a city, I typically do not drink much water due to quality concerns and also because the raw foods I eat already contain high-quality water. My water consumption ranges between 0.5 liters and 1.5 liters per day. I used to

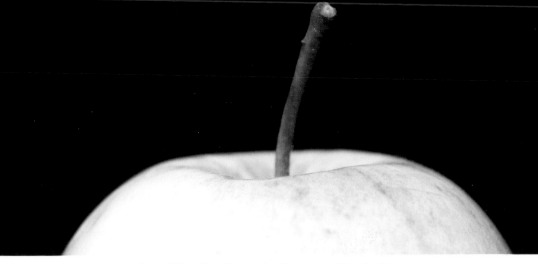

One of the planet's greatest treasures: The Apple.
This was a wild one picked in Canada.

consume distilled water and found it lifeless and depleting after several years. One positive benefit of distilled water is that it is uncontaminated "blank tape" that can be re-enlivened. I learned to add substances to it to bring distilled water (or any bottled water) back to life such as lemon, lime, blades of grass, green herbs, sea or rock salts, MSM powder and/or Dr. Patrick Flanagan's Crystal Energy (a mineral product that makes water wetter).

Whenever possible, I store my water in a clay egg container per the recommendation and design of Viktor Schauberger. When I remember, I take a moment and bless my water before drinking it. I also write the word "love" on my water drinking glasses; this may sound like a wild "New Age" idea, but it has been scientifically shown by Dr. Emoto to favorably alter the structure of water. Part of my core philosophy is to stack the odds in my favor whenever possible.

Whenever possible, avoid distilled water bottled in plastic. Distilled water is "mineral hungry" and tends to draw substances including plastic into itself. Plastic mimics estrogen (the female sex hormone) inside the body. Summit Springs or Raw Water from Maine is my personal favorite commercially available bottled spring water (available in glass). Other spring waters (such as high-end Grander water) bottled in glass are great.

Gardening

By eating raw plant foods, I believe you will become deeply interested in gardening as I have. Gardening cultivates an intimate connection between you, the plants, the Sun and the Earth. Gardening nourishes us twice: once by the exercise involved in creating the garden, and again when we eat the food. In my own life, my garden continues to show me new ways to experience and explore the Earth's mysteries.

Growing plants compels us to eat our food in its natural, raw state, because of all the energy we have put into harvesting the food. It compels us to compost our food scraps and to improve the soil each year. Growing our own food decreases pollution because it reduces our participation in the transportation and/or packaging challenges incurred by shipping food.

In the great outdoors you can never grow bored nor weary, but will remain content and joyful. "All my ills my garden spade," wrote Emerson. The most contented and happy people are those who breathe in the rich vapors of their home garden. I know that is where I feel best.

The essence of my entire message is found in growing gardens, living as close to Nature as possible and in making friends with the animals. It is in doing those things that all may be learned. I am reminded of the maxim, "Before a person may govern a city, s/he must first be able to govern a garden." I find gardening one of life's greatest pleasures and watching fruit trees grow from seed to maturity one of the secrets of longevity.

The greatest books I have ever discovered in the field of gardening include: **Secrets of the Soil** by Christopher Bird and Peter Tompkins, **Sea Energy Agriculture** by Dr. Maynard Murray, **The Fertile Earth** by Callum Coats (about Viktor Schauberger) and **Paramagnetism** by Philip Callahan.

MY PERSONAL DIET

1   My challenge for this lesson is for you to begin bringing plants into your life. Start with simple house plants, sprouting trays, a greenhouse and/or a backyard garden.

2   Eating raw plant food is the way to live in total harmony with the Earth. What if you took all the fruit and vegetable remnants left over from what you ate and, instead of throwing them away, you used them to fertilize your plants?

3   Make your home beautiful. The abode of the Sunfoodist is rich and luxuriant; it is filled in one place with exotic fruit trees and garden herbs — all fertilized by the compost of a plentiful Sunfood lifestyle. It is recognized as a special place of massive abundance.

4   Become a fully activated human being. Read and take action on the information contained in the gardening books mentioned on the previous page.

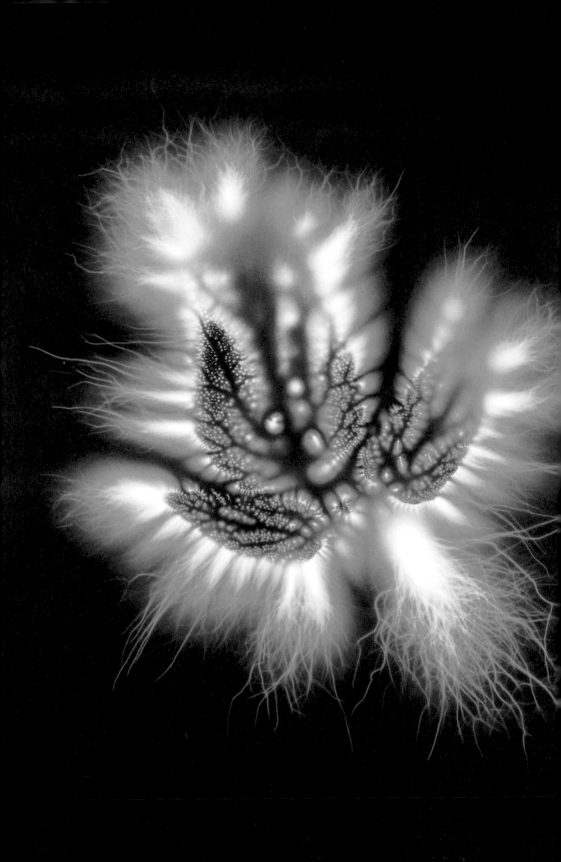

18

100% RAW

"THE PARADISICAL DIET IS NOT ONLY SUFFICIENT, BUT IT
BRINGS YOU HIGHER AND HIGHER, INTO PHYSICAL AND MENTAL
CONDITIONS NEVER BEFORE EXPERIENCED."
— *Professor Arnold Ehret*

"THE GREATEST VALUE OF THE RAW-FOOD DIET IS ITS
TRANSFORMATIVE VALUE. TO A GREAT EXTENT, WHEN YOU
TAKE UP THE RAW-FOOD DIET, YOU BECOME A NEW
AND DIFFERENT AND BETTER PERSON. YOU DON'T JUST STAY
THE SAME OLD PERSON ONLY A LITTLE HEALTHIER. YOU BECOME,
TO A GREAT EXTENT, A NEW BEING WITH NEW INTERESTS,
A NEW PHILOSOPHY AND OUTLOOK ON LIFE, NEW GOALS
AND NEW DESIRES. YOU BECOME MORE OF YOUR ESSENCE,
YOUR TRUE NATURAL SELF. YOU BECOME A PERSON WHO IS
MORE A PART OF THE ONE GREAT LIFE OF NATURE AND LESS
OF THE CONFUSED HUMAN WORLD. YOU BECOME LESS
'OF THE WORLD' AND MORE 'OF THE EARTH.'"
— *Joe Alexander, Blatant Raw-Foodist Propaganda*

"FOR EVERY DISCIPLINED EFFORT, THERE IS A MULTIPLE REWARD."
— *Jim Rohn, success philosopher*

I feel it is an essential part of my purpose on Earth to let people know that they can eat 100% raw food — that it is possible, magical and sustainable. For me, eating 100% raw has allowed me to master many of the lessons necessary to achieve an absolutely extraordinary level of health and to open wide the doors of hidden possibility. It has not been easy.

Is 100% raw extreme? To humans… yes. But not to wild animals in nature. It is the way food has always been done. Raw is the way Mother Earth prepares food for her children. Remember: life is extreme. It's life or death. If you want extreme transformations in your life, you need to start taking extreme actions. This is no dress rehearsal; this is the real thing. People are dying. The major diseases in America are related to the way people eat. People are looking for the answers. People are sick and tired of being lied to (figuratively and literally). The Earth is being trashed with pollution and it can be reversed by simple fundamental changes. Permit this challenge: get out on a limb, you will discover that is where all the fruit is!

Anything that would tend to limit your greatest gift — the power to think and reason clearly — should be eliminated above all things. Any quantity of demineralized, weak and/or unhealthy food, clouds the mind to some degree and leaves a residue of debris in the body that dampens the electrical circuitry in the brain.

The time is upon us to become more discerning in our food choices. The threat of pesticides, the danger of animal products, soil demineralization and genetic engineering can no longer be ignored. Yesterday's cooked-food diet won't cut it today. The standard animal food, processed diet is a gamble; we never know what is truly in the food.

Let's look at this process as starting a new diet while avoiding implied limitations. This is not about denial. 99.99% of all the food on Earth is raw plant food. Eating a natural food diet is the ultimate freedom. There is such a variety of raw plant foods on this Earth it is astonishing. Have you ever tried a black sapote, cherimoya, durian, eggfruit, elderberry, galia melon, habanero pepper, jackfruit, lemonade berry, loquat, lychee, mamey, mountain apple, pomegranate, prickly pear, sapodilla, suriname cherry, or white sapote? Have you ever tried butterleaf lettuce, chicory, dandelion, dinosaur kale, fennel, lamb's quarters, lemon grass, miner's lettuce, nopal cactus, sorrel, watercress, wild mustard, wild onion or wintercress? Obviously I have only just touched on some of the variety of edible plants that are out there. You could try a new fruit and vegetable every single day for the rest of your life and not even come remotely close to trying them all!! There is too much abundance!!

For me, a 100% raw-Sunfood diet is the ultimate high. People are intelligent and they understand that they should be feeling great all the time. The depressing effects of cooked foods and animal products are a major reason why people resort to intoxicating liquors and drugs.

The question of going 100% raw is a question of cleverness, metabolism, persistence and spiritual certainty. We cannot be healthy by denying ourselves or feeling guilt. Have the maturity to adjust your lifestyle to accommodate your diet while enjoying the process. I often tell my seminar listeners, "The old habits die hard, but they do die!"

It may be best to stabilize at 70% raw, then 80% raw, and continue on from there if you choose. We want to avoid the "yo-yo effect" — doing 100% raw and then binge eating and then returning to 100% raw. We also want to avoid eating excessive amounts of nuts, seeds, sweet fruit, or prepared raw food in order to meet our current fuel (calorie) needs to stay 100% raw. One must critically evaluate whether 100% is realistic based on one's current fuel (calorie) requirements (eating raw radically decreases calorie sources which may be healing, yet unbalancing in the short or long term). Set a level of raw, organic food consumption that is appropriate and realistic for you now.

When you reach a stable level of 95% raw, it will be fantastic. You may experience that the body eventually starts to push towards letting go of all cooked foods in the diet — and this is in the natural course of things. After many years on a high-raw, but not all-raw diet, the body becomes more refined and goes into an immediate "detox mode" as soon as any cooked food is ingested, leaving one functioning at less than optimal capacity.

My experience had been that by eating 95% raw food, I received 95% of the amazing results. After being comfortably eating 100% raw food for several years, it seemed that I was receiving 1,000% of the results.

A 100% raw diet is a wonderful goal if it is appropriate for you. I feel blessed to know that it is possible. I know many people who have been eating 100%

raw foods for 5, 10, 20, 30, even 40 years and longer, and who have attained an incredible level of health and vitality. I know many people who have been eating 70–80% raw foods for 20, 30, even 40 years who have also attained an incredible level of health and vitality. Once I had set the goal, I did not go 100% raw foods immediately. I went 95% raw overnight and then gradually weaned myself off the last 5%. Previously, I had been eating an 80% raw organic vegan diet.

In general, I have found it is better to give individuals shorter-range goals, such as going one day, one week or one month 100% raw. And this is great for cleansing. It is best to envision that goal, than to envision going a lifetime without cooked food. Once the initial pattern is established, then one can duplicate that pattern — it becomes a blueprint for success.

As I mentioned in **Lesson 12: Transition Diet**, the key to transitioning to raw food is to experiment on a small scale. First, set a goal to go raw for three days, then expand that to a week the next time, then a month; keep expanding all the time. Write your raw goals down and commit to them. Then see, after achieving your goals, how much further you can go. Make a commitment that requires you to surpass your physical and emotional obstacles. Refuse to consider any other option except your goal of vibrant health.

What is fascinating is that the temptations of cooked food begin to lose their strength. The former "pleasures" associated with cooked food will automatically reverse as one continues to step outside of the old comfort zone into the raw realm. It is not that one has to discipline oneself forever to stay away from the "pleasures" of cooked food, it is that one is no longer attracted to those foods. They are often discovered to be no longer pleasurable, but instead lifeless and devoid of nutritional and spiritual strength.

The best time to begin is always right now. Teddy Roosevelt's most famous saying was: "Do what you can, with what you have, where you are." The best place on Earth, the greatest opportunity in the world, is right where you happen to be right now. You are sitting on your own fortune — your own "Acres of Diamonds."

Let's make the change now! Your life is too important to allow your diet to fall to a point where it finally takes your desire for survival to overcome your appetite for "poor" foods.

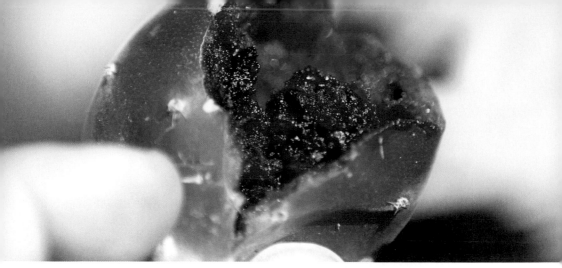

The fruit of a rare Sonoran desert plant: Night-blooming Cereus.
This is one of my favorite desert (dessert) foods!

There are many things you do now which would have seemed difficult to you ten years ago. Those things themselves did not change, but your idea of your-self changed. What if you were to think things differently today?

It is going to take courage. Where there is no joy there can be no courage; and without courage all other virtues are meaningless. Enjoy the process and let Nature take its course. Nature's smile is for the joyful, the courageous, the disci-plined and the all-daring.

Complacency is the great enemy of possibility. Just keep taking action. Focus all your energy, not on fighting the old, but on building the new habits.

It is going to take a view to the long-term. The ability to think long-term, to be long-sighted, depends on the ability to delay gratification. The ability to delay gratification determines how much spiritual power we have over our physical body. Delaying gratification is a sign of wisdom and maturity. By delaying food gratification you start making incredible strides.

Self-discipline has been defined as the ability to make yourself do what you should do, when you should do it, whether you feel like doing it or not.

To become a raw-foodist, you must have the desire. You must be willing to pay the price. The price may be much or it may be little, but you must condition your mind to pay it (and pay it gladly!), regardless of the cost. Remember Andrew Carnegie's saying, "Anything worth having is worth working for."

As you find yourself ready, it is time to cross the border; to sail out into an unknown sea; to commit to reaching a 100% organic, mineral-rich, balanced, raw, Sunfood diet. As you'll see, you will not fall off the edge of the world. You will have to overcome the stormy seas of negativity and the waves of peer pressure, the perilous storms of accusation and the scurvy-ridden sailors of mediocrity, the glide down the wave-crests into the wave-valleys of detoxification, but afterwards it all will appear before you a new land, a land transformed into a paradise, a land explored thus far by only the curious and the brave! You may well discover the timeless truth that when you change, the world changes automatically. You will look through different eyes. You will be transformed into a new being! Commit! There is no strength in compromise.

If you choose, you can reach a point where you are able to do all you need to do in the external world (social food visits with friends, business luncheons, etc.), yet have no inner food conflicts because you will have attained a new consciousness. Your insights will be powerful. You will make statements with great certainty without knowing how it happened. Uncanny events will become commonplace.

When I let go of cooked food, life became even more exciting. After many years of eating exclusively raw foods, my mindset became more resolute, flexible, clear, free of doubt; my body became lithe, supple, sensitive and filled with energy. My yoga practice was completely transformed. I gained a proficiency to push myself beyond all perceived physical, mental, emotional and spiritual boundaries.

I woke up after napping in my backyard one day with a bird bouncing around my head and face. We just looked at each other. When you go raw, the animals do not look at you as something strange anymore, you do not carry the obvious smell of civilization's diet. You become more of the continuum of life — one with the animals. What price can you put on a unified connection with Nature? It is priceless.

100% RAW

1 Many raw-foodists ask me why people do not go 100% raw. 100% raw does present challenges. These challenges may be overcome through knowledge, persistence, effort and discipline. I have discovered the following 10 reasons why people do not eat 100% raw:

1) They are not ready, their body and mind has not adjusted. Their favorite cooked foods still taste better than their favorite raw foods. With time, the taste buds change, the body acclimates to new, cleaner foods, and progress with raw food becomes easier. Everyone should transition at a pace that is outside their comfort zone, but not in their shock zone.

2) They do not have the metabolism for eating all raw foods and are unable to find a balance point even though they are well educated on the subject and have tried many different approaches over many years. This is natural and normal. The information in this book is not the truth. It is my best approximation based on years of research and experience. As long as we are conscious about our food choices, eating organic, mineral-rich raw food and seeking out that perfect health balance, we are making progress. An 80% raw plant diet seems to be a more workable approach to more people and is, in fact, enough to save the planet.

3) They require more education on the subject. They don't realize the importance of eating 100% raw plant foods and the magic in it.

4) They simply are not serious. They talk, but never do. They want to make an improvement in their life, but they are not willing to make the necessary effort.

5) They don't know how; they are confused by conflicting opinions on diet. They don't understand the idea of eating 100% raw plant food.

6) They haven't accepted 100% responsibility for their lives and their health, happiness and longevity. They don't feel they are worthy enough to be extraordinarily healthy. They don't feel they deserve it.

7) They don't go 100% raw because of the fear of rejection. They fear their friends and family will reject them and their new lifestyle and/or that the opposite sex will reject them.

8) They fear the unknown. Eating 100% raw is the unknown for most people, and for that reason, they fear it instead of embrace it! Eventually, we have nowhere to go, but into the unknown. Which do you prefer?

A known hell or a strange heaven? The way you are going now is leading down a specific path — a destiny. One day you will arrive...the question is where?

9) They get unbalanced because they do not exercise and/or eat a healthy combination of green-leafy vegetables, sweet fruits and fatty foods. Thus they return back to familiar food habits.

10) The inability to face their suppressed emotional issues when they arise. One of the major challenges I have seen in people going 100% raw is facing suppressed emotional trauma. A 100% raw plant-food diet presents your emotional issues to you — it brings them right to your consciousness. These issues often involve one or both parents. To win through, one must have the courage to face these emotional issues squarely and release them. Holding on to 10% "comfort foods" in the diet can be helpful, as it will slow the emotional traumas from arising too rapidly.

2   Get out your journal. Do any of these ten reasons apply to you and why? How will you face or overcome these challenges? Record the answers in writing in your journal.

3   Remember: Going 100% raw is great, but it is also beautiful to give a 100% effort. 100% raw is not for everyone. Decide what works for you in your lifestyle.

Opposite: a magnificent Kirlian photograph of a speck of organic raw cacao powder.

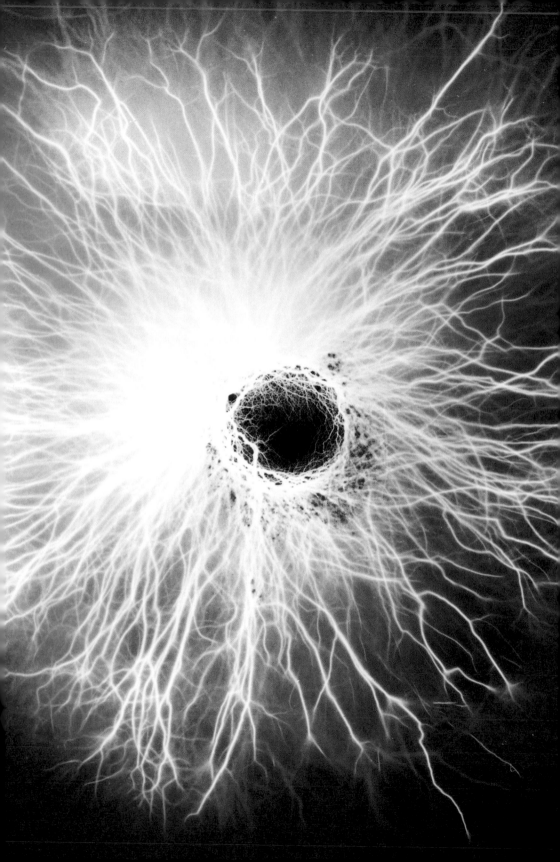

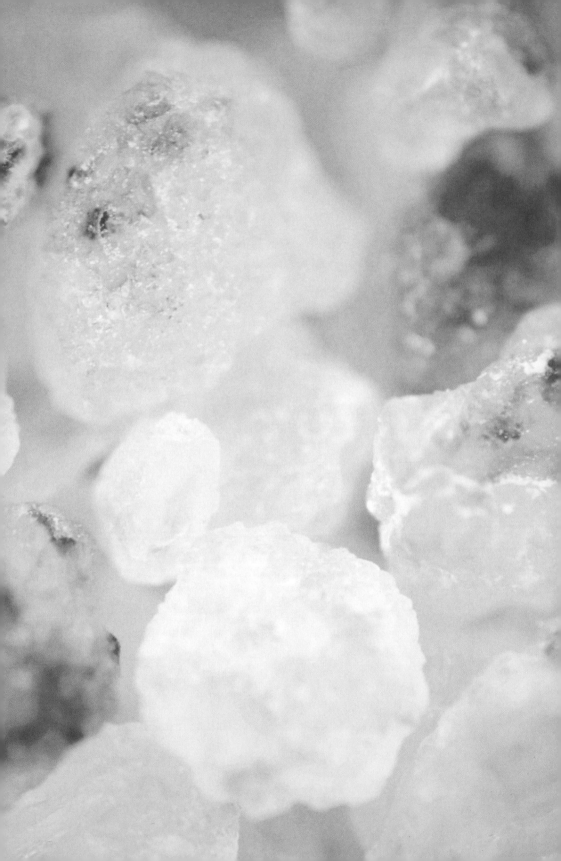

19

MINERAL TRADE-OUT

Vitamins are never an issue when eating raw plant foods. All raw plant foods, even if not of an excellent quality, are abundant in all the vitamins we need to thrive. For instance, the B vitamins may be found in deep-green leafy vegetables, nuts, seeds, bee pollen, royal jelly, spirulina and fermented plants. Vitamin B12 was addressed in **Lesson 16: Wild Food**. Vitamin C is found in many fruits, especially citrus fruits and peppers of all kinds. The best source of vitamin E is the avocado, olives, and mechanically separated raw rice bran.

This lesson is about minerals, because it has been my experience, in studying nutrition, that minerals are far more important than vitamins.

Colloids are the mineral building blocks of the body. A colloid is a mineral suspended in solution with energy. They are extremely small and resist the pull of gravity. They conduct electricity throughout the body.

The Sun evaporates water from the leaves of plants, concentrating the protoplasm solution. Thus, due to osmosis (the movement of water from an area of greater concentration to an area of lesser concentration), water containing soluble minerals is spirally suctioned up from the roots into the leaves of the plant. In this way the protoplasm is continuously concentrated and the leaves become loaded with colloidal minerals suspended with Sun and Earth energies. Each plant mines a different spectrum of minerals from the soil and provides a different nutrition to the body. Calcium (lime), however, is the primary leaf mineral. Interestingly, calcium also makes up about 50% of the alkaline earth mineral matter of the human body, and is found in all bodily tissues, but chiefly in the bones, teeth and the muscles. The importance of leaf minerals for the human body cannot be overstated. When we consume plant leaves we are provided with fresh colloidal minerals with which to construct our bodies.

We can see the colloidal leaf minerals precipitate out of freshly-made, green juices if we allow the juice to sit and lose energy. As a juice loses energy (zeta potential), it begins to change from an alkaline medium to an acid medium; it no longer has the energy to hold minerals in suspension. This is what happens to the blood as it acidifies from poor nutrition. The blood no longer has the energy to hold minerals in solution and thus minerals precipitate out in all the wrong places, such as the muscle tissue, joints, bones, etc. causing arthritis, weakness, bone spurs, etc.

Some types of arthritis occur when the blood's acidity is high. High blood acidity means low blood energy and low blood solubility. During this state, minerals are not held in solution and thus precipitate improperly. Arthritis is typically the result of a meat-based diet. Meat, raw or cooked, is extremely acidic, thus, meat lowers the blood's energy, causing improper mineral precipitation.

Some types of arthritis are definitely linked with an overabundance of cooked, acid-forming elements in the body (from meat), and some types are also linked to irritants introduced into the body by eating cooked nightshade plants (tomato sauce, french fries, baked potatoes, fried eggplant, tobacco, etc.). For those with an exacerbated arthritic condition I recommend against eating any meat, and to avoid all nightshades (chilies, eggplants, peppers, potatoes, tobacco, tomatilloes, tomatoes), even if eaten raw. I have noticed with some individuals that sensitivities to cooked nightshades may continue even when nightshades are eaten raw.

Osteoporosis also occurs when the blood's acidity is high due to an excess of acid-forming foods in the diet. Remember: the quality of the food entering the body directs the quality of the blood and lymph. To balance an acid condition in the body, the blood must draw alkaline minerals from the bones. Dairy products are alkaline (based on their minerals) but acid-forming once the body no longer has the enzymes and vital energy necessary to metabolize them. An acid-forming diet, over the long term, will leach minerals from the bones, leading to osteoporosis. To begin to address an osteoporosis condition, please reference **Lesson 14: Alkaline and Acid**. Consistently introduce significantly more alkaline-residue foods into your diet, such as lettuce, kale, collards, oranges, figs, broccoli, etc. in combination with specific seeds (flax seed, pumpkin seed, hemp seed).

Additional help with osteoporosis can come from adding progesterone supporting nutritional supplements or foods into the diet. Coconut oil and maca powder are two excellent foods to help support the building up of progesterone for increasing overall hormone production.

In conjunction with nutrition, weight-bearing exercise is important for healing osteoporosis. Horsetail (*Equisetum arvense*) tea also seems to be highly effective in helping increase bone density.

Trade-Out

After eating Sunfoods under the Sun for a sufficient period of time, the body begins removing everything that is improper. This process will continue for several years until you become a rejuvenated being. As you continue eating raw, you will eventually replace every cell and restructure every tissue using the high-quality minerals, nutrients and positive energy that you are putting in your body.

After a sufficient period of eating Sunfoods at a 100% level (usually between six months to three years), the body will begin to purge acids and replace minerals. Mineral trade-out can be instigated by herbal cleanses which tend to stir up toxic, acidic residues in the body and intestines. If one is eating a diet high in demineralized raw food, sweet fruit with low green-leafy vegetables, mineral trade-out may occur sooner (usually less than six months). This is when the teeth problems arise, which is indicative of the body purging acids and also indicative of a lack of minerals in the body and diet, especially calcium, magnesium, iron and silicon. At the point of mineral trade-out, one needs to take in at least 2.5 pounds (1.1 kg) of green-leafed vegetables daily (one-third eaten, two-thirds juiced), increase the intake of sea vegetables, use up to ten tablespoons of green super-foods (powdered grasses and algae) per day, include more seeds to help synergize and utilize the green foods and simultaneously cut down on eating hybridized sweet fruit and high-fat, acid-forming nuts.

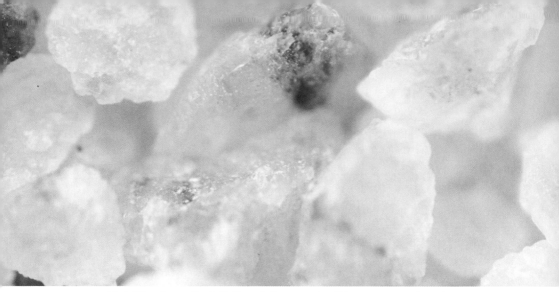

Pink Himalayan Rock Salt contains over 80 different trace minerals.
This salt deposit was laid down in the distant past by an ancient ocean.

Mineral trade-out signals to you that a deep cleaning and healing of the body tissues is taking place. It means your body has really gotten to the core tissues for replacement. This is a process of the "good" pushing out the "bad."

When you notice that your teeth are becoming stronger this usually means you are past the period of mineral trade-out, which typically passes within a few weeks or months, even though it takes many years of eating highly-mineralized food to become remineralized. If you are unsure or confused on this issue, always err on the side of taking in more green juice and superfoods. And because teeth issues often arise when minerals are out of balance, always maintain excellent dental hygiene.

The lesson of mineral trade-out is that eating highly-mineralized food grown in highly-mineralized soil is essential to achieve extraordinary health.

When you eat, always go for the highest-quality, highest mineral-content foods available to you. Unfortunately, most commercial fruit trees are short-lived and are shallow feeders. The fuller and richer the taste of the fruit, the more minerals it contains. The roots of wild fruit trees go down from 10 to 25 feet (3.0 to 7.5 meters) where there has been no soil depletion. The nut trees, that live for decades, send roots 40 to 50 feet (12 to 15 meters) deep to mine the Earth. Planting fruit and nut trees will help remineralize the Earth because they pull minerals from down deep and deposit them on the surface in the form of falling leaves, fruits, and nuts creating a fertile bed for gardening vegetables. (See

Chart: Tree Mineralization in **Lesson 7: The Sunfood Diet**).

Remineralization

> "GOD SLEEPS IN STONE, BREATHES IN PLANTS,
> DREAMS IN ANIMALS AND AWAKENS IN MAN." — *Hindu proverb*

The yield, strength and mineral content of raw plant foods — whether they are commercial, organic or wild — is improved by remineralization. Remineralization is the process of loading the soil with crushed and pulverized rocks which restore the full spectrum of mineral elements. The soil microbes, earthworms and plant roots are directly nourished by an abundance of soil minerals.

The research is in with soil expert and raw-foodist Don Weaver. Don Weaver has demonstrated conclusively in the book, **The Survival Of Civilization**, which he co-authored with John Hamaker, that plants and trees depend far more on the soil and its mineral content than they depend on climate to produce high quality leaves and fruits.

Insects always infest trees and other plants (as pathogens invade people) that are weakened by malnutrition and no longer have resistance to their natural enemies. The hybridized commercial crops grown today in weak demineralized soils are heavily sprayed with pesticides to keep the insects from overrunning the whole show.

John Hamaker writes:
"This question of the proper feeding of the soil is the crux of the whole food situation, for if the soil starves so does the plant and so do we. We cannot have healthy human beings without healthy food crops, and these depend entirely upon the healthy feeding of the soil."
"High yields depend on loading the soil with both a large surface area of available minerals and organic matter."
"Examine a stone, other than limestone, in the soil. Crack it open. Under a very drab demineralized exterior 'skin' you will see the minerals. That skin represents the depth which the microorganisms have been able to penetrate the crystal structure of the stone."

When the rock is ground to dust, more "skin" is exposed to feed the soil microbes. One of the best fertilizers for trees and plants is crushed rock. When rock is pulverized, exponentially more of its surface area is exposed and more minerals are available to the micro-organisms in the soil. In one pound (0.45 kg) of finely ground gravel you have about ten acres (four hectares) of surface area for the microorganisms to feed on.

The mineralized rock dust you combine with your plant soil will eventually show up as a major difference in the size, taste quality and texture of the food grown therefrom. Any rock dust mixture that will give good growth and is found locally is preferred.

Another substance containing fantastic remineralization qualities is dilute ocean water. Ocean water contains 90 minerals and un-assayable monoatomic mineral elements. Ocean water is perhaps the most highly mineralized substance on Earth. Ocean water can be added to soils in 20 to 1 (20 parts pure water to 1 part ocean water) or 30 to 1 or 40 to 1 concentrations. Even more dilute homeopathic applications can be tried (such 100 to 1 or 1,000 to 1 ratios). Interestingly, both Rudolf Steiner and Viktor Schauberger seem to favor homeopathic methods for healing weak soils.

MINERAL TRADE-OUT

1 Discover rock dust. Visit your local gravel quarry, ask for the chemist, get several bags of rock dust (they should be free), and throw and sprinkle the dust directly into the soil around your trees and garden. If local rock dust is not available or if you would love more information about rock dust, please visit www.remineralize.org. They can provide you with the best information and the most economical sources of rock dust available world-wide.

2 Discover the power of using dilute ocean water on your soils, gardens and indoor plants and sprouts.

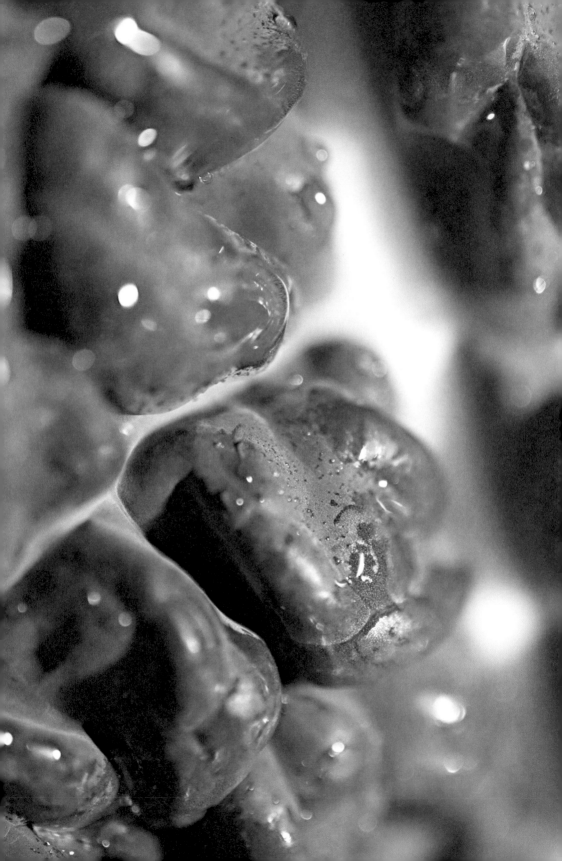

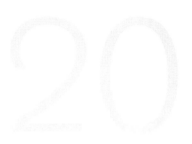

LESSON

TEETH

One of the ways anthropologists date human fossils is by looking at skull teeth. The more modern the fossil, the more tooth decay. Analyses of striations on fossilized teeth show no decay or premature wear when hominids ate a raw-vegetation diet. Most paleontologists agree that tooth decay coincided with the discovery of fire and accelerated with the advent of agriculture.

An unbalanced, cooked diet lacking in alkaline minerals (calcium, magnesium, silicon) and high in sugar and acid-forming minerals (phosphorus, chlorine) damages teeth formation. Because the "buds" that become the teeth are formed in the pre-natal stage, the diet of the mother has a lifelong influence. Due to improper nutrition, the body does not have the energy or minerals with which to properly control the eruption of teeth into the mouth. Poor nutrition results in crowded and malformed teeth, along with an altered bite. These structural dental challenges begin essentially as birth defects and are exacerbated by continuous improper nutrition. T.C. Fry reported in an article entitled, "The Myth Of Health In America" which appeared in Dr. Shelton's **Hygienic Review** (37:7, p. 150-152) that 98.5% of the US population suffers from dental problems of one type or another. These may often be reversed and corrected in one or more generations of eating significantly more mineral-rich organic green-leafed vegetables, grass (wheatgrass), certain herbs (horsetail tea or bamboo sap) and other raw foods in general.

The average adult human has 32 teeth: 4 canines (the dullest of any primate),

8 incisors, 20 molars: 12.5% dull canines, 25% incisor teeth, 62.5% grinding teeth. This indicates that the majority of what we should eat is food which must be chewed (ground up), such as fibrous plant matter and seeds.

Calcium combines with phosphorus to form calcium phosphate crystals that build the structure of bones and teeth. These crystals are incredibly light and are formed into a pattern similar to that found in a diamond. They have a weight-bearing capacity four times greater than an equal amount of reinforced concrete.

Teeth and bones are dynamic living tissues that are constantly being replaced and rebuilt. To support this process, both calcium and phosphorus are required in a 1:1 ratio. Most people follow a diet high in phosphorus (foods such as: cooked rice or grains, nuts, potato and corn chips and meat), but they do not balance their diet with easy to assimilate calcium-rich foods (green-leafed vegetables). This creates an acid-condition that leaches calcium from the bones, and especially the teeth, to neutralize the acid, thus leading to tooth weakening and decay.

Meats, nuts and grains are the heaviest foods in acid-forming minerals. Undoubtedly, the introduction of milk products (high in calcium) into the human diet coincided with the explosion in meat and grain consumption when humans domesticated grazing animals and wild grains. Because pasteurized (cooked) milk products are not suitable for human consumption (and for other reasons mentioned in earlier lessons), calcium should come primarily from green-leafy vegetables and/or their juices.

Contrary to the belief that fruits are alkaline, many fruits are slightly acidic in their end-mineral breakdown, meaning they contain slightly more phosphorus than calcium (reference **Lesson 14: Alkaline and Acid**). Even alkaline fruits, such as oranges, have such a strong citric acid content that, if eaten excessively, may damage tooth enamel, unless the teeth are cleaned with a brush and an antimicrobial substance (i.e. colloidal silver or essential oils) or green leaves after a meal. Raw-foodists and fruit enthusiasts can develop dental challenges if green leaves are not included in the diet in adequate proportions to provide alkalinity and an excellent calcium-phosphorus balance.

Green-leafy vegetables help clean sugar from the teeth. The harmful effects of refined and processed sugars on the teeth have been well established, but even excessive fruit sugar can damage the teeth, although not to the degree as these other types.

The body best assimilates calcium, when both magnesium and manganese are present together. Green-leafy vegetables are high in magnesium, manganese, and silicon. Spinach is the best source of all three of these minerals together. When eating, one should daily consume 1,000 mg of calcium, 300 mg of magnesium, and 5 mg of manganese (one to two pounds of whole or juiced green-leafy vegetables will be adequate).

Silicon-residue foods play a major role in bone and teeth formation in the body. A high-intake of silicon-residue foods has been shown to heal broken bones at an accelerated rate (see Louis Kervran's book **Biological Transmutations**). Silicon-residue foods include: bamboo sap/shoots, horsetail (an herb), hemp leaf, oats, cucumbers, lettuce, nopales (prickly-pear cactus leaves), okra, ripe bell peppers, radishes and tomatoes.

Chewing green leaves helps clean and repair the teeth. I like to say in my seminars, "A few days of 'leafarianism' (eating leaves) naturally brushes the teeth and helps heal mineral deficiencies."

Wadging like the primates is an excellent way to heal the mouth of pyorrhea, gum disease and cavities. Wadging means to load your mouth with greens and chew and compress the pulpy matter into the teeth and gums like a ball-player who chews tobacco. Continue to chew and compress the pulpy matter in the mouth for 30 to 45 minutes without swallowing. Years ago I did this every day for weeks at a time for lunch by chewing on mouthfuls of wild malva for 20-30 minutes — wadging with wild food heightens the healing potential.

Having said all that, the coup de grace of tooth health and healing comes back to the simple logic of observing nature. Which animals possess the strongest teeth? The ruminants. The cow, horse, zebra, goat, wildebeest, etc. These animals are primarily grass eaters. I have made light of this observation and in my experience, nothing works better for strengthening teeth than chewing wild grasses.

Be sure to maintain excellent dental hygiene by doing the following:

1. Be sure to daily floss between all of the teeth. Unlike a natural animal's teeth, the average person's teeth are crowded together.

2. Brush your teeth daily. Be sure to also brush your gums and tongue. The apes are often seen cleaning their teeth with small chewed up branches rich with resin, much as we use a toothbrush. Consider using 3% food-grade hydrogen peroxide, sea salt and/or essential oils instead of toothpaste. Brush your teeth, rinse and gargle with fresh ocean water if at all possible. I do not use toothpaste and have not since 1992. I used to brush my teeth with sea salt and/or essential oils. Since I have had the metal taken out of my mouth, I now always use food-grade 3% hydrogen peroxide in a spray bottle for my dental hygiene. If you have metal fillings in your mouth, do not use hydrogen peroxide as it can draw metal and mercury ions into your salivary environment, thus degrading fillings and exposing one to heavy metal toxicity. Of important note here is that a mouth environment of high acidity and a diet high in sugar are relatively incapable of damaging teeth without the aid of plaque-forming streptococci bacteria. Certain essential oils and especially hydrogen peroxide kill these bacteria.

3. Eat green-leafy vegetables and chew on grasses. Green leaves and grass blades are the best source of calcium and mineral salts. Chlorophyll is a mineralized medicine. Our teeth are living bones whose primary minerals are calcium and phosphorus aided by silicon, magnesium and manganese.

4. In my experience working with people, I have found that fasting is a good way to heal a minor toothache. A minor toothache may be the body's signal that it needs a rest from the constant food bombardment, so that it may heal. After fasting on water for a few days, brush your teeth clean and then consider giving your gums a complete physiological rest from food and brushing for several more days. If you have severe pain in a tooth, have lost a tooth, have an infection, have a chipped tooth, have bleeding gums, or if teeth problems persist, please see a holistic dentist.

TEETH

1   As you begin The Sunfood Diet, set up an appointment to have your teeth cleaned by a dental hygienist. Have all the excess residue removed from your teeth. This will help give you a fresh start.

2   Have mercury amalgam fillings removed from your mouth as soon and as safely as you are capable. Mercury is one of the most toxic substances known and should not be in our mouths. I know individuals and friends who were close to death from mercury poisoning due to leaching amalgam fillings. They had the mercury removed, discovered eating raw plant foods, sought other alternative healing methodologies and healed. Consult a holistic dentist for proper removal and replacement. Be sure you are protected from mercury amalgam dust by a "rubber dam" when you have your fillings removed.

   The presence of metals in the mouth causes an 'electrical short circuit' of the vital nerve energies. This is true not only for the specific area where the metal is located, but will also be reflected in other parts of the organism that correspond to that area of the body's circuitry. Thus an amalgam filling in the lower, left molar(s) may affect the sigmoid colon, or an amalgam filling in the "eye tooth" may affect the eye, etc.

3   Read **Whole Body Dentistry** by Mark Breiner, DDS and **It's All In Your Head** by Dr. Hal Huggins.

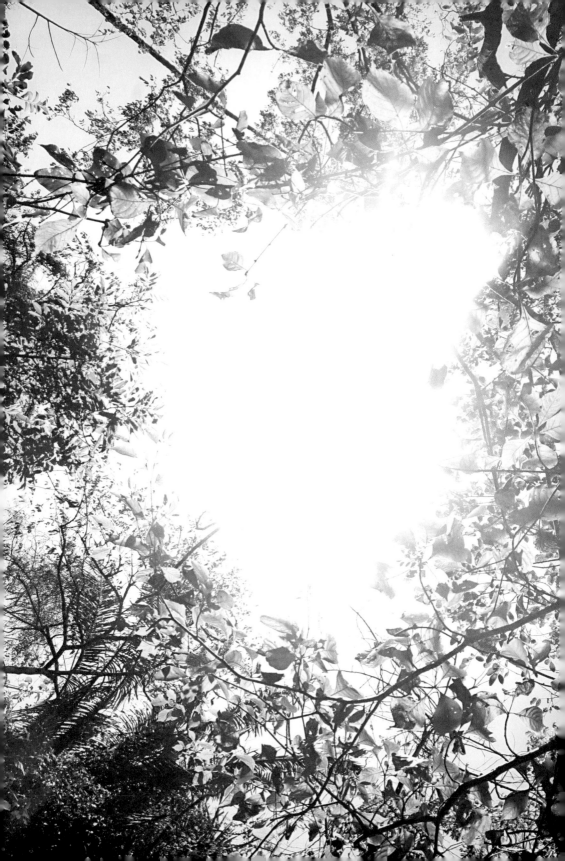

21

SUN

"WE CHOOSE THE GOD-LIKE SPLENDOR
OF THE BEST-LOVED SUN
TO INSPIRE US;
MAY THE SHINING SUN
BRIGHTEN YOUR LIFE!"
— *Ramayana*

"IF GORILLAS HAD A RELIGION, THEY WOULD SURELY BE
SUN WORSHIPPERS." — *Dr. George Schaller, Year Of The Gorilla*

Have you discovered absorbing nutrition directly from the elements — the air, the soil, the water, the Sun?

All life on this planet derives from our great Sun. The Sun beats like a great heart through every living organism. They say the molecules that make up our bodies were born in the great infernos of our superabundant star.

The air we breathe is transformed Sun energy. During photosynthesis, as plants absorb Sun energy, they transform carbon dioxide (CO_2) into vital oxygen (O_2) for animals to breathe. Here, at the first step, Nature dictates the necessity of animal life upon the underlying matrix of Sun-imbued plant life — animal respiration depends specifically on solar energy.

The foods we eat are energy reservoirs of transformed Sun energy. Through photosynthesis, plants capture energy from the Sun and lock that power into their stems, leaves, seeds, roots and fruits. All animals are transformed plants. The body of the zebra is nothing more than grass. The body of the lion is also grass, as it preys on the grass-eaters.

To a great extent we are heliovores — beings nourished directly by Sun energy. Sunlight can transform your health. The human body, with many capillaries in the skin surface, draws in Sunlight that is converted directly into nourishment by hemoglobin in the blood, just as chlorophyll converts Sunlight into nourishment in the plant. Remember, hemoglobin and chlorophyll are identical except for one mineral. Hemoglobin contains iron, chlorophyll contains magnesium.

Sunlight makes us bright and cheery. It cultivates a healthy positive attitude. A lack of Sunlight has the opposite effect. We see that people in colder climates who stay indoors all winter are often afflicted by a seasonal depression which has been attributed to a lack of Sunshine during the winter months.

The same elements in green-leafed vegetables which protect the leaves from ultra-violet radiation also protect you when you ingest those leaves. One of these substances is beta-carotene, literally shielding the nucleus of each cell.

The benefits of Sunshine are improved by eating correctly as the Sun and fresh air act like magnets in drawing toxic matter to the skin. When the body is clean and internally protected with antioxidant plant compounds you will be amazed at how long you can be in the Sun and how well you tan. Antioxidants are found naturally in richly-pigmented foods such as algae, cacao beans, all types of berries, grapes and dark-green leaves. When people eat correctly and are detoxified, reasonable exposure to the Sun cannot lead to skin cancer.

A diet high in cooked fat (free radicals) and chemicals, and low in green leaves and antioxidant plant compounds has been positively linked to skin cancer. This is because free radicals and toxins in the unprotected skin are baked and mutated by the Sun's rays. Researchers at Baylor College of Medicine found that people on a low-cooked-fat diet had a greatly reduced risk of developing pre-malignant growths and non-melanoma skin cancers.

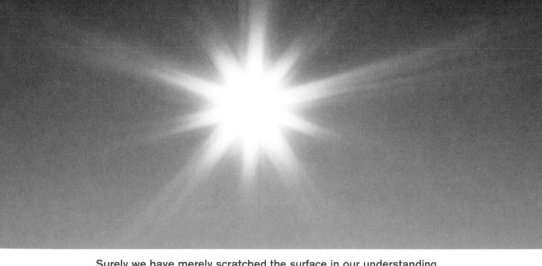

**Surely we have merely scratched the surface in our understanding
of what the Sun actually is.**

Sunlight improves our health in many different ways.

A good Sunbath is an incredible waste eliminator, as it draws toxins out of the skin. The skin is the body's largest eliminative organ.

Dr. Kime tells us in his wonderful book **Sunlight**:
"Cholesterol [formed by the body, not foreign cholesterol] turns to vitamin D — a vitamin needed for proper bone formation — when Sunlight or ultraviolet light strikes the skin. Without this vitamin the bones do not become calcified and will bend easily. This condition is called rickets."

Dr. Kime describes that Sunlight builds the immune system and increases the oxygenation of the skin.

Dr. Kime writes:
"A study of the results of combined Sunlight and exercise, showed that group that was getting the Sunlight treatments with exercise, had improved almost twice as much as shown by their electrocardiograms, as had those who only exercised, even though both groups were on a general health resort treatment program."

Sunlight lowers blood sugar. It is a natural insulin. A diet high in sweet fruit must also be accompanied by Sunshine on the skin to help metabolize the sugar. Sunlight helps to store the sugar as glycogen in the liver, muscles and cells for later use.

Exposing the skin to the Sun stimulates the capillaries and brings more blood to the skin surface. This helps to heal cuts, bruises and rashes. In World War II it was discovered that exposing abrasions, open wounds and broken bones to direct Sunlight led to quicker healing.

Many types of molds and fungi are destroyed by direct Sunlight. Candida cannot survive in direct Sunlight. A good step towards overcoming candida is Sunlight on the naked body (reference **Lesson 13: How To Use The Sunfood Triangle**, Eating To Overcome Candida).

Sunlight increases the strength of digestion. Sunlight increases the body's internal "fire." In Chinese oriental medicine we find the concept of yin-yang balance and we see that "cold" raw foods may be balanced with hot Sun energy.

Sunlight improves the eyesight, regulates the hormones and increases mineralization potential. Bringing direct Sunlight into the eyes (Sun-gazing) unmitigated by glasses, windows or filters at dawn and dusk has been part of the doctrine of breatharianism (living on energies other than food) for thousands of years. At dawn and dusk, more atmosphere is present between us and the Sun, splitting the light like a prism into more wavelengths to activate unknown elements of consciousness. This extra atmospheric cushion also provides more protection so that one does not burn one's retina.

The practice of Sun gazing should begin with 30 seconds in the morning and evening and then increase to longer periods as one acclimates. Adepts at this practice are said to Sun gaze for as long as 45 minutes at dusk and dawn.

Sunlight directly on the skin, especially on the breasts and reproductive organs heals impotence and dysfunction in those areas. A contributing cause of challenges in those areas is restrictive clothing and a lack of Sunshine.

SUN

1   Try cacao butter, coconut oil or fresh aloe vera gel as a Sun lotion. Cacao
    butter is the best natural sunscreen that is a whole food.

    By following The Sunfood Diet your resistance to ultraviolet (UV) radiation
    and Sunburns will increase. Due to the antioxidants in my raw-food diet it
    is difficult for me to get burned under the Sun; even if I have not been in
    the Sun for several weeks. The best UV protection is inner protection.

    Commercial sunscreens disable the body's natural sunburn alarm mecha-
    nism. Most suntan lotions, creams and butters are made of chemicals
    mixed with cooked-fats which produce free radicals in the skin just like
    dietary cooked fats. For these reasons I do not recommend commercial
    sunscreens — purchase only organic, high-quality sunscreens containing
    stable oils.

2   Seek out at least 30 minutes of direct Sunlight each day on as much of
    your body as possible. No matter where one lives, the practice of simply
    allowing the Sunlight to reach one's exposed face will provide benefits.

    There is no mistake in Nature. We are designed for a life of "Fun in the
    Sun!" Enjoy the abundance Nature has to offer — soak in the golden rays
    of life. Sunlight is good mood food.

    Consider the following: "Everyone, ill or well, looks better, feels better, gets
    healthier and functions more gracefully after exposing every part of their
    naked bodies to the beautiful Sunshine. Sunbathe each moment you can.
    It enlivens you in every possible way!"

3   Whenever possible and whenever you remember, practice the art of Sun
    gazing at dusk and dawn.

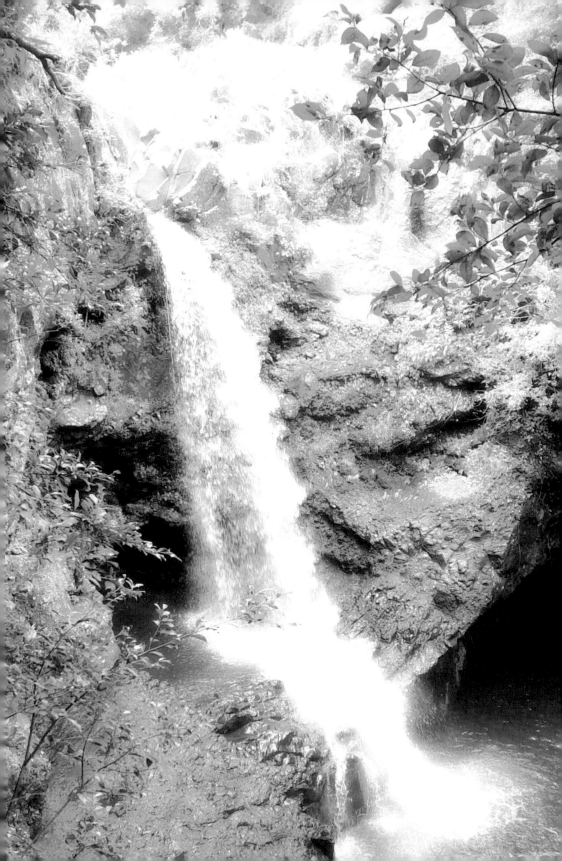

22

BREATHING (PRANAYAMA)

"AND THE LORD GOD FORMED MAN OF THE DUST OF
THE GROUND AND BREATHED INTO HIS NOSTRILS THE BREATH
OF LIFE; AND MAN BECAME A LIVING SOUL."
— *Genesis 2:7*

"FOR THE RHYTHM OF THY BREATH IS THE KEY
OF KNOWLEDGE WHICH DOTH REVEAL THE HOLY LAW."
— *The Essene Gospel of Peace, Book I*

I have provided you thus far with a detailed treatise on how to lighten the diet to liberate more energy for achievement, but before I go further, let me tell you: Do not be deceived — little energy comes from food — stimulation comes from food. The digestion of food takes energy away from the body. Energy comes first from the spirit, and then primarily from the air — from oxygen — and from a lack of obstructions in the body. A lack of oxygen makes people weak, and food is what they turn to for strength (stimulation). For more energy, start breathing!

All scientific considerations aside, air contains some life principle (prana) that keeps the human body functioning. Prana is not oxygen, but etherealized monoatomic elements or something even more exotic. These etherealized elements are spirally unzipped out of the air and into our bodies by the act of breathing. Isn't that fascinating?

When you sleep you automatically breathe, but you do not automatically eat! One can live for weeks without eating, for days without drinking, but only fleeting minutes without breathing. Yet breathing is the most neglected science in the health field. All other organs operate to keep the lungs functioning. The lungs, in turn, keep the internal organs healthy by pushing and squeezing them, allowing the fluids to move around, within and through them.

Every breath contains more air by weight than would be eaten at a typical meal, and we are taking thousands of breaths a day! One is just as poisoned by toxic air as by toxic food.

The power of breath is four-fold:

First and foremost, the breath controls the energy level in the body. We know that everything is energy — matter is just a form of frozen energy. The more oxygen and etherealized matter available to your cells, the more energy you have to accomplish your goals and the less food you desire. Many people overeat because they are not breathing deeply.

If you feel hungry, sick, tired or worn out, a good way for you to quickly rejuvenate yourself is to go outside and take 30 deep diaphragmatic breaths.

Second is the fact that the lungs play a major role in the human immune system. The lungs are the pump for the lymph system. There is four times as much lymph fluid in the body as blood; lymph bathes every cell of the body. As long as the lymph is kept clean and pumping through the body in an orderly fashion by daily deep breathing, the immune system will become incredibly strong.

Deep breathing alkalizes the body by removing carbonic acid (dissolved carbon dioxide) from the blood and lymph.

Third, controlling the breath allows you to begin to also control the so-called autonomic (automatic) functions of the body (i.e. heart rate, blood flow, body temperature, etc.). The yogis of India have long-known that every state of the mind and body is associated with a corresponding respiration pattern. Long slow breaths slow the heart (that is why Ehret called the heart a valve, not a pump). Deep breathing warms you up. If you feel cold by eating raw foods, then

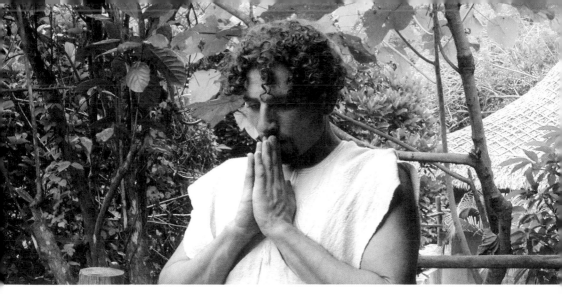

The control of breath is the first essence of yoga.

take deep breaths to warm your body. Take deep breaths to increase your inner "fire" energy.

Fourth, oxygen eliminates pain. Pain in the body is always associated with a lack of oxygen in that area. Athletes who strain a muscle often continue to play, in fact prefer to play, because by staying active the strained muscle remains oxygenated and will be less painful. One can find relief from backaches and sore muscles by deep breathing.

It is the control we exert over our own breath that most distinguishes humans from the other primates. The primary mammal groups that can control their breath are those with aquatic characteristics, such as the dolphin, the hippo, the seal, the whale and even the elephant.

Longevity is associated with slowing the breath. Those species that breathe very slowly live the longest. The giant tortoise breathes only four times a minute. Humans in comparison, breathe 18 times a minute, and a restless monkey 32 times a minute.

While breathing in through your nose, hold your mouth lightly closed, and leave your tongue comfortably pressed to the roof of your mouth. Ideas and inspiration come to us by breathing through the nose. Experiment with making your breathing so slow that it would not disturb a feather on your nose.

Exhaling is more important than inhaling. To fully help detoxify the body, blow out all the air from the bottom of the lungs then hold your breath. The vacuum produced in the lungs will exert a drawing force that pulls poisons from the blood into the lungs for elimination.

A rarely discussed reason why people become addicted to smoking cigarettes derives from the breath control that smoking entails. When someone smokes a cigarette they fall into a habitual breathing pattern that fundamentally alters their state and energy level until they feel "relaxed." Practicing deep breathing helps overcome addictions to smoking.

By breathing deeper and more rhythmically, you become calmer and can concentrate and work better. Slow, deep diaphragmatic breathing was the first health discipline I really practiced consistently for years. I credit late-night deep breathing exercises with improving my performance in college when I was studying engineering. I often would need an additional two extra hours every night to do work, so at midnight I would go outside and do at least ten deep diaphragmatic breaths in the 1:4:2 ratio described on the next page. From this practice my mind would clear and my energy would soar.

We are breathing all night as we sleep and the exhaled carbon dioxide accumulates in stuffy homes. Keep your home windows open as much as possible, especially at night to allow fresh oxygen to continuously revitalize you. Consider, bringing a plethora of house plants into your bedroom and home to provide you with fresh oxygen.

Breathing is our most vital experience. Be silent, breathe deep. Silence is power. Silence is an art. Long life is a matter of deep rhythmic breathing and keeping extremely quiet. Be silent and you allow your conscious, doubting, warring mind to listen. The best performers have the calmest breathing and quietest minds during the moment of truth.

BREATHING (PRANAYAMA)

1 In my opinion, the best pattern for deep diaphragmatic breathing, which I have used daily since age 19, is the following 1:4:2 ratio:
• Breathe in (through the nose), for a multiple of one count. The nose simultaneously filters and humidifies the air we breathe. The cribriform plate above the septum in the nose also regulates the temperature of the air entering the lungs.
• Hold that breath, for a multiple of four counts. This fully oxygenates and stimulates the body.
• Breathe out (through the mouth), for a multiple of two counts. The out breath releases toxins.

An example of this breathing ratio:
• Breathe in for 6 seconds.
• Hold that breath for 24 seconds.
• Breathe out for 12 seconds.

2 I have also had much success with the following 1:1:1:1 yogic breath ratio:
• Breathe in (through the nose), for a multiple of one count.
• Hold that breath, for a multiple of one count.
• Breathe out (through the mouth), for a multiple of one count.
• Hold the lungs empty, for a multiple of one count. This creates a vacuum suction that draws toxins out of the tissues on the following inhalation.

An example of this breathing ratio: Breathe in for 6 seconds.
• Hold that breath for 6 seconds.
• Breathe out for 6 seconds.
• Hold the lungs empty for 6 seconds.

3 Practice 30 deep diaphragmatic breaths each day following either of these patterns, or both. Tune your lungs to these patterns. Initially, some dizziness and light-headedness may be experienced by breathing in this fashion as the brain becomes fully oxygenated; but this phenomena will pass as the body grows accustomed to deep breathing practices.

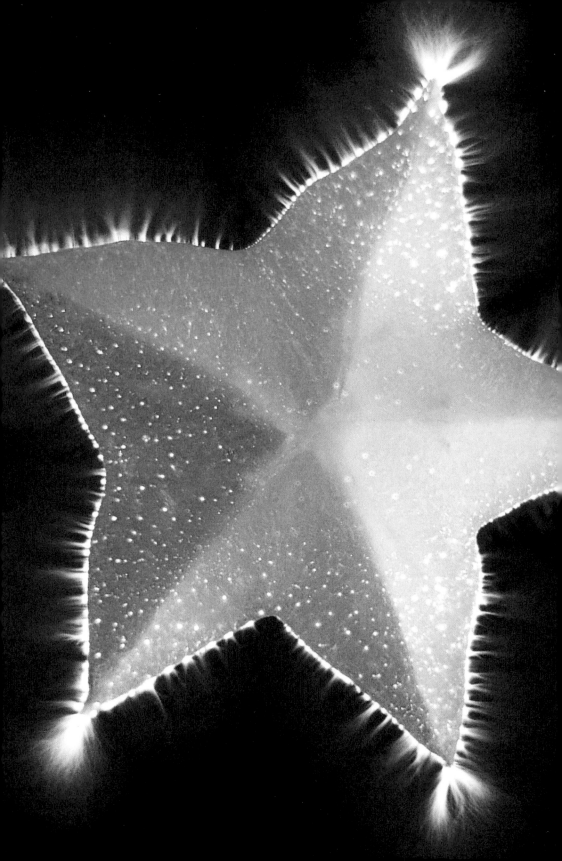

23

THE PHYSIOLOGY OF EXCELLENCE

"THE HIGHER YOUR ENERGY LEVEL, THE MORE EFFICIENT YOUR BODY.
THE MORE EFFICIENT YOUR BODY, THE BETTER YOU FEEL
AND THE MORE YOU WILL USE YOUR TALENT TO PRODUCE
OUTSTANDING RESULTS." — *Anthony Robbins*

Excellence is a habit. Good health is an achievement — there are certain things you have to do. When your health improves, every other aspect of your life improves simultaneously. The ways you view your potential and the world improve too.

Physiological things, such as muscle tension, what we eat, how we breathe and our posture all have a huge impact on our mental imagery, emotional state and spiritual strength. A physiology of vibrant health produces a mindset, emotional attitude and spiritual power of vibrant health. A physiology of vibrant health has an uncanny knack of attracting the right people, foods and exercises that we need, right when we need them. That is the law: things produce after their own kind.

The As If Principle

We are physical, mental, emotional and spiritual beings — it is a four-part scale with each dramatically influencing the other. The As If Principle demonstrates that we can use physiology (the way we are holding and moving our

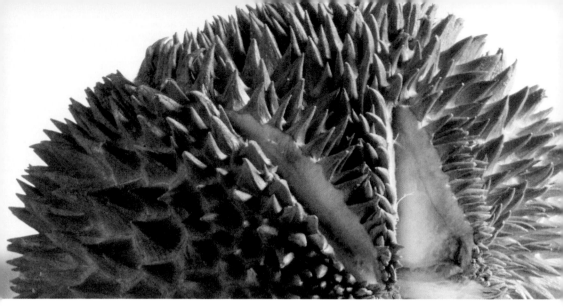

Simply smelling the durian fruit (pictured above) will immediately cause a shift in your physiology.

physical body) to influence our mental, emotional and spiritual states. The As If Principle is invoked by taking on the physiology of the state we wish to reach.

Stand up tall and proud. Smile like you have never smiled before, from ear to ear. Breathe in deep. Now, try to get depressed. But do not stop smiling and do not change your physiology. Go ahead, try and feel sad. You cannot do it without changing your physiology. Every mental, emotional and spiritual state is associated with a certain physiology.

Excellence is a state of physiology. Excellence is created by the way you carry yourself. Robust deep breathing, a knowing smile, a confident stride and good posture, all create excellence.

Act as if you felt more energized, powerful and resourceful than you ever have before and pretty soon you begin to become that way. When you act like a winner, you become a winner. Act as if you already are one of the healthiest individuals on the planet and pretty soon you begin to become that way.

If you ever feel mental, emotional or spiritual trauma, change the way you are moving your physical body. You can change the way you are using the muscles in your face, the way you are moving your eyes, the way you are carrying your entire muscular system. Anthony Robbins tells us: "Emotion is created by motion." You are in control of your mental, emotional and spiritual state. Tell yourself: "I am the master of my state. Nothing or no one can change how I feel except me. Through motion, breathing and posture, I alter my state in a moment."

Eating food at the physical level accesses different mental, emotional and spiritual states. Beautiful food accesses beautiful states of consciousness. The great thing about The Sunfood Diet is that it is something you can physically do. You just take action and the mental, emotional and spiritual benefits automatically arise.

Empower Your Physiology

In addition to diet, the more exercise and stretching you do, the greater will be your health, and the more you will empower your physiology. Those who are in excellent physical shape are more in tune with their bodies. They have more control over their bodies and, as a result, are better able to control their mental, emotional and spiritual states.

Fitness and health are not the same. Fitness is the ability to perform athletic feats. Health is a state of overall well-being, excellent digestion and vibrant aliveness. Many professional athletes have excellent fitness, but poor health. This is why we often see some former athletes ending up as physical wrecks after illustrious careers.

Daily exercise and stretching are as essential to excellent health as diet. Exercise and stretching move the lymph fluid and elevate the immune system. Low-impact lymphatic exercises, such as jumping on a trampoline or rebounder, are particularly powerful because they softly exercise each cell against the pull of gravity. Also wonderful and smooth is the use of walking poles during hiking which gently strengthens the upper body and creates a cross-country cardiovascular feel.

Exercise consists of two elements: endurance and strength. Endurance has to do with inner cleanliness. The less obstructions you carry around inside of you, the greater is your endurance. Strength has to do with overall muscular power. Muscular power is built by consistent yet varied training. I learned years ago to consistently "surprise my muscles" to overcome plateaus.

Stretching consists of two elements: flexibility and alignment. Both are developed and enhanced by yoga.

When you combine raw foods with yoga, you tune into a phenomenal state of being. The Sunfood Diet transforms your metabolism and the biochemistry of your body. Yoga reforms physiology by the consistent practice of different stretching-spiritual poses (asanas). Yoga helps squeeze toxins out of the tissues, opens up tensions and improves the mechanical functioning of the body. Yoga is about "letting go" to increase flexibility. Yoga will get the spine straight beginning with opening up the hips and sacrum. Practice yoga stretching after sleeping, sitting or walking. If you have chronic back pain, start looking into yoga and eating more green-leafy vegetables to get your body alkaline (also consider sleeping without a pillow to allow the spine to rest in its natural position).

To achieve your true potential, you must cleanse your body of tension, free your mind of stagnant knowledge, and open your spirit to the physiology of pure excellence.

THE PHYSIOLOGY OF EXCELLENCE

1   Begin exercising daily. Engage in the type of exercise you enjoy, whether it be: walking, swimming, cycling, weight lifting, jumping on a rebounder, etc. Exercise outside in Nature whenever possible.

2   Enroll in a yoga class today. Read books on the subject; rent yoga videos; find an experienced teacher. Attend one of our raw-food yoga retreats and experience physically transformative magic.

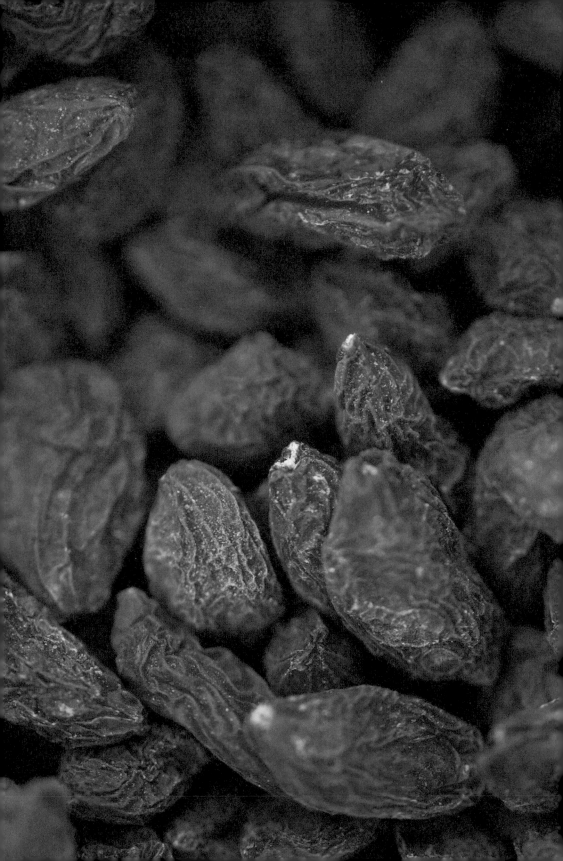

24

THE POWER OF ASSOCIATION

"No success is possible without a change
in your peer group." — *Peter Lowe, success philosopher*

"Burn bridges, not your food." — *Raw Aphorism*

Your mind is like a garden. The visiting birds and bees and bugs and winds are like television, radio, computers, friends and relatives. If you fail to control and carefully plant the seeds of positive thought in your garden-mind with positive media, friends, or relatives, then negative seeds will grow by default.

Computer programmers know GIGO: Garbage In, Garbage Out. It is just as hazardous to feed junk information to your mind as it is to feed junk food to your body.

If we do not provide our minds with the programming we desire, others will provide that programming for us. Control your suggestive environment carefully. Cultural tendencies seem to favor more of a never-ending deluge of negativity, laziness and chaos.

You are greatly influenced by your immediate suggestive environment. Anything that gets through to your conscious mind is influencing you. Are these influences helping or hindering the unfolding of the flowering potential within you? If they are hindering, you must decide to remove those influences, or remove yourself from such influences.

Unhealthy people are like sponges. They will try to gain energy from whomever they can. They draw the energy out of others. Since their energy is low, and they do not know how to create it on their own, they will try to take it from those around them. These are the people who steal your most valuable asset: your vital life energy. You know who they are. They are always ready to criticize rather than compliment. They are full of subtle verbal abuse and softly negative comments. They constantly try to keep you indebted to them. When they go into their routine, turn away. Disassociate from these people. Love them from afar. The power to walk away from negative people is the best gift you can give to yourself.

Napoleon Hill has pointed out that the most common weakness of all human beings is the habit of leaving their minds open to the negative influence of other people. You must remove yourself from the range of influence of every person and every circumstance that has even the slightest tendency to cause you to feel inferior or incapable of obtaining the object of your purpose.

It takes a lot of energy to achieve your goals. You cannot afford to have negative people around you who drain your energy. Even if you make tremendous efforts in improving the quality of the information reaching you, if you still allow the same negative people in close, you will stumble. Select the people you associate with carefully — whether they be in person, on the phone or on the Internet.

Join an inspiring crowd. The people around you are a reflection of yourself.

In **Unlimited Power** Anthony Robbins writes: "If you can surround yourself with people who will never let you settle for less than you can be, you have the greatest gift that anyone can hope for. Association is a powerful tool. Make sure the people you surround yourself with make you a better person by your association with them."

Only through the harmonious relationships with other living things may an individual have full, unhindered, complete use of all physical, mental, emotional and spiritual faculties.

Weed your life of negative influences. Protect your garden. Develop a garden so rich, so abundant, that after many years you won't need to weed it at all; it will be perpetually growing so many positive beautiful plants and offering forth such incredibly vibrant fruits that a weed will not be capable of growing in it.

THE POWER OF ASSOCIATION

1   Surround yourself with plants, animals, people, books, pictures, motivational
    mottoes and other suggestive reminders of your beauty and greatness.
    Build around yourself an impenetrable atmosphere of prosperity and
    achievement. Saturate your life in every way and by all means available,
    with those people, places and things that promote your visions and goals.
    Make each day one continuous positive affirmation. The only things we
    have in life are our moment-to-moment experiences. Make each moment
    a sensational joy.

2   Take a page in your journal and draw a line down the middle of it. On the
    left side, list 6 people with whom you are willing to spend less time with
    due to their negative influence on you. On the right side, list 6 people with
    whom you would like to spend more time with due to their positive influ-
    ence on you. Make this page a goal; act on it immediately.

**A magnificent Kirlian photograph
of an organic goji berry.
The goji berry contains 18 amino acids and over 20 trace
minerals. The goji berry is the richest source of beta-
carotene found in any food/herb. This amazing little fruit
is considered the number one
food/herb in Chinese medicine.
It synergistically makes all other herbs work better
when it is added to herbal formulas.**

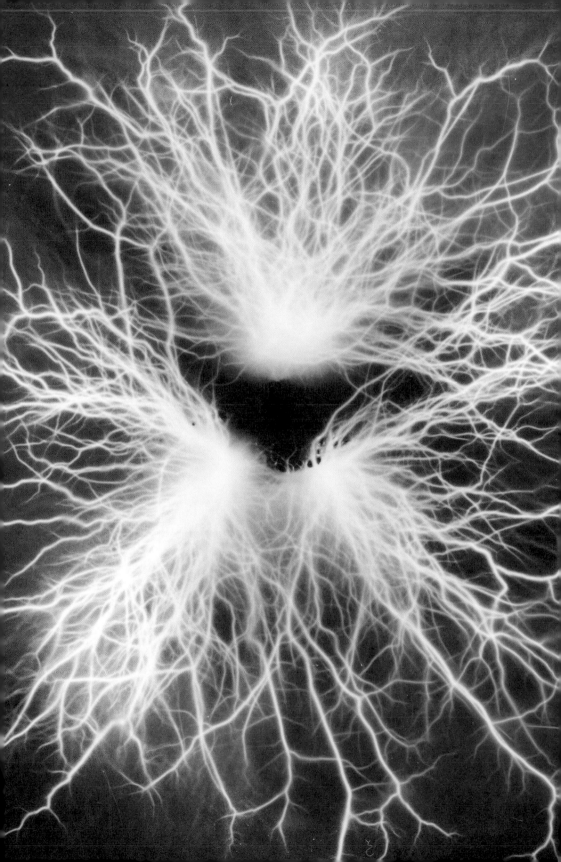

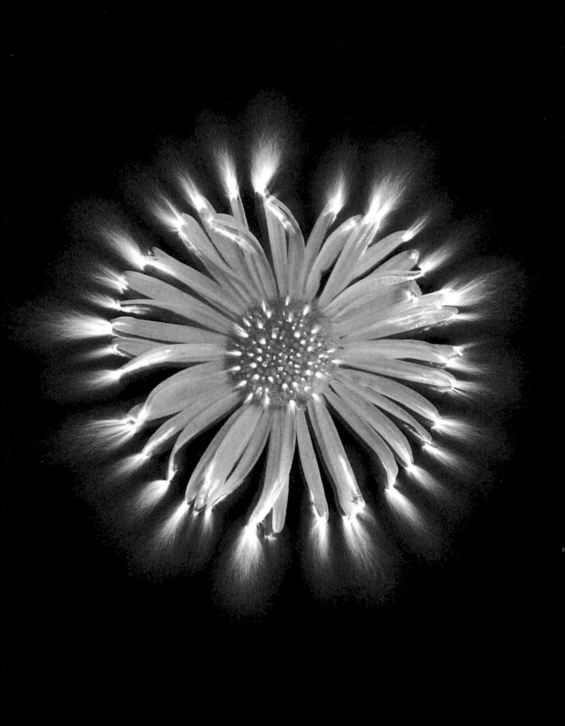

25

SATURATION POINT

"INFORMATION IS THE COMMODITY OF KINGS." — *Anthony Robbins*

We live in an era where all knowledge is available to all those who seek it out.

There is an abundance of useful information out there in the world. We are at the source. We can choose. We may tune into any frequency we like. We can learn anything we desire.

Learning is never what one expects. Every step of learning is a new task. Learning is an unending quest. There is something for you to learn from every experience, every individual you encounter, every book you read, every audio, DVD and video recording you listen to or watch.

A commitment to life-long learning is an essential part of health. Positive information is to the mind what Sunfood is to the body. A malnourished body cannot thrive. Neither can a malnourished mind. A body fed by the negative energy of unconscious "hit-or-miss" food becomes ill. A mind fed by negative energy and wrong thoughts becomes ill. A diet based on raw food is necessary to health, but if the mind is not also given pure food, the body will suffer. A mind fed evil, unkind thoughts of destructive criticism, condemnation, hate, jealousy, fear and doubt will reproduce such emotions in the physical body, leading to illness.

You are made or unmade by your own education. You are at the source; you can control what information you are allowing to enter your awareness. You may study anything you desire. You can recapture a child's ability to learn by becoming inspired by new information. Studies presented in progressive educational books, such as **The Learning Brain** by Gorden Dryden and Jeannette Vos, prove that learning causes the brain to physically grow and rewire itself in a whole new way.

We learn in many ways: by repetition, by emotional impact, but the absolutely most powerful way to learn and master any subject is by saturation.

In my experience, the entire secret of success is saturation. Start bombarding yourself with words and pictures consistent with your goals. Just have fun. Read books that forward you in the direction you are headed. Listen to success tapes in your car. Listen to success tapes while you eat. Watch educational videotapes at the end of the day. Attend seminars that provide additional inspiration to accelerate your goal achievement. I guarantee that, when you start this program of massive saturation, you will dramatically improve your entire life and begin to rapidly manifest your dreams.

The most successful individuals in any field remain so by continuously adding to their own stock of knowledge by appropriating the thoughts, phrases and ideas of geniuses through a program of information saturation. A mind nourished continuously by the ideas of genius minds will remain alert, brilliant, flexible and receptive. If this renewal is neglected, the mind will stagnate — we see this in musicians who seem to have lost their "edge." "If you don't use it, you lose it," is a common phrase of simple yet profound truth — it is in strict accordance with the cosmic laws.

The way to make a radical change in your life is to consistently bombard your brain with a new stream of personal-development information, presented by different people, and presented in different formats. Since your number one goal is to be totally healthy, all the information entering your mind should be furthering that goal and none of the information should be detracting from it.

To achieve vibrant health, educate yourself on the subject of gardening, herbs, natural living, raw foods and related subjects through reading. This has been, and continues to be, a major factor in my own health.

Saturation means attending every health seminar possible. Attend every success seminar possible. Attend every seminar given in your specialty area. Each speaker can provide you with wonderful distinctions that can transform your life. Any one speaker might say something you have heard before, but in a slightly different way, a way which immediately applies to you. The energy of a live performance cannot be matched. Go to success seminars for fun.

When you are healthy, and your suggestive environment is cleared, you can accelerate your success by converting all information entering your mind into one focused field — the field in which you desire to excel. Make all information input positive, uplifting and focused on the items necessary in this field for your goal achievement. You can become an expert in any field in less than five years, and if you truly saturate yourself in the way I have advised, you can become an expert in any field in two or three years.

If you want health, you have to study health. If you want success, you have to study success. In my own life, I have made a study of superior health and incredible success because they are favorite subjects. I am fascinated by vibrant health. I am fascinated when I see someone who is totally alive. I am intrigued by phenomenal success. I love hearing success stories. It is so interesting to hear the stories behind mega-music bands, such as The Beatles or The Bee Gees or ABBA. Saturating my mind with the secrets of health and the stories of super success has revolutionized my life. The mystery of incredible success is unlocked when one's fascination is met with saturation.

Reading

If you want to get good at something, read a book on it. Read many books on it. More is better.

The successful individual with a purpose in life makes it a business, a responsibility and an exciting and fun use of time to read books relating to that purpose. In that way, important knowledge is acquired which comes from the experiences of others who have gone before.

An individual's reading program should be as carefully chosen as the daily diet. Reading is a food, without which mental growth will stagnate.

Business philosopher Jim Rohn says, "Miss a meal, but don't you miss your reading." What excellent advice! Reading a book written by a person you admire puts you in a mental and emotional state similar to theirs. Those with a purpose devour books like paradisical fruits.

We intuitively know that readers are achievers. Leaders read. Feed your mind with good reading.

Success philosopher Brian Tracy describes that one hour of reading in your chosen field each day will make you an authority in that field in three years, a national authority in that field in five years, and an international authority in that field in seven years. Just reading alone!

READ

Do you want to lead?
Read.
Do you have a mind to feed?
Read.

Read every chance,
During each snippet of time.
Choose a variety of
Prose and Rhyme.

"The Secrets of the Ages
Are found on written pages."

Five years hence,
You'll be the same as now,
Except for the people you meet,
And the books you browse.

Learn from those
Who've gone before.
Find out how
They opened the door.

Discover wild stories,
Get a new feel.
Don't spend your time,
Reinventing the wheel.

Take notes on your books
And write them all down.
The results you reap
Will amaze and astound.

The answers to your questions
Have already been found,
They exist somewhere —
Written down.

Read every page on your bookshelf,
You'll laugh out loud
And attract brilliant wealth.
You'll cry without sound,
And breathe in new health!

Words through your eyes,
Deeply impress;
Transformed they become
The thoughts you express.

Read an hour a' day,
In the field you choose.
With persistent action,
You can't lose!

Everything you read
Is a marvelous seed!
Which explodes into fortunes
And inspires great deeds.

I once had read, "Success leaves clues."
So I asked a genius, "What do you do?"
After much probing, the genius did say:
"Well, I read three books a day."

There is a vast world
To explore,
If you'll just read —
A little bit more!

How To Begin Saturating Your Mind

Ideally, your entire day should be one continuous bombardment of positive, uplifting information.

The first waking hour sets the pace of the day. Whatever you do, listen to, or read in that first hour stays with you all day long. Have you ever woke to a song, and that song was in your head throughout the day? This is the principle in action. What if you awoke each morning to the most uplifting music, or the most powerful success literature possible? It is great to feel those inspirations coursing through the body all day long.

The alpha-wave state of the brain is the state of highest mental activity. It is the state you are in when you awaken in the morning and right before you sleep at night. You may achieve the alpha-wave state by taking ten long, deep breaths. You may achieve higher performance on tests or in physical competitions by saturating the mind (through positive affirmations, goal writing, goal reviewing, reading, success audio listening, etc.) when the brain is in the alpha state.

Begin each morning with empowering messages and then continue the bombardment throughout the day. Raw foods action supplemented by daily self-improvement information saturation is a success formula that cannot be topped.

Chaos theory teaches us that even tiny differences of input could quickly become overwhelming differences in output — a phenomenon mathematicians have termed "sensitive dependent on initial conditions." In weather this translates into what is known as the "Butterfly Effect" — the notion that a butterfly stirring the air today in Peking can transform storm systems next month in New York. Since this is true, imagine how a massive difference in mind input through focused information saturation will equate into an extraordinary difference in output. The Butterfly Effect would become a Phoenix Effect.

SATURATION POINT

1. Everyone has their own way of learning things. Find out what works best for you. My preference is for reading and audio tapes. What is the best learning modality for you? If this is not clear, ask yourself: "How can I figure out what learning modality works best for me?" Try different approaches. Try alternative learning strategies.

2. Invest in good books. Invest your money in your personal growth and your family's education. Find the best health books and read them!

3. Make plans this week to attend a health or success seminar in your area.

4. Record all good ideas in your journal. Become a collector of good ideas you have gathered from live seminars, books, audio tapes, videos and personal experiences.

5. Become a success-tape addict. Listen to success tapes while driving, eating or exercising. Dispose of cooked-food addiction and replace it with success-tape addiction.

6. During your first waking moments each morning, listen to a song that inspires you and that will keep you charged throughout the day. During the first 30-60 minutes each day, read success books or listen to empowering audio tapes while doing yoga.

7. Tape a new motivational quote to your nightstand or bathroom mirror every week.

8. Organize to save time on the Internet. Make an outline of what you plan on exploring before you get online.

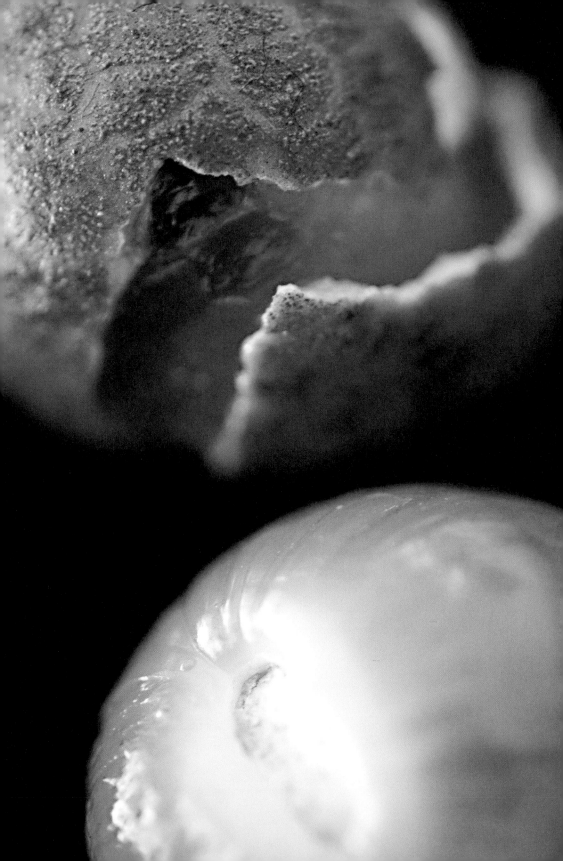

26

THE INVERSE PARANOID

VERILY THE MOST NECESSARY THING IS CONTENTMENT UNDER
ALL CIRCUMSTANCES; BY THIS, ONE IS PRESERVED FROM
MORBID CONDITIONS AND FROM LASSITUDE. YIELD NOT TO GRIEF
AND SORROW: THEY CAUSE THE GREATEST MISERY. JEALOUSY CONSUMETH
THE BODY AND ANGER DOTH BURN THE LIVER:
AVOID THESE TWO AS YOU WOULD A LION." — *Baha'u'llah*

"NOTHING HAS ANY POWER OVER ME OTHER THAN THAT WHICH
I GIVE IT THROUGH MY CONSCIOUS THOUGHTS."— *Anthony Robbins*

"ALL BAD THINGS MUST COME TO AN END." — *Raw Aphorism*

In order for you to remain in the "flow" all the time, in order for you to achieve the health levels you desire daily, you must be able to convert negative thoughts into positive thoughts.

You can create an aura of positive energy around you by a positive mental attitude. A positive outlook means confidently expecting to learn and benefit from every situation. When you are in the right frame of mind, any obstacle may be transformed in a moment into greater effort that will bring you closer to the massive success of which you are capable.

Attitude is everything. A bad attitude does not come by chance — it is constructed by negative thoughts and emotions.

Negative emotions are always harmful. They serve no useful purpose. They poison and acidify the body. Negative emotions are the primary reason why people fail to achieve the highest levels of material and spiritual success. Feelings of doubt and fear always lead to failure.

If you experience negative emotions in your life, let them flow through you rather than bottle them within you. You can dispel negative emotions physically by: hitting, kicking, yelling and/or biting. Dispel anger by driving a golf ball, kicking a football, screaming aloud and/or chewing dark green-leafy vegetables or grasses. Let the anger pass through you into the physical object. Transmute anger into positive action.

You can dispel negative emotions through normal exercise (although not as quickly as through the methods mentioned above). Dancing, lifting weights, surfing or walking are all effective ways to manage negativity.

You can also dispel negative emotions mentally by reframing the experience, by changing what the experience means to you. When you look for the good in any situation, then the good looks for you and you dispel negativity.

All experiences may be transmuted into useful service. No experience need be a negative mental liability. Through the power of thought, one may transform sadness to happiness in a nano-second. Your ability to reframe any situation, to find the positive benefit, is unlimited.

It is not what happens to you, but your reaction to what happens to you that counts. No mental challenge is stressful in itself, only your response to a mental challenge can cause stress.

Nothing is entirely good or bad for you until you say so. If you believe that everything which happens to you in life contains some good within it, then everything will come forth to strengthen you and help you to rise to another level of consciousness.

Problems are challenges; challenges are good; challenges are inevitable. Every challenge in your life is heaven-sent to teach you a valuable physical and spiritual lesson. Every challenge contains its gift.

Use your willpower to keep any disappointment from dampening your spirit. Every disappointment builds character, knowledge, strength and stamina. Use each setback as a stepping-stone for advancement.

Accept defeat as an inspiration to greater effort and carry on with the belief that you will succeed. Convert defeat into a challenge to greater effort.

Most people sense intuitively that there is another side to life — a better way. But when they advance towards it, they are struck by a bombardment of contradictory information and negativity that stumbles them. This is the test you must pass to achieve success. Napoleon Hill discovered in researching his **Laws Of Success** that the greatest achievers he interviewed found their greatest successes just beyond their greatest failures. So, even following an enormous perceived failure, keep yourself in a state of total resourcefulness and you will eventually succeed. Success lies on the far side of failure.

There is one unbeatable rule for mastering frustrations and disappointments, and that is to accept the lesson learned and continue to work diligently and intently towards one's goals. Use strong emotions, whether positive or negative, to inspire the creation of ideas through your imagination, then take action upon those ideas.

You are in control. You either make yourself miserable, or you make yourself strong. The amount of work is the same. In fact, it takes even more energy to be miserable than to be strong. It takes more energy to be a "paranoid" than to be an "inverse paranoid." Consider this: it takes 13 muscles to smile and 112 muscles to frown.

An inverse paranoid is someone who believes the universe is conspiring to do them good. The personality of the inverse paranoid is characterized by a positive mental attitude. A positive mental attitude is one of the best indicators of how healthy a person really is. Due to a positive mental attitude, the inverse paranoid is always more likely to succeed.

The inverse paranoid expects to win and is always swift to make decisions based on intuitive feeling without fear or regret. My experience has been to always trust my gut feeling.

The inverse paranoid trusts her/his instincts — with "instinct" as a direct download of information from infinite intelligence.

The inverse paranoid continues to smile and expect the best results, in even the worst situations. The mind of the inverse paranoid is a transformer that takes all challenges and transmutes them into creative opportunities. Every discordant word and thought becomes transformed into greater things.

The inverse paranoid calls upon spiritual powers through which obstacles may be removed at will. That spiritual power changes the biochemistry of the mind and body to access greater resources to overcome any challenge.

In my journal I have written the following: "Nature is conspiring to do me good, to keep me young, and to place me at the top of the world." That is the attitude of the inverse paranoid.

Indian philosophy explains that once we state something ten thousand times it becomes a mantra, a thought form that shapes the future. The word "mantra" in its Sanskrit derivation is a combination of two words "man" (thought) and "tra" (liberation). A mantra should be a thought of liberation. The slogan, mantra, or motto of the inverse paranoid is: "Today is the best day ever!" Try saying that aloud or to yourself ten thousand times! I have — and the results are revolutionary.

THE INVERSE PARANOID

1   Understand the messages of failure and pain. Failure and pain speak one
    language — they directly communicate to us what kind of change must
    take place. They tell you where you have gone wrong and where you have
    gone right. They chart your course and tell you when and where you are
    off target.

2   The next time you are faced with a boring, stressful, intense, extreme,
    hilarious or silly situation, say to yourself: "Today is the best day ever."
    Repeat this over and over in your mind as much as possible.

DON'T WORRY ABOUT IT, EMBRACE IT

From:
Frustration to
Fascination.
Bust to
Boom.

Misery to
Magic,
Thrilled,
And Ecstatic.

Disgust to
Delight.
Heavy to
Light.
Weakness to
Might.

Shadow to
Sun.
Fear to
Fun.

By power of mind
You'll discover and find
You can go from:
Vanquished to
Victorious.
Drab to
Glorious.
Tense to
Joyous.

Don't worry about it,
Embrace it.
Every adversity carries,
A seed of great benefit.

Substitute good thoughts
For bad.
Happy thoughts
For sad.
Rule your brain,
Join the few.
You can only think:
One thought, not two!

Go from:
Devastation to
Procreation.
Labor to
Recreation.
Irritation to
Innovation.
Desperation to
Inspiration.

Turn it around,
You're in control.
Why not happily attain
Your every goal?

Worse is better.

From anger
To laughter,
And sorrow
To smiles.
Go from rags to riches
In the shortest of
Whiles.

Don't hate,
Feel great.
Lift yourself up to
The highest state.
You are the master, of
Your fate.

Failure to
Success.
Insult to
Jest.
Worst to
Best!

Don't grieve,
But perceive:
What happens,
Happened.
Its already the past.
Only in your mind,
Can an event last.
Stress won't ever change it.
Don't worry about it —
Embrace it.

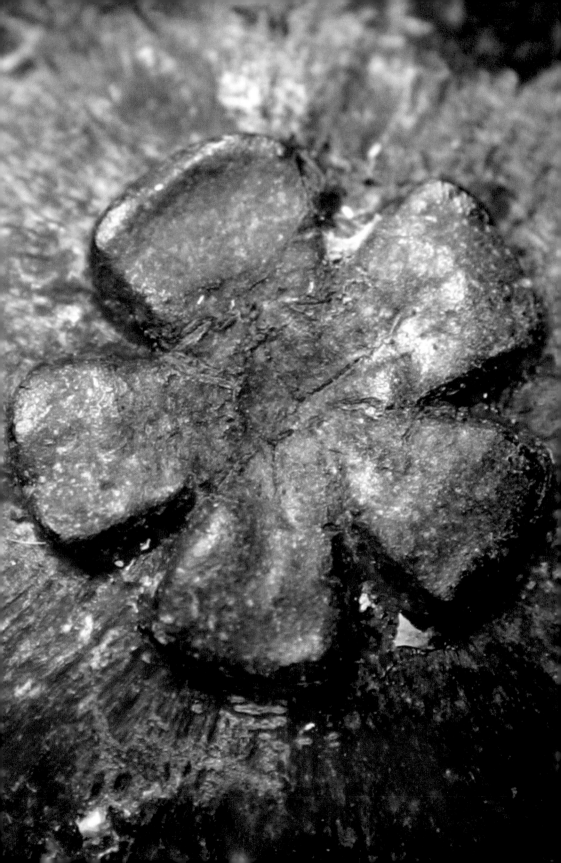

27

TAPPING INFINITE INTELLIGENCE

Spiders have always constructed their webs as they do now, and each type weaves its own style of web. They were never taught nor needed any experience. From where does this knowledge arise?

Birds have always built their nests as they do now, and each type constructs its own style of nest. They were never taught nor needed any experience. From where does this knowledge arise?

Science has no reasonable answers to these questions. Science says these creatures are guided by "instinct." But science fails to explain what "instinct" is, how it arises and where it is stored. It is more intuitive to look at a spider and understand that it is a perfectly tuned being accessing infinite intelligence through an unobstructed nervous system when it spins a perfect web during its first try. An unobstructed nervous system is connected with the ability to tap infinite intelligence. The cleaner the body, the purer the instinct; instinct is infinite intelligence working through the living being.

Based on studies of the neocortex region of the brain, researchers at Stanford University concluded the average person uses only about 2 percent of her or his mental powers! Why are so few people tapping their mental abilities? Perhaps it is because they are constantly poisoning themselves with improper foods, associations, thought patterns and ideas. When you clean away the poison, you open up dormant areas of your brain capacity. Your true potential is vast.

Within you is a vast genetic library containing all the wisdom you need to accomplish everything you desire. The essence of your spirit has the capability to tap infinite intelligence.

Infinite intelligence is the ether, the storehouse of eternal knowledge, the sum of all thoughts past, present and future. It is likened to a "cosmic circuit board" we may tap into through specific questions, silence, and pure living. It is the spiritual energy that turns seeds into plants and plants into flowers. It arcs flowers into the lovely face of the Sun. Though it may be quiet and extremely subtle, it is there and it stays there, never to be underestimated.

When you purify your body after several months or years of wholistic health practices and raw-food nutrition you seemingly become more in touch with infinite intelligence. This is, in my opinion, the greatest value of eating raw plant foods. The proper diet can literally unlock dormant genius as it allows one to increase the intensity of thought to the point where one can freely communicate with sources of knowledge not accessible to the average person. By the process of fine-tuning the body into its natural state, The Sunfood Diet allows you to tap into the resource of "cosmic vibrations."

How does this happen? Consider Dr. Norman Walker's words in **Colon Health: The Key To A Vibrant Life**:

"The entire universe is composed of an infinite number of vibrations which, by their very condensed numbers, form matter, substance, or intangible things, much like the thousands of individual threads in a weaver's loom form a piece of cloth by the warp and woof — or crossing and re-crossing — of the threads. Cosmic energy vibrations are vibrations (or wave lengths) in the universe of inconceivably astronomical numbers per millimeter in length or per second in time."

Dr. Walker also describes the cosmic energy receiver or antenna, the hypothalamus.

"The human organism is a mysterious, miraculous electronic computer administered by a tiny gland, the hypothalamus, located in the mid-brain. Nothing goes on in the human organism that is not watched over, controlled and administered by the hypothalamus."

"Considering the fact that nerves spread out to every part of the brain from the hypothalamus, and that the cleaner the body is, the higher the cosmic energy vibrations available to the brain, it certainly pays to cleanse the body and keep the colon in a constantly clean and healthy condition...The hypothalamus is a transformer which lowers the cosmic energy vibrations of the universe from untold millions of volts down to the degree of energy-voltage which the individual needs from moment to moment."

It is now understood that the pineal gland governs parts of the hypothalamus, making the pineal gland another master gland. On a diet of processed food, the pineal gland calcifies and hardens. The brain becomes dense and obstructed with waste matter which would have distorted the cosmic receiver and blocked out the cosmic life energies. A diet of alkaline-plant food dissolves these obstructions and deposits, freeing the flow of energy. Thus we see that the cleaner your body, the greater your latent powers of mind.

After you go on a raw diet, and especially when you fast, moments of inspiration from infinite intelligence will drop into your mind, sometimes at random. As you tune your physical body, inspirational moments will occur more and more often. The mind becomes tuned to the broadcasting signals of infinite intelligence. Through purification you can tap a mighty power you never knew you possessed.

Consider what Henry David Thoreau wrote in **Walden**, "...Every man who has ever been earnest to preserve his higher poetic faculties in the best condition, has been particularly inclined to abstain from animal food, or from much food of any kind."

Let your body become a receiver through which the energy of the cosmos can flow. When you feel pure intelligence flowing into you, rays of genius will strike you — follow these intuitions. From infinite intelligence come the solutions to all challenges. Each ray of its divine radiance is an idea which may illuminate the world. When we align ourselves through diet, through belief, through focus, through optimal physiology, we are in contact with infinite intelligence. The goal is to live in contact with infinite intelligence at all times while flowing from grace to grace.

Embrace the infinite intelligence that bathes all of the Earth's life. Every individual is a receiver and a broadcaster within this realm of intelligence. As such, the individual has no limitations on what information s/he can tap into, except those accepted and set up by the individual in her/his own subconscious mind.

The subconscious mind is the connecting link between the conscious mind and infinite intelligence. It is a pump through which thought power may flow. The pump is activated by thoughts inspired by emotional and spiritual feelings.

Self-discipline means using your will-power to focus on only those emotional thoughts which fulfill your desires so as to begin the flow of infinite intelligence into the conscious mind, and to eliminate those emotional thoughts which lead to self-doubt and ruin.

Professor Arnold Ehret described that the lungs are a pump (they actually move the blood and lymph) and the heart is the valve that is stimulated by the flow. In the same way, the subconscious mind is a pump, which (by its control through self-discipline) moves infinite intelligence. The conscious mind is the valve that receives and is stimulated by the flow. If the body is obstructed physically through inappropriate diet and lack of exercise, the lungs will be hindered and the blood will not flow cleanly into the heart. In the same way, if the subconscious mind is troubled, infinite intelligence will not flow clearly into the conscious mind.

After you emotionally drive an idea into the subconscious mind for a long enough period of time, the tables will turn and the idea will begin to drive you effortlessly!

Tapping infinite intelligence allows you to tap into the frequencies of other minds. Napoleon Hill described in his book, **The Master Key To Riches**, that our brains contain a vibration center, which is comparable to a sensitive radio broadcasting and receiving center. It is tuned into the life-force energy surrounding us. This powerful center projects thoughts and feelings, and receives unending swarms of vital messages. It is a tireless two-way communication system of infinite capacity. One mind can broadcast, and the thunder of that communication echoes through the cosmos, whereby it is picked up by those tuned to the same frequency and they share in the vibrations of that thought.

Synchronous living —
An antenna in your mind.

Broadcast to the world
And everything you'll find.

The flow of infinite intelligence is accelerated by what Napoleon Hill originally called "The Mastermind Principle." He defined it as "an alliance of two or more minds blended in a spirit of perfect harmony and co-operating for the attainment of a definite purpose." This principle is invoked when another mind, operating at the same frequency as the first — with identical hopes, aims and purposes as the first — is brought into communication with the first. When this synchronicity occurs, a third intangible cooperative mind is formed within the sphere of infinite intelligence. He discovered this to be one of the greatest secrets of success for the super-prosperous.

TAPPING INFINITE INTELLIGENCE

1   Be sure to have your journal ready, near your bed or on your person, so that you may record your insights.

2   The flow of infinite intelligence is accelerated even further when a Mastermind Alliance is formed between two or more minds purified by eating raw plant foods. Attract others on the path of eating raw plant foods and join with them in activities, business ventures, family gatherings, etc.

**A Kirlian photograph of a whole organic cacao bean.
Cacao beans are perhaps the most sacred food substance
in the world. All chocolate is made from cacao beans.
You cannot have chocolate without cacao.
Cacao beans are the raw form of chocolate.**

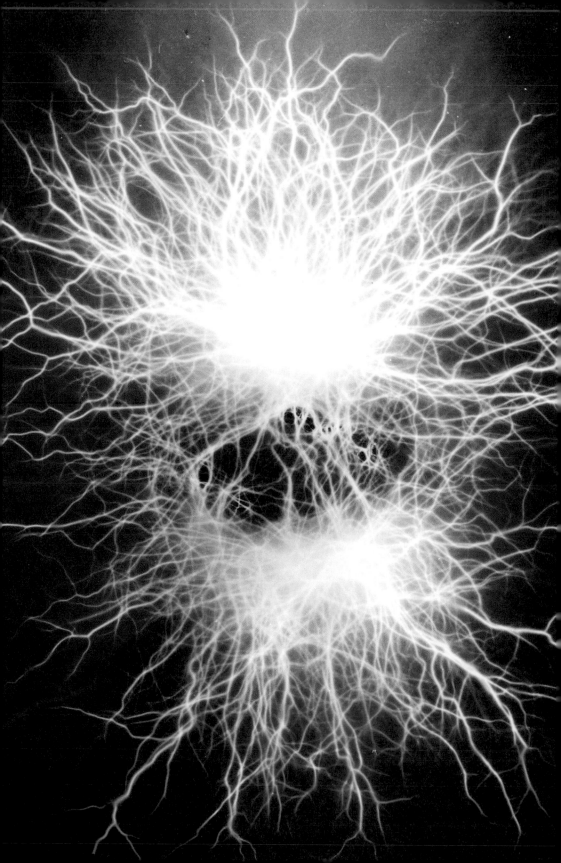

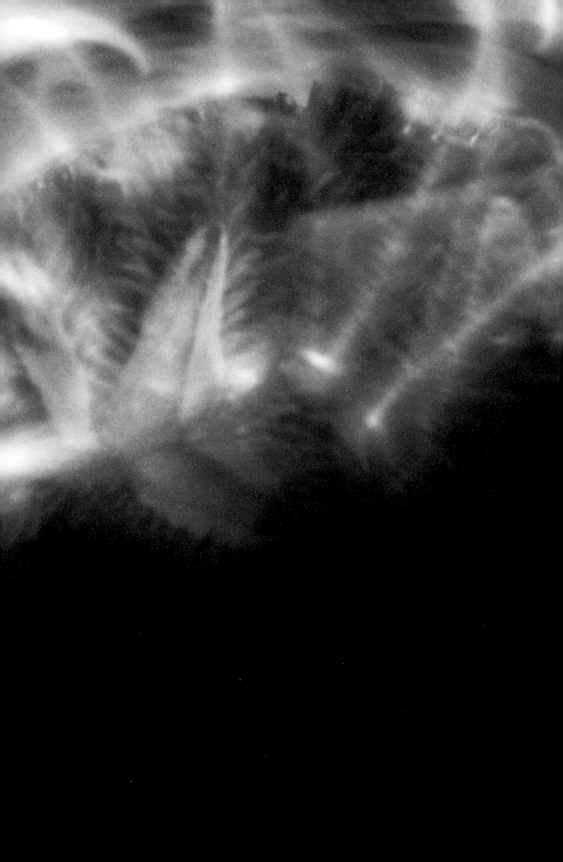

28

QUESTIONS ARE ANSWERS

It is amazing what one can receive simply by asking for it.

"Ask and it shall be given you; seek and ye shall find; knock and it shall be opened unto you. For everyone that asketh receiveth; and he that seeketh findeth; and to him that knocketh it shall be opened." (Matthew 7:7-8)

How do you get whatever you want?...Ask! Ask yourself or others. Ask your superconscious mind. Ask specifically. Ask with emotion! Asking creates possibilities. Asking questions is how you change your own focus and the focus of others. If you ask for a dollar, you will receive a dollar. If you ask for the highest joy possible, you will get that too.

The challenge is not to find the right answers, but to find the right questions. Depending on how you ask the question, you get a more empowering answer.

Richard Bach wrote in **Illusions**, "Isn't it strange how much we know if only we ask ourselves instead of somebody else?"

Between your ears lies the most incredible computer on Earth. When you ask your brain specific empowering questions, it will — every time — come up with precise answers. By asking your brain questions you are able to tap infinite intelligence (the innernet) which consists of all knowledge past, present and future.

Years ago, I gave a health seminar to a corporate group. Afterwards, when people congregated around me, a young gentleman approached and asked a most potent, yet succinct question. To this man's question I gave a poignant answer, although at the time, I didn't realize its profoundness. I still often think about the answer to that question. In reference to the world's challenges, he asked, "So what is the solution to all this craziness?" I stood there a moment and replied, "Grow your own food."

When a question is asked, the answer will make its appearance.

Stop for a moment and look around you. The world is filled with overflowing abundance. All you have to do is have the courage to ask for your share of the infinite.

Do you remember the song?
"When you wish upon a star,
Makes no difference who you are,
Like a bird, out of the blue,
Your dream comes true."

Manifest your wonderful wishes by asking for them.

Why do people not ask for what they want? Because of the fear of rejection. Always remember: rejection is never final. Fear is conquered by acts of raw courage.

If you ask for anything in the world with enough commitment, courage, desire and persistence, you will get it. In their wonderful book of the same title, Mark Victor Hansen and Jack Canfield call this principle **The Aladdin Factor**. Everyone who asks receives — it is decreed by cosmic law.

QUESTIONS ARE ANSWERS

1   Ask yourself the following questions daily:

2   What specific actions can I make today to powerfully increase my energy levels?

3   How can I attain a state of health perfection while enjoying the process?

4   What can I enjoy doing that will greatly increase the beauty of the world and which is in harmony with my purpose for being on Earth?

5   How surprised would I be to discover incredible abundance in my life?

6   How can I improve the value of life for everyone I encounter each day?

When you feel moved, write down the answers to these questions in your journal.

QUESTIONS ARE ANSWERS

Ask yourself questions
That uplift and empower.
Ask your brain questions,
And answers will soon flower.

How do you tap into:
All that you've learned
All that you've seen
Every page you have turned.

It's all still recorded
In your subconscious mind.
It's all still there,
But difficult to find.

Ask yourself questions
Specific and distinct.
Draw out ideas from,
your deepest memory link.

No open-loop questions, like:
Why does this happen to me?
What kind of answers,
Would you expect to receive?

An answer comes at will,
If the question is asked right.
An answer written down,
Will let you sleep at night.

Answer with a question
No problem is unsolved,
Asking empowering questions
Is how your brain evolved.

Questions are the answer
To all life's maladies
The wisdom of the body
Is in your memories.

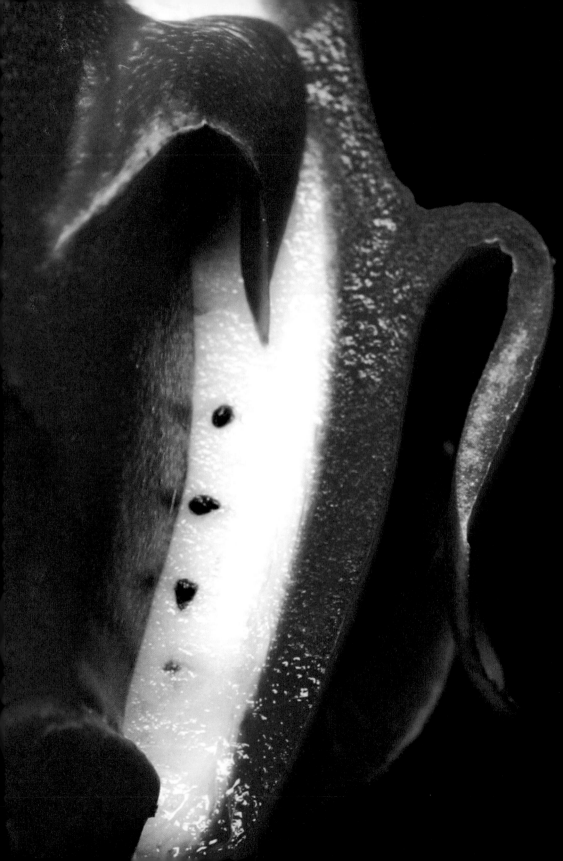

29

THE LAW OF ATTRACTION

"To bring anything into your life, imagine
that it's already there." — *Richard Bach, Illusions*

The Law of Attraction is:
1. Universal — it operates everywhere.
2. Eternal — it is ongoing.
3. Absolute — it operates whether you know it or not.

Your mind is a living magnet. You automatically draw people, things and circumstances into your life in harmony with your dominant thoughts and desires. Every person, all the animals in your life and every object you have are here because you have chosen to draw them here.

The Law of Attraction demonstrates that you will experience whatever you hold in your conscious mind long enough and deeply enough. Whatever your goals, whomever you want to meet, the law will magnetize them into your life. The more emotional and spiritual intensity you attach to your thoughts, the quicker that desire becomes reality.

Recall the following words from **Lesson 1: The Principle Of Life Transformation**: "Health is not something we can get; rather, it is something we attract, by the person we become. If we chase after health, it will elude us like a butterfly. However, if we calmly attract health by becoming the type of person who can be radiantly healthy, it will land upon us with a most radiant flutter."

Health attracts health. Happiness attracts happiness. Prosperity attracts prosperity. This is in absolute harmony with the foundational law that things produce more of their own kind. The happier you are, the happier are the people around you.

Things do not balance out. Success breeds more success. Failure breeds more failure. Like attracts like, it is the cosmic law again. Each produces more of its own kind.

We can only attract to ourselves a vibration that mirrors our present consciousness. Your present environment is a mirror reflection of yourself at this time. Your surrounding environment is constantly being recreated as your life progresses. Everything you have in your life right now is only a duplication of what you subconsciously believe you deserve.

You were created in the divine image and you possess within you the spark of that creative power with which, consciously or unconsciously, you create the conditions around you. You are always a creator of circumstance and never a creature of circumstance. You are at the cause, not at the effect.

Those people who feel they will be alone eating raw foods, might want to think things differently. Most people think at the "effect" side of things. They believe there are no other raw-foodists out there, so they can excuse themselves from going all the way. Or they excuse themselves by claiming high-quality organic fruits and vegetables are not available. The truth is, they are always on the "cause" side of things, and by the Law of Attraction they are in every moment attracting to them the reality they expect. If you eat raw, then you would attract other raw-foodists, and not before. If they committed to finding the highest quality organic food, they would attract it, and not before.

The change must first come within you and then you will attract what you need.

Highly advanced beings in all fields walk the planet Earth. How do you meet them? How do you learn from them? You must learn to match their frequency and attract them into your life.

I have heard the stories of many people all over the world who persisted forward. They felt lonely, isolated by their diet and thus created that reality. However, as they persisted, and the Sunfood delivered its effect, their vibration changed, as did their consciousness. Even in the most remote locations other raw-foodists would show up in their lives. You will be absolutely astonished by how many people are into raw-foods, or are willing to go raw with you when you reach the right frame of mind!

You attract into your life those with a message for you. The message that "when one is ready for a thing, it presents itself" is proved by the indisputable fact that you have picked up this book and that you have found me at precisely the right time for you.

Embrace the Law Of Attraction. Accelerate your transition. Become more social, meet new dynamic people. Attract into your life beautiful people and relationships by becoming beautiful inside. Pair up with those (especially a lover) who are headed in the same direction as yourself. Employ The Mastermind Principle as discussed in **Lesson 27**.

The most attractive thing you can do is smile. Everyone knows that a beautifully happy being is a sight to behold. A smile profoundly affects all who see and feel it. Like the Sun, a smile brightens the entire day.

The most powerful vibration you can send out is love. Love is the very essence of the Law of Attraction. The most blessed, beautiful people are those who continually send out love vibrations towards all the living plants and creatures around them. By sending out love you always make the world a better place to live for all of the Earth's precious creatures.

Learn to love. Love helps heal every injury, every illness. Let love emanate from your being. Let your spirit sing with a new-found love for Life. Love is magical. It is the greatest gift and the most powerful force in the universe.

Love withheld, in the past or present, lies somewhere at the root of all psychosomatic illness. Attempting to compensate for the lack of love causes erratic, neurotic behavior. Love withheld cascades down from the emotional body into the mental body, causing neuroses and from there it slides into the physical body in the form of illness. In simple terms, love deprivation causes sickness.

Love is necessary to our being. It is our most vital Sunfood. It supports us, sustains us, gives us the power to overcome. You never can tell what a loving word can mean to someone. Speak loving, caring words to friends and family members, especially when they are ill, and they will become healthier. They will be physically, mentally, emotionally and spiritually uplifted!

Send out waves of loving energy. We know by the Laws of Karma that what we put out comes back to us — multiplied. As much love as you put into your interactions, that is how much love comes directly back to you.

To be loved, we have to love ourselves. Loving yourself is very healthy. Only when we love ourselves do we have enough love to give away. By giving love we then receive love.

THE LAW OF ATTRACTION

1   Two key points to live by daily:
    Stop chasing, start attracting.
    Stop striving, start arriving.

2   Ask yourself: "What will it take for me to love myself completely in every facet of my being?" Record the answer in your journal. When you love yourself, your journey through life will be so much more enjoyable and you can start to love others as well.

3   Stop taking everything so seriously. A "seriousness addiction" plunders the joy of life.

THE LAW OF ATTRACTION

It is operating always
In greater or lesser forms.
It directs the roaring majesty
Of deep-blue tropical storms.

It masters mighty mountains
And rolls each grain of sand.
It alters the course of rivers
And pulls the tide to land.

It summons bee to flower
And drone to honey queen.
It is felt by primal wisdom
But rarely is ever seen.

It may shift its shape
And shape its shift
To bring two, eye to eye.
Try to grasp its power:
It eludes,
Like a butterfly.

It calls the bird to the tree;
It lays the eggs in the nest.
It turns the tides of fortune
And never does it rest.

It lingers in the mortal world
And filters through the dust.
To bond a fated pair
It takes the form of lust.

The Law is organic power
Captured by clean living;
Drawing forth Nature's favor,
When love is what you're giving.

Like and like beget,
'Birds of a feather' attract.
That purer bodies captivate
Is the ever-certain fact.

Success attracts success
Fortunes rising higher.
People, places, things
In harmony with your desire.

When you are ready,
For what you want.
When you truly believe
You deserve it.
All the resources will show up
With the people to support it.

Help is ever on the way,
Drawn by your conviction.
When you are absolutely certain,
You call the cosmic law to action.

The Law is eternal —
A mysterious, magical charm.
Multiplying Life:
It creates a jungle from a farm.

Nothing circumvents its pull.
Not one escapes its force.
Nothing is by chance.
It is part of every source.

It brings a hand to hand;
It touches a paw to paw.
Primal love vibrations —
The Mistress of Cosmic Law.

It magnetizes masterminds
And shapes the destiny of worlds.
It spins the cosmic froth about,
And giggles in little girls.

It is Nature's gravitation,
Method of motivation,
Modus of procreation,
Concept of creation.

The Law of Attraction —
The Logic of the Spheres.
Desire a thing deep enough,
And it suddenly appears.

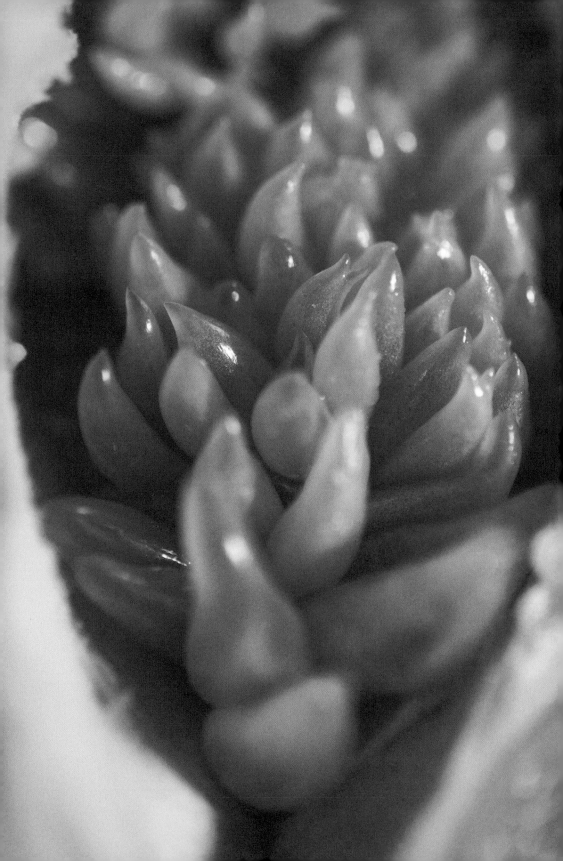

30

THE MYSTERY OF SEX TRANSMUTATION REVISITED (SEEDS MUST LIVE)

"...The 'forbidden food' in the midst of fruits and herbs (Garden of Eden) is their seed, which if eaten destroys their own purpose of reproduction, and makes man and woman 'go to seed'..." — Dr. Johnny Lovewisdom, Spiritualizing Dietetics: Vitarianism

The drive for sex is one of the most powerful of all desires. Success philosopher Napoleon Hill found that when driven by this desire, people develop keenness of imagination, courage, will power, persistence and a creative ability unknown to them at other times. He found that the desire for sexual expression is so powerful that people will run the risk of life and reputation to engage in it. He concluded that when harnessed and transmuted into other channels, the driving force of sex energy maintains all of its motivating attributes which may be used as powerful creative forces in literature, art or in any other profession or calling, including the accumulation of wealth. What Napoleon Hill revealed was that those who had achieved incredible accomplishments had a high degree of sexual charisma. They had learned to channel their sex energy into success — they had mastered the art of sexual transmutation.

Napoleon Hill also discovered that those who experienced great successes in their life did not achieve those lofty heights until the age of forty or beyond. He attributed this to the ability, with age and experience, to transmute the sexual impulse into areas of creativity and achievement. Now this is possible to do without having to wait for age and experience to bring the sexual drive under control. The sex drive can be transmuted through the right use of diet.

Proper use of diet allows us to channel energies used for sex up the spine into the brain for superior mental performance. This is a secret of creative ability. Transmuted sex energy lifts the mind into a higher sphere, allowing communication with infinite intelligence.

A pure diet of fruits, green-leafed vegetables and certain other raw foods, (but no nuts, seeds or eggs) allows one to better control the sex drive. Foods that contain seeds (such as cucumbers) are okay to eat, however, the eating of individual nuts and seeds (e.g. almonds, pumpkin seeds, rice, etc.) is to be avoided for a planned period of time. The teachings of herbalism (the Doctrine of Signatures) demonstrate that eating seeds causes us to "go to seed." The hormones in nuts, seeds and eggs drive the sexual organs.

To sublimate the sex impulse and use it to drive you forward and upward in great health, wealth (business and sales skills), and vitality, stop eating nuts and seeds of any type for a specific period of time. A pure seedless diet automatically sublimates the sex energies. Sexual sublimation cues up the mind so it works rapidly, efficiently, clearly, with real inspiration. The control of the physical side of sex expands the imagination. It lends mighty power to the creative faculties.

Male sexual fluids have extraordinarily high levels of trace minerals. For males, excessive ejaculation — "spilling the seed" — without nutritionally replacing what is lost, drains minerals and life-force energy from the body, which causes premature aging, leads to an accelerated loss of hair in men and contributes to impotence. Men can replace sexual fluids by specifically eating nuts, seeds, wild coconuts, coconut oil, cacao (raw chocolate), maca root, seaweeds, avocados, olives and bee pollen. Breathing pure air and Sunbathing nude will also help restore sexual fluids and energy.

Due to the mineral deficit and toxicity caused by the standard diet, men often experience a "crash" or a mood swing after ejaculation, which is typically not pleasing to the sexual partner. This will reverse and may be totally eliminated once the diet is mineralized and purified by eating a healthy balance of high-

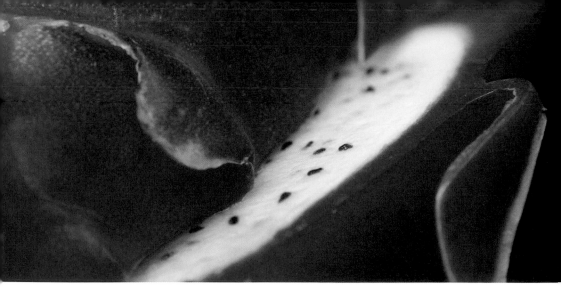

Creativity in Nature is most closely associated with the reproductive elements of plants: The flowers, the fruits and the seeds. Pictured above is Dragon fruit.

quality raw plant foods.

The books and articles I have read on diet, spirituality and sex generally agree that between 25% and 40% of the life-force energy men accumulate from breathing, eating, Sunlight, spiritual power, etc. is transmuted into sexual energy, which is stored physically in male sperm. A single ejaculation contains 200 to 500 million sperm cells. If we consider each sperm cell as a potential human being, there are sufficient sperm cells for a man in a few days to generate the current population of the Earth. That is the power of semen.

Complementary to dietary considerations, there is a Taoist technique for redirection of the sexual energy called the "big draw." This technique involves drawing back the discharge of sexual energy and redirecting it up the spine to the brain by drawing in the breath at the moment one is nearing sexual climax. Through practice one can develop this retention ability. The increase in sexual potency that follows is quite remarkable in that it creates great libido, more subtle sexual enjoyment, remarkable capacity and progressively increasing sensitivity.

For men, the point is to have sex, but not to ejaculate every time. Sex is essential to excellent health as it restores imbalances in the body chemistry, excites the sex hormones and balances the other major glands (the adrenal, thymus, thyroid, pituitary, hypothalamus, and pineal). Sex clears the mind, frees the spirit and helps build a wonderful relationship with one's partner.

A healthy body is a sexual body. Sexual people have a bountiful supply of attractive magnetism.

Two tuned beings consciously uniting their physical bodies invoke a powerful spiritual energy. There is no substitute for spiritual sex. Sharing pleasure and love unconditionally with another adds a new meaning to existence. In my opinion, sex as a raw-foodist with a raw-foodist is a more amazing experience than anything I had known before.

How To Increase The Sex Drive

"Having sex with another is usually more pleasurable if the person smells appetizing, tastes and looks good (just like food)."
— *Joshua Rainbow, Biotrophic Protocol*

To increase the sex drive, eat nuts, seeds, wild coconuts, coconut oil, cacao, goji berries and maca. Eating nuts and seeds stimulates the desire "to go to seed!" From personal experience I have found watermelon seeds to be quite an aphrodisiac. I am also convinced that the stamen-center of the cherimoya fruit has aphrodisiac qualities. Other raw plant foods that excite the sex impulse are: avocados, olives, raw organic olive oil, raw dulse (seaweed), pollen (pollen from the male date palm tree is an aphrodisiac for women), onions, garlic and hot peppers (the yogis of India have long-known that spicy foods excite the sexual passions). By eating significantly more of all these foods, males will see a major increase in sperm count and females will experience a greater sex drive. (Eat organic food only. Pesticides, when absorbed into the body, end up in the sexual fluids; they decrease sexual vitality and cause sterility.)

THE MYSTERY OF SEX TRANSMUTATION
REVISITED (SEEDS MUST LIVE)

1   Set a period of one month aside to use the power of sexual transmuta-
    tion. For that one month eat no nuts, seeds or eggs of any type. This will
    automatically sublimate the sexual energies and provide you with more
    creative abilities in other areas. Use that time to complete a project at
    home, with the family, or in business.

2   For men: experiment with having sex without ejaculation and with drawing
    the sexual energy up the spine into the brain.

3   For women: cleverly include some aphrodisiac foods into you and your
    partner's smoothie each morning (cacao beans, maca root powder and
    coconut oil are recommended). Expect extraordinary results.

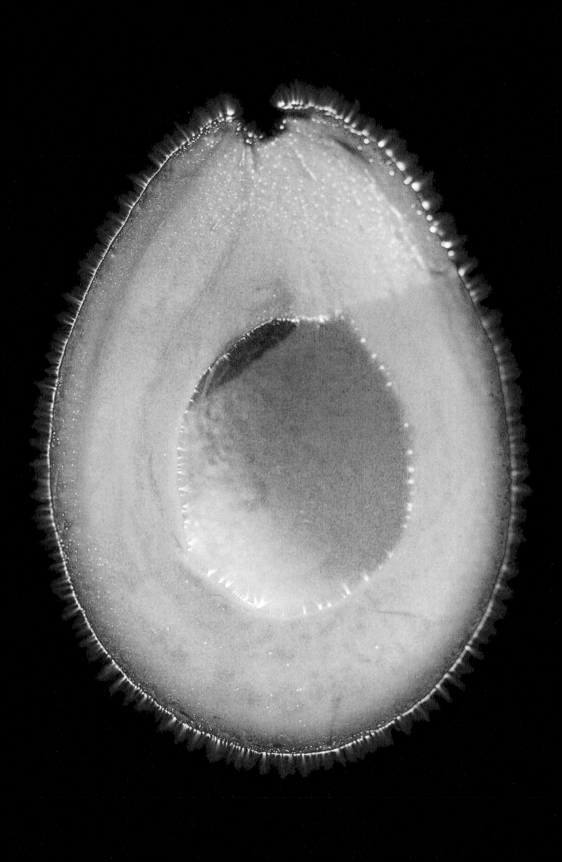

31

AVOCADOS (PERSEA AMERICANA)

Aboriginal to Mexico and Central America, the avocado tree has migrated its way into North America, and has since spread throughout the world.

In English, avocados have been known by over forty different names, including: Alligator Pear, Butter Fruit, Butter Pear, Custard Apple, Laurel Peach, Midshipman's Butter, Shell Pear, Spanish Pear, Subaltern's Butter, Testicle Fruit, and Vegetable Marrow.

In the nutrition reference book, **Whole Foods Companion**, it is written, "The English word avocado is a corruption of the Nahuatlan Mexican ahuacatl, itself an Aztec shortening of ahuacacuahatl, which means testicle tree. The Aztecs explained that their ahuacatl was given the name not only because the fruit resembled a testicle and grew in pairs, but because it greatly excited sexual passion."

The avocado is the new world olive. It is the fatty fruit that dominates the Americas as the olive dominates the Mediterranean world.

The avocado has a huge variety of tastes and flavors — over 500 different types have been identified. Avocados very rarely ripen on the tree. They ripen on the ground as most fatty fruits do. Each variety in and upon itself is very sensitive to environmental conditions and picks up a superior taste when grown in mineral-rich soil and is left to ripen naturally. Some of the heavier varieties, such

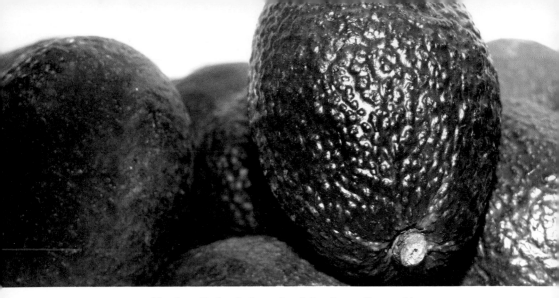

**The favorite food of raw-foodists all over the world:
The Avocado.**

as Reed, Cannonball, Pinkerton, etc. should be left on the tree for at least one year to allow their true oil content to set in.

Avocados are a rich, emerald cream. The gentle flavor, high-fat content, smooth texture and natural oils within them make avocados an ideal beauty food, and an excellent baby food.

There is no doubt about it, avocados are the best transition food from a cooked-food diet to a raw-food diet. Fatty raw plant foods are remarkably satisfying. Fatty foods in general (nuts, seeds, coconuts, avocados, olives, durians, etc.) transition you from cooked foods to raw foods — they are the bridge.

The avocado is in ascendancy right now worldwide; more and more people are discovering its secrets. You want to know how powerful the avocado is? The avocado can help save the human race because avocado fat replaces meat and dairy fat. The avocado replaces resource-depleting animal products in the diet. Keep in mind: at least 260 million acres (1.05 million square kilometers) of United States' forests have been cleared for cropland to fuel the meat-centered diet; the percentage of U.S. topsoil loss directly attributable to livestock raising is 85%; more than half the water used in the U.S. is used for livestock production; 2,500 gallons of water is required to produce one pound (0.45 kg) of meat. Avocado trees not only provide food, they also create clean air, beautify topsoil and provide homes for wildlife.

Many raw foodists I have met have eaten one to three avocados nearly every day since they started on a program of natural nutrition. Most seem to never get tired of them! I know raw-foodists who have been eating one avocado nearly every day for five, ten, even twenty years.

One day I was at the beach looking for a place to surf while eating an avocado. A gentleman walked by, looked at me, and commented, "soul food." He was right. Avocados are soul food. They feed our essence.

Sometimes rich fatty raw food is challenging on an individual with a compromised liver or with weak digestion. The digestive energy required to digest rich fatty raw food is eased when these foods are blended in smoothies, raw soups or when eaten with green leaves. Digestive enzymes rich in lipase also assist with fat digestion.

Almost every raw foodist I have ever met is an avid fan of the avocado. But, some wonder whether or not they are addicted to the fruit. What they are feeling is not an addiction per se, but a manifestation of the body's desire for fat. To get off avocados, simply replace them with another fatty plant food. Soft, young coconuts make an excellent replacement. Nuts and seeds work great. Sun-ripened olives are also an ideal fatty food. Optimally, I think it is excellent to move around the fat category eating macadamia nuts for several weeks, then olives for several months, eating some avocados, bringing in some durian, then pecans. This is how I have come to eat raw plant fats. This gives your body some variety and makes your diet easier on the digestive organs, especially the liver.

AVOCADO

A New World treasure —
Never found?
Which ripens amongst
Leaves on the ground?

The smooth, rich taste
The Mayan fruit.
The raw-wild flavor
Behind Pan's flute.

Sexual passion
An instantaneous connection.
Smooth, clear skin
A perfect complexion.

The emerald idol
An erotic oil
The polished leaves
From exotic soil.

Indulge your lips
In fertile cream.
Awaken to a
Wonderful dream.

The misty forest
The secret delight.
Urban fruit foragers
In avo-groves at night.

They gaze upon
The twilight sky
As silver jewels
Sway nearby.

The bass, the beat,
The tribal drum,
The Sunfooder singing:
"I've got to have one."

The dictated cry, that:
"Thin is in"
Can never bring forth
The beauty within.
"Fat's where it's at!"
Says the tribal man.
A filled luscious body
Is Nature's plan.

Sensual compassion
The Avocado transition;
The jungle fruit
Has come to fruition.

The searching masses
With food to burn
Perhaps one day
Will listen then learn
That the golden secret
Of El Dorado
May be found within
The Avocado.

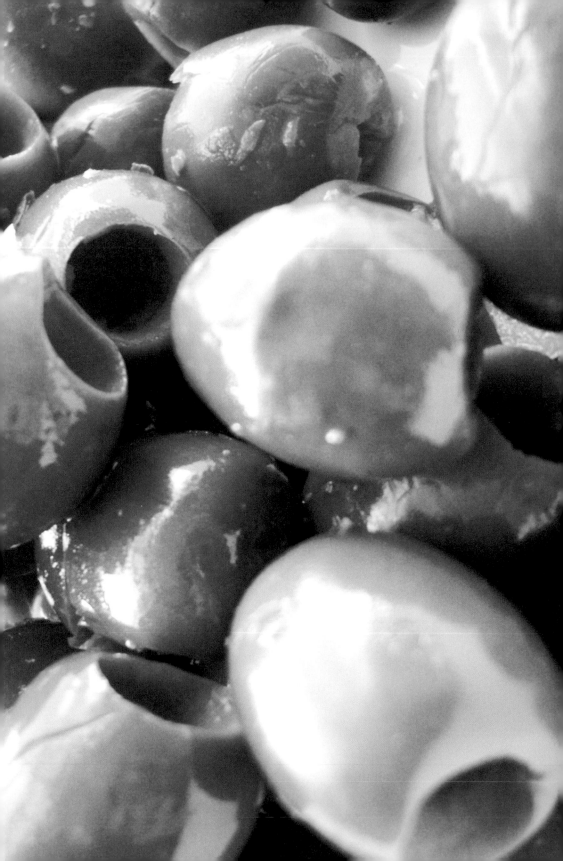

32

THE OLIVE (OLEA EUROPEA)

"Olives — Their lubricating, cleansing, beautifying and rejuvenative power is the greatest among all fruits."
— *Vera Richter, The Cook-Less Book*

Olives are quite possibly the world's most perfect food. Olives are a biblical fruit associated in the scriptures with symbols of goodness, happiness, purity, and prosperity. In ancient Greece, during the height of their culture, Solon, the great law-giver, enacted laws protecting all olive trees. He made it a capital offense to kill a tree or to cut one down.

The Romans believed the olive to be an incredibly sexual fruit, an aphrodisiac, especially when eaten in large quantities. The Romans were the first to perfect the stone-press with which they extracted the olive's oil.

If I had to pick one fruit to live on for the rest of my life, it would be the olive. Once you delve into the olive, you will become privy to the great Mediterranean secret of health, happiness and longevity. The olive is a magical fruit. But the olive remains a mystery to almost everyone I know, including other raw-foodists. Few people know how to eat an olive naturally.

It took me several years to unravel the olive's mystery. The first clue I discovered about olives is that they are a type of fruit that ripens on the ground. Avocados, dates, cherimoyas, and even citrus fruits fall into this category (I have noticed citrus fruits reach their peak maturity after weeks, or even months, on the ground in the Sun. If you buy citrus fruits in the store, leave them outside under the Sun if possible, or in the windowsill to allow them to reach their full ripeness).

Olives must be picked fresh and Sun-ripened. As the olive ripens in the Sun, the bitter component (oleuropein) is converted and the fruit suddenly becomes edible! The black olives commonly grown in the United States and the Mediterranean reach their ripe maturity when the fruit softens and the internal flesh of the fruit changes from white or red to brown or black. The olive skin may begin wrinkling at this stage as well. Though there are these markers to watch for, olives are a food you acquire a "feel" for. From experience, I can look at an olive under a tree or pick one up and know if it is ripe or not, even if it has not undergone obvious external changes.

The second clue I unraveled was that olives taste best and are most digestible in their juicy ripened state before they become too dry. Although olives are an ancient biblical fruit, very few people have eaten them in their juicy ripened natural state. Juicy Sun-ripened olives are beyond description. The olive has such a marvelous variety of flavors. I might eat ten in a row, all from the same tree, while noticing a different flavor in each olive. I usually do not stop with ten; I might eat 50 olives with a salad for dinner. On some days as many as 100 have passed my lips! (Here I am referring to wild Mission olives growing in Southern California. When eating bigger, raw Sun-ripened Peruvian olives, quantities eaten are typically one-third of the Mission olives).

I recommend avoiding high quantities of vinegar-soaked olives as they are acid forming (which can help assist the digestion of vegetables, yet can upset the stomach if eaten excessively). Canned black olives have been pasteurized and soaked in ferrous gluconate (an iron compound which darkens them) and should be avoided. Excellent cured olives include "water-cured" or "raw sea-salt and/or olive-oil cured" olives (these should be eaten moderately because of their high-salt content, e.g. not more than fifteen with a salad). Aside from picking them from under the tree, the best choice to eat olives is to find thick, juicy Sun-ripened olives.

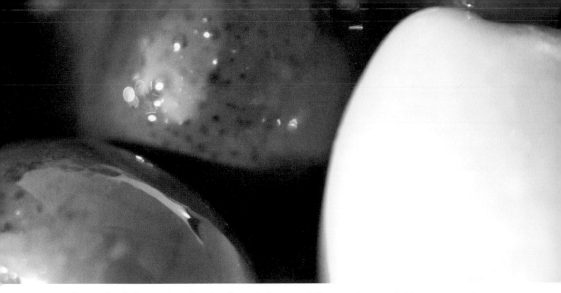

Olives (and the entire olive tree) contain one of the most powerful immune system supporting substances known. This substance is concentrated in olive leaf extract.

Olive trees are now ubiquitous in the southwestern United States as well as throughout the Mediterranean world, the Middle East and India. Olives grow abundantly in California, especially in Southern California. They were originally planted there by the Spanish and have essentially become naturalized — and even grow wildly, having been spread by the birds. I have also seen olives growing abundantly in southern Nevada, especially in the Las Vegas area. They grow throughout Arizona as well. They love the desert.

Consider the power and benefits of the olive. The raw olive is:
1. The fruit richest in minerals.
2. The fruit richest in calcium. Olives contain twice as much calcium as oranges by weight.
3. High in magnesium.
4. High in amino acids, including leucine, aspartic acid and glutaminic acid.
5. An alkaline fruit.
6. A fatty fruit (mostly monounsaturated fat).
7. An alkaline fat source.
8. Loaded with beneficial omega-3 and omega-6 fatty acids.
9. High in vitamins A (carotene) and E.
10. In possession of many antioxidant properties. Antioxidants deactivate free radicals allowing us to live longer, overcome illness and maintain more acute mental and muscular faculties.
11. Available in different varieties, which fruit all year around.
12. Pressable into a powerful oil, usable in a limitless number of ways all year around.

13. Able to soothe the mucous membranes with its oil.

Olives have the greatest propensity of any fruit to dissolve toxic mucus in the system (in fact, they are three times more powerful than oranges in that respect). In Arnold Ehret's classic book, **Mucusless Diet Healing System**, he reprints Ragnar Berg's Table which organizes different foods by their acid-binding or acid-forming potential. The higher the food's acid-binding potential, the greater its ability to dissolve mucus and cooked-food residues in the body. The olive, it turns out, is the highest mucus dissolver of any fruit. It rates with a value of 30.56 with figs following behind at 27.81, no other fruit in the chart ranks above 20.00. To give you an idea of how high these values are, the orange, an excellent mucus-dissolver, ranks at 9.61.

Olive oil is a soothing fat for damaged and dry skin, hair and nails. It can be used to soothe the skin after shaving. Olive oil may be used on baby skin instead of the harsh "baby oil" brands available in stores.

Some olive oils are devoid of lipase (the fat-splitting enzyme), probably because they are made from unripe olives. This is why I recommend only stone-crushed, cold-pressed extra virgin organic American or European brands in dark bottles (oils are light sensitive). I find Greek and Italian olive oils to be slightly better in taste and quality because they adhere to higher quality standards. The cold-pressed, stone-crushed olive oils of the ancients are available today from a select group of growers who adhere to the ancient ways.

THE OLIVE

The mysterious little fruit
Few can understand
Was there overseeing
Achilles last stand.

It rode the tides of war
Traveled the Odyssey,
Even to be crowned as:
Athena's sacred tree.

A tree so rich with jewels
To cause an army to invade.
The bravery of Lycurgus
Can ever it...fade?

The prize, the wise
Would realize.
Is the food of the divine.
Ripened from soil,
Made to oil,
Valued more than wine.

Grown erratic,
Rough between stones.
Dropping fruit which:
Builds strong bones.

Clearing the complexion
Building affection
Creating a fertile,
Instantaneous connection.

The symbol fruit of
Massive abundance.
The startling
Charisma of the ancients.

Across the seas,
For the royals,
Thales' secret,
To carry the oils.

The sea-farer's bed,
The sacred union,
It is time for a:
Mediterranean reunion.

The gnarled tree,
Grown by the seas,
Reveals the wisdom
This world needs.

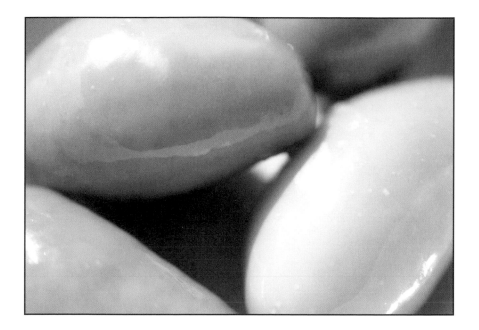

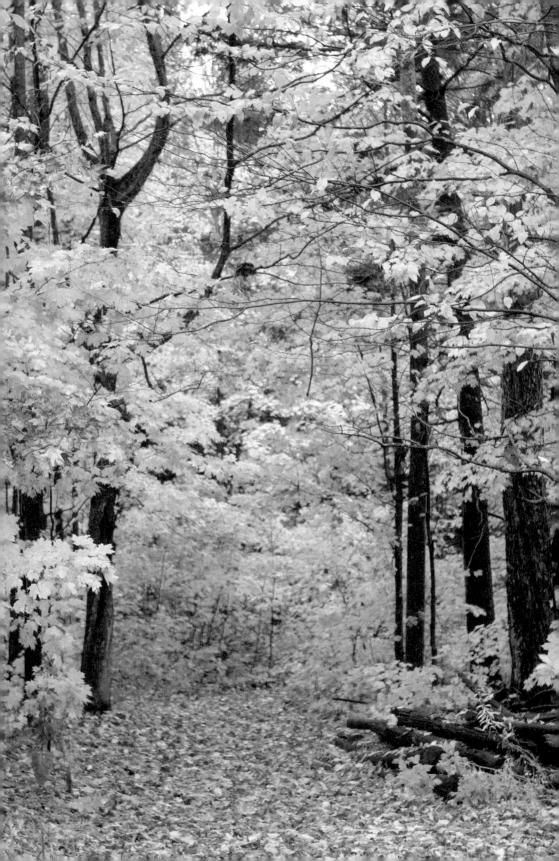

33

TIME MANAGEMENT THROUGH FASTING

"FASTING IS AT ONCE A JOURNEY NEAR AND
YET SO FAR. BY UNDERGOING ONE, MORE WILL BE LEARNT
FROM IT THAN ALL THE LANDS YOU VISITED OR BOOKS
YOU HAVE READ." — *Morris Krok*

Fasting (resting the body from food) is part of life. People fast every night when they go to sleep; this abstainment from food and liquid may last eight to ten hours or longer. Now if humans lived in a normal and natural way, each night's repose would be adequate, but because humans live so far away from the natural state, the nightly nocturnal fast is not sufficient to completely rest or purify the body.

Isn't it interesting that the major religions of the world teach the benefits of fasting? I find that fascinating.

The journey into fasting is about becoming a finely-tuned spiritual instrument. Fasting is mentioned as part of nearly every religion on Earth. Fasting on water is a spiritual practice. Undertaking a fast measures self-discipline and self-control. Fasting tests the will.

Fasting is Nature's foundational law of all healing and revitalization. Nature's healing command is: "Don't eat, lie down, hide, be quiet." Fasting seems to be a part of every answer. Are you confused? Fast. Feeling ill? Fast. Sick to your stomach? Fast. Those who fast regularly know that not eating has a cleansing effect on all areas of the mind, body and spirit.

Fasting enables the body to start healing itself. The amazing thing about fasting is that it is Nature's supreme medicine. When one begins to fast, the elimination process is set in motion and the entire body commences a cleansing program. During a fast, the body can focus its enzyme power to autolyze (dissolve) tumorous formations and toxic residues.

While fasting, the blood thins (recall **Lesson 10: Detoxification** where we learned how the quality of the blood is formed at the intestinal villi). This allows the thick mucus trapped in the lymph to diffuse out into the blood for elimination. This is the process of diffusion, elements move from areas of greater concentration to areas of lesser concentration.

Orange, grapefruit, lime and lemon juices dissolve toxicity, mucus and excess calcite deposits so they may be washed out and eliminated. I recommend including the pith (the white inside of the rind) with your citrus juices, especially when fasting. The pith contains bioflavonoids, fiber and calcium.

Case studies conducted by fasting doctors over this last century prove that the longer you fast, the more centered you become, the better you heal, the higher your intellectual activity and the younger you appear. The pancreas secretes enzyme-rich digestive juices when the stomach and duodenum are empty. These fluids travel into the intestinal tract, are absorbed by the intestinal villi and then enter into the blood and lymph to digest undigested fats, carbohydrates and proteins.

When your body is cleaned and tuned through fasting, you will experience a continuous flow of vibrant health, electric energy and mental strength. This will enable you to perform at levels you never thought possible. Time will slow down, but your brain will speed up. You will feel amazingly calm. Your consciousness will glow as ideas flow through you exactly when you need them.

Fasting is an art. One masters fasting by developing the ability to raise the functions of the body while the blood sugar is low.

If we are living with passion and with a purpose, then fasting is exciting, never boring.

Let us not lose sight of the truth: food is a means to an end, not an end in itself. The paradox of The Sunfood Diet is that food is not an issue. As long as the food is raw plant food, eat what you need for fuel and get on with accomplishing your goals. Be so busy accomplishing your goals that you don't spend any time even thinking about food. Use the secrets of diet and fasting to help you advance in all areas of life including, spiritual pursuits, relationships, business and emotional poise. Get more done in less time.

The best time to get tedious, organizational work done is during a fast. Time management is best accomplished through fasting. Eating food is a tremendous consumer of time.

How To Fast

One must be careful with fasting. There are health conditions that do not react well to fasting. For instance, a fast is not recommended for diabetics who have taken insulin for more than two years. Those taking certain medications or recreational drugs should also not fast, until they have detoxified their body, eaten a mineral-rich, organic diet and stopped the intake of all chemicals. Otherwise, fasting may cause too much poison to flow out of the lymph fluid into the blood too quickly.

One should build up stores of natural amino acids (superfoods), chlorophyll (greens), sugars (fruit), and raw plant fats in the system for at least 6 months before undertaking a fast of two days or longer.

To begin fasting, try the no breakfast plan initially — no break-fasting. Then go one day and continue further.

Preferentially arrange to fast when the seasons change or on the full moon; these times are when the body cleanses the strongest. During each change of seasons, Nature does its house-cleaning by expelling poisons; this is why people experience the flu (detoxification) during the seasonal changes. When the moon is full, the tidal energies are pulled, "levity" energies are higher and the body is triggered to detoxify.

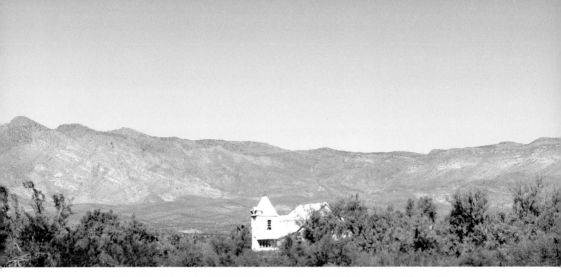

One should preferably fast at a sanctuary in Nature away from the attendant responsibilities of household duties.

I recommend fasting on fresh spring water mixed with fresh lemon juice. The lemon juice acts as an internal soap by dissolving mucus and cooked-food residues. The fasting I recommend for accelerated healing is designed to keep the blood sugar low — as a low-sugar fruit, lemon works perfectly.

The fasting I recommend for time management can include coconut water, fruit juice and/or green-vegetable juices, but may also be done just on water with lemon juice. When you are fasting for time management, small fasts of two or three days may serve your purpose. I typically will fast on water all day, while working at my business, then accomplish an incredible amount of work in the evening and at night (reading or writing), wake up after five hours of sleep at 5:00 am and work three or four more hours before breaking the fast and eating something the following morning.

If you are new to Sunfoods, fasts should be undertaken with care. Ease into them. For those who are inexperienced, fast for small intervals (one or two days). Go on an adventure with a trustworthy friend or family member. Spend a day fasting out in Nature in a forest, at a pond or near a waterfall, consuming only pure water.

As you begin to undertake longer fasts, you will recognize that the body first uses up the sugar in your system for fuel, then, after three days, clicks over to glycogen stored in the cells and liver. The body will eventually tap into the body fat and begin converting that to fuel until it is depleted. Protein breakdown is the last thing the body turns to for fuel.

During a fast, an individual should be concerned about bowel movements. The bowels may not move when they need to. If you feel a bowel movement is necessary while you are fasting, administer an enema to yourself or visit a colon hydrotherapist. Colon hydrotherapy while fasting is very cleansing and tremendously healing.

The amount of water you drink during a fast should be dictated by thirst. Four quarts (four liters or one gallon) of water or juice each day should be adequate. The less fluids you take in, the more aggressive (and hazardous) will be the fast. Do not push yourself beyond the bounds of reason, if you feel dizzy, weary, extremely thirsty and/or experience pain in the kidneys (outer lower back) drink more water, add fresh juice or even return to eating very light raw food (a cucumber, berries, cherries or an apple).

As you are fasting, read books on the subject to keep you focused and motivated. During a fast my motivation is renewed whenever I read Arnold Ehret's book, **Rational Fasting**. Arnold Ehret brings up a crucial point in his writings: how you break a fast determines to a large extent the value of the fast and the degree of rejuvenation. Remember the rule that however many days you fast, it takes the same amount of additional days to fully recover. If you fast for ten days, then it will take ten additional days after the fast to return to normal eating and lifestyle patterns. Preferentially break a fast with a juicy alkaline fruit, such as a papaya or cucumber; fresh figs, grapes, or cherries also work quite well. Breaking a water fast with wild coconut water is also quite magical. The introduction of alkaline fruit will cause a peristaltic wave and a flush of all the dislodged toxins throughout the body. Keep in mind the stomach will shrink from days of fasting. Wait at least two hours before eating something else to allow the full cleansing peristaltic wave to sweep through the body (peristalsis is a muscular contraction which flows wave-like through the colon helping to expel waste). The next meal may consist of heavier foods, preferably blended, such as fruits and avocados mixed together. After one or more days, whole green leaves may be reintroduced into the body. Cooked food should be avoided following a fast. One the other hand, superfoods (blue-green algae or spirulina) can be helpful to add not only during the fast, but after as well.

Generally, the more toxic a person is, the more weight they will lose during a fast. Weight and size lost during a fast can be regained with no detrimental effects if desired; the body retains a "memory" as to its normal proportions. I have found that at this point I can fast four to five days on water with almost no weight loss.

What I Learned From The Yaqui Medicine Man

I once met a Yaqui Indian medicine man of the same race and ethnicity as Don Juan from the Carlos Castaneda books. He was a robust man who radiated an extraordinary vitality, grace and simple gusto for life. I believe he was 82-years-young when I met him. But his age was unguessable to anyone who did not know. He looked in some ways as if he were ten years old; he had many of the features of a young boy. I looked at his hands closely and noticed no wrinkles and no liver spots.

He has followed a vegan diet since birth, as taught to him by his mother (overturning the false idea that indigenous peoples are not vegetarians or vegans). Only three times in his life has he eaten animal foods (raw rattlesnake twice, as a ceremonial experience; and turtle soup once). His friends told me he could identify thousands of herbs.

He told me the story of how he crossed the Desert of Silence in the State of Sonora Mexico. He crossed without food or water for eight days all the while sucking on a small pebble.

He described that fasting was the key to spiritual awakening. He fasts two days a week, taking in very little water. He also fasts three days every full moon.

Breatharianism

Recall **Lesson 2: The Foundational Law** — things produce after their kind. When you overeat one day, you are hungrier the next. The more you eat, the more you want to eat; the less you eat, the less you want to eat. The more you fast, the easier it is and the less you desire food. Fasting becomes easier the more you do it.

I am of the opinion that when the body is finely tuned and totally purified on all levels (physically, mentally, emotionally and spiritually), one can fast for an extremely long time.

In his fascinating book **Spiritualizing Dietetics: Vitarianism**, Dr. Johnny Lovewisdom describes exactly how he fasted for seven months and seven days on 99% distilled water (the other 1% consisting of citrus, tomato or green juice), and then, four months later, again fasted for six months and 17 days on 99% distilled water.

Jasmuheen of Australia, founder of The Self-Empowerment Academy, describes in her book **Living On Light** how she has lived on herbal teas and very little food since June 1993. She writes, "It is not about fasting, it is about allowing, trusting, clicking into an energy pattern of knowing that our true sustenance is provided by Cosmic Light, which sustains many beings from many Universes, and is a possibility offered to us here and now. Nor is it a process of denial..."

I know Jasmuheen personally. She has stayed at my home in Southern California. She eats very little — less than anyone I personally know. Every day spent with her demonstrated to me that her energy levels were high and balanced. She is a lot of fun. While staying with me she spent two to four hours meditating each morning and evening. I got the impression that her lifestyle is easy for her.

In my estimation, the end goal of natural nutrition and mind-mastery is "breatharianism" — a lifestyle involving yoga, meditation, laughing, regular long fasts and a pure, frugal diet.

TIME MANAGEMENT THROUGH FASTING

1   After eating plenty of raw foods for at least 6 months, prepare and under-
    take your first fast. While fasting, read books on fasting. This will help
    strengthen your resolve. I recommend **Rational Fasting** by Professor
    Arnold Ehret, **Fasting Can Save Your Life** by Dr. Herbert Shelton and
    The Miracle Of Fasting by Paul Bragg.

2   As a healthy life discipline, make routine fasting part of your life. Fast
    three to seven days on water, fruit juice and or vegetable juice during the
    change of seasons. Fast when you attend seminars. Fast for time
    management. Fast for fun!

**Opposite: a magnificent Kirlian photograph of
organic cacao butter (cocoa butter).
Fasting may mean going without food, however, it does
not mean going without sensual skin nutrition!**

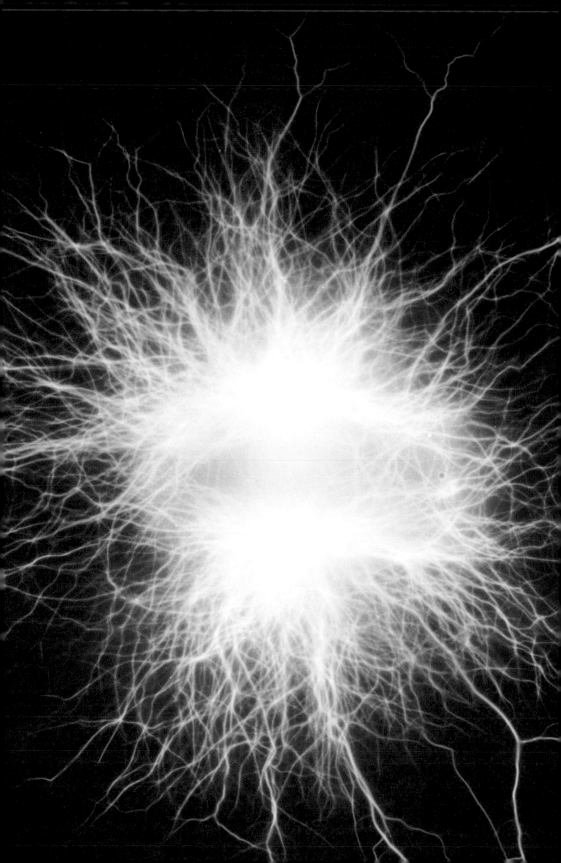

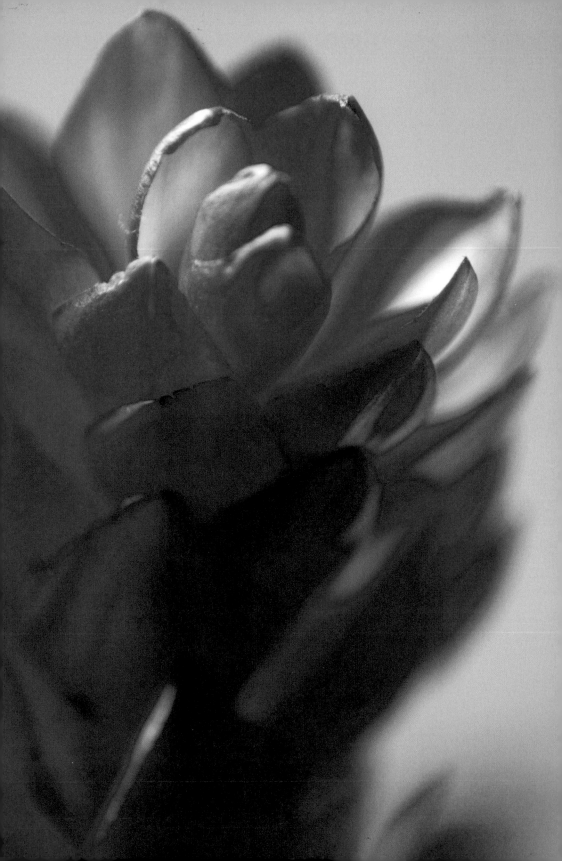

34

DO WHAT YOU LOVE TO DO

"INDEED, THERE IS NO SUCH THING AS TRUTH IN ITSELF:
THERE CAN ONLY EXIST THE PROCESS OF LIVING TRULY — IN SO
LIVING AS TO CONSTANTLY MANIFEST THE FULLNESS OF
ONE'S BEING — IN SO LIVING THAT THE ACTUAL PROCESS OF
ONE'S LIFE REFLECTS FULLY THE WHOLENESS OF
THE GREATER COSMIC PROCESS." — *Michael Tobin*

"IF IT MAKES YOUR HEART SING, DO IT!" — *Jasmuheen*

You are here on Earth to become exceptional, to make a majestic contribution and to help achieve something wonderful which uplifts all living things. You are part of a great plan set in motion by the divine hand. Every obstacle you face is filled with indispensable experience points which lead you to higher and higher skill levels. Every adversity you face is exactly what you need to face in order to allow you to rise further up.

You were put on this Earth for a reason. Everything has its place and purpose, and so do you. Each individual has their own assignment. Your existence is not random. You are endowed with a gift that only you have. Within you is a Strong Exciting Essence Desire (SEED). Nourish it, make your contribution.

You exist to fulfill the destiny conceived at your inception. Your destiny is not something you can get; it is something you already know.

Find your area of excellence and channel all of your abilities, your entire focus into becoming the best there is in that field. Choose your garden and start planting. Get bent on a specific purpose in life and do only that which furthers the accomplishment of that purpose.

When you find your purpose in life — the job you were designed for — then you will be able to do it without even thinking of money or food. You will be able to do it with great joy and effervescence even while fasting — that is how you know.

The greatest successes in the world have found their area of excellence and focused all their resources into that area. There are no exceptions to this rule.

Those who are doing what they were meant to do have the wisdom to keep their own counsel, and do not waste their time trying to discourage others. Healthy individuals seek only to lift their fellows to a new level of progress. They are so busily engaged in promoting their purpose on Earth that they have no time to waste with anyone or anything that does not contribute in one way or another to that purpose. This is not a self-centered mode of living, because those who do what they love to do are so good at what they do, they give others exactly what they want.

We are here to serve others. How is it that we may best serve others? By fulfilling our assignment on Earth. That is why this book is in your hands now — I am fulfilling my assignment. We always contribute to the betterment of all by focusing on what is best for our own state of mind and the Earth's integrity.

Your contribution is a spiritual force that has more power than your own brain. It has the power to live on, grow and expand, even after you are long gone.

You will always feel happiest and most spiritually fulfilled by doing what you love to do no matter what the financial rewards. And you are in control of determining your financial rewards by answering the question: How can I do what I love to do and create financial abundance while doing it?

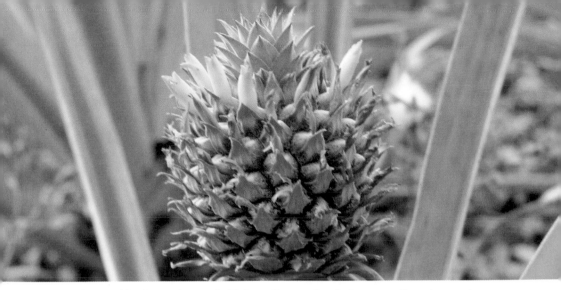

Competition is rarely seen in Nature. Cooperation is far more often observed with all parts working together to achieve a greater whole.

Just as you deserve an abundance of physical, mental, emotional and spiritual health, you deserve an abundance of financial health. Money in itself is neither good nor bad, it is neutral. Financial abundance can be used to support tremendous projects to help save tortured animals, grow trees, protect the land, develop environmentally-friendly free-energy implosion technology and heal the planet.

One common attribute of self-made millionaires is that they are doing what they love to do. They love what they do so much that they challenge themselves continuously to achieve the highest levels of success in their field, and the financial abundance follows.

The best, most fun and most exciting way to attract financial abundance is to find out what you really enjoy doing in life, the thing you have always loved doing, the thing you always wanted to spend all your time on, and then leverage your mind to figure out how to attract money while doing it. Make your favorite hobby your livelihood. When you are greatly enjoying what you are doing, people will be glad to invest their money with you! Turn what you have in your heart into something thousands, even millions, of people can enjoy, and you may use your rewards to live an abundant life spiritually, emotionally, mentally, physically and financially. Remember: wherever your heart is, there you will find your treasures.

What you do for a living each day should be enjoyable for you. If it is not, you are on the wrong track. If you are stuck doing something each day you do not like to do, you must figure out a plan of how to stop doing it, and how to start doing what you like to do.

All of Nature is part of a single giant organism in which every living creature has her or his own place and purpose. When you undertake The Sunfood Diet you will become more connected to the great workings of Nature and your true place and purpose will become more obvious to you. You will be "compelled" to let it unfold. Eating raw "compels" you to get into your own true pattern of life.

Zero-based thinking states: If the situation is wrong for you, if it is emotionally draining you, get out. Anything which emotionally drains you can cause you to do unhealthy things. This is why a pure diet and lifestyle compels you to get into situations that are right for you.

Would you be surprised to discover that one of the keys to health is to do what you love to do? Doing what you love to do is actually the easiest way to become, not only wealthy, but healthy as well!

Destiny

No two lives are alike, each attempts to unfold a divine pattern, a great and holy destiny, a unique form of abundance. As you live true to your own deeply-known destiny, you will radiate as perfectly and as beautifully as the most divine wild fruit tree. No one can stop you from reaching your highest potential, if you will but follow your own true pattern of life.

Wasted is every thought, feeling or vibration which is out of harmony with your true pattern of life. Learn to live by the pattern of life that is contained within you. You already know what it is. Now it is time for you to remember.

I have found my own true pattern of life is not that of an ascetic peace-lover wandering in bliss. I am animated by strong Sun-fired passions. I am driven by an overpowering internal fire. I will draw the line and take a stand. I feel that this is true to who I am and to try and be otherwise, based on some model of cooked spirituality, is not true for me. I live my life with a great intensity to bring this beautiful raw-vegetarian lifestyle to the world.

There is a force that wants you to realize your destiny; it tickles your appetite with a taste of success. For it is not only possible that you have your dream — it is necessary.

The closer you get to realizing your destiny, the more your destiny becomes your true reason for being. When your desire is highest in intensity, then you are closest to the true spirit of the world. When you want something so powerfully that literally nothing can stop you, then you have found your mission on Earth and all the universe will conspire to help you achieve it.

Life is generous to those who pursue their destiny. Those who live out their destiny know everything they need to know. Pursue your aspirations and goals in every moment, and one day your destiny will be realized!

To attract health, wealth, peace of mind, emotional beauty and spiritual fulfillment, do — all the time — what you do best. That is the path to incredible success in life, and is always the path of least resistance. You are more apt to succeed when you do what comes naturally. Develop your life's dreams along the line of least resistance. Is this not how the potent seedling sunders the cement?

Tilt your head and listen, now is the time to finally hear the unmistakable invitation ringing down the years — the call of your destiny. For the sake of a future for us all here on Earth...DO ONLY WHAT YOU WERE PUT HERE TO DO!

DO WHAT YOU LOVE TO DO

1   To uncover your true path in life, there are many things you can do; begin by answering the following questions on paper and recording them in your journal:

a)   Begin by thinking about your childhood. Tap into your subconscious mind. What did you really love to do between the ages of seven and fourteen? What captivated your attention? What still captivates your attention? Write these ideas down in your journal.

b)   Make a list of the twenty things you enjoy doing most in life. What gives you the greatest excitement? This will stimulate the creative action mechanism within your subconscious mind into revealing your purpose. Write your answers down in your journal.

c)   The subconscious mind may also be activated by reading. Start reading everything you can, this will help you uncover your purpose more quickly. Which books will you read this month to help you discover your life's passion? Write down at least three books you will read this month.

d)   Ask yourself: Where will I be and what will I be doing ten years from today if I keep doing what I am doing now? Record this answer in your journal.

e)   Ask yourself: In what area do I express an extraordinary passion? When you know the answer to that question, then you know what you need to be doing. Record this answer in your journal.

f)   Ask yourself: How can I do what I love to do and create financial abundance while doing it? Record this answer in your journal.

HEIGHTENED PROSPERITY

Each one
Teach one.
Each one
Reach one.
Each one
Grasp more.
Each one
Reach for
The most
Of what you can be.
The best
Of what you can see.

Each one
Teach fun.
Each one
Love Sun.

What excites you
You should do.

Each one
Reach back.
Each one
Heal lack.

Each one
Release strife,
Each one
Live more life!

Be alive,
Happily achieve.
It's all yours
If you believe.

Each day
Plan a way.
Each night,
Plan a site.
That you will see
When your dreams become —
Reality.

Each dawn
Listen long
To an uplifting book
An enchanting song.

Set the pace,
Win the race,
Give to all,
A smiling face.

Each life
Touch deep.
Bigger dreams
Less sleep.

Break bounds,
Become the best.
Leverage your mind
Surpass the rest.

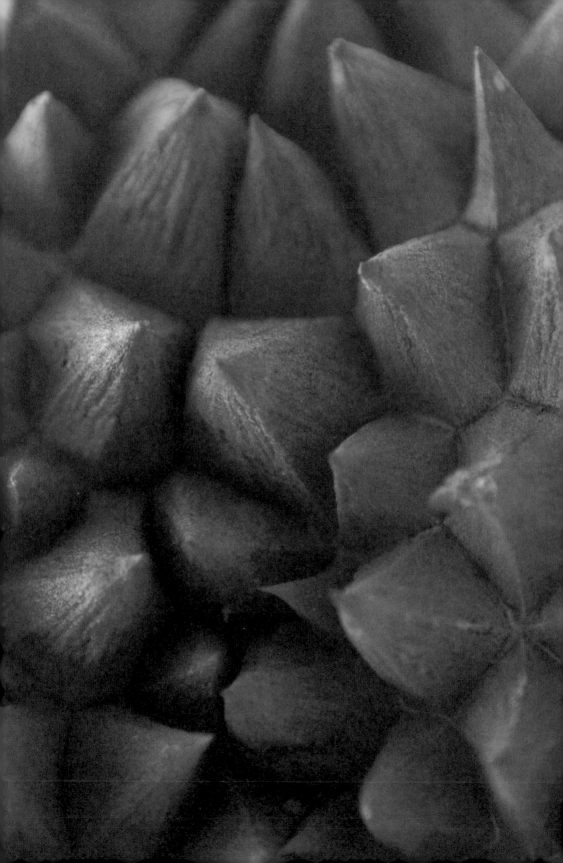

35

PERSISTENCE

BEGIN AGAIN — YOU CAN, YOU KNOW.
SEEK OUT A BETTER WAY TO GO.
FORGET THE PAST — THE PAST IS DEAD,
AND ALL TOMORROW LIES AHEAD!
THERE'S NEVER A TIME TOO LATE TO START
TO BRING TO FRUITION THAT DREAM IN YOUR HEART.
BEGIN AGAIN NOW, THIS MINUTE, THIS DAY!
A NEW LIFE IS WAITING — DON'T WISH IT AWAY!
— *Author Unknown*

"DO THE THING AND YOU SHALL HAVE THE POWER." — *Emerson*

"BY BEING PERSISTENT YOU ARE
DEMONSTRATING FAITH." — *Earl Nightingale*

"ALL GREAT SUCCESS IN LIFE IS PRECEDED BY LONG, SUSTAINED
PERIODS OF FOCUSED EFFORT ON A SINGLE GOAL, THE
MOST IMPORTANT GOAL, WITH THE DETERMINATION TO STAY WITH
IT UNTIL IT IS COMPLETE. THROUGHOUT HISTORY, WE FIND
THAT EVERY MAN OR WOMAN WHO ACHIEVED ANYTHING LASTING
AND WORTHWHILE, HAD ENGAGED IN LONG OFTEN UNAPPRECIATED
HOURS, WEEKS, MONTHS AND EVEN YEARS OF CONCENTRATED,
DISCIPLINED WORK, IN A PARTICULAR DIRECTION. FORTUNATELY,
THE QUALITY OF SELF-DISCIPLINE IS SOMETHING THAT YOU CAN

LEARN BY CONTINUOUS PRACTICE, OVER AND OVER, UNTIL
YOU MASTER IT. ONCE YOU HAVE MASTERED THE ABILITY TO DELAY
GRATIFICATION, THE ABILITY TO DISCIPLINE YOURSELF TO
KEEP YOUR ATTENTION FOCUSED ON THE MOST IMPORTANT TASK
IN FRONT OF YOU, THERE IS VIRTUALLY NO GOAL THAT YOU
CANNOT ACCOMPLISH AND NO TASK THAT YOU
CANNOT COMPLETE." — *Anonymous*

There is a rite of passage all must pass before they enter the hallowed halls of immortality. To pass those gates, one must possess the one key that opens all doors. A key that eludes all those who have yet to align their lives with their divine blueprint. A key that only opens the gates of fate when one has committed oneself entirely. That key is persistence — relentless persistence.

Before persistence, no army can stand, no wall can hold, no limit can remain. Absolutely nothing can take the place of persistence. There is a magical place awaiting those who will persevere. Persistence pays off.

Don't quit, no matter what. Decide to hold on in advance.

When Buster Douglas knocked out Mike Tyson it was the biggest upset in boxing history. When Buster Douglas was knocked down in that fight, it was time for his test. Before that fight ever started, he had decided he was getting up no matter what — he had committed himself to go all the way. He had just gotten out of an alcohol recovery center, his mother had just died, his wife was going down with disease. He was considered a nothing, a bum. When he got knocked down, Buster Douglas had a reason to get back up. He got back up and knocked Mike Tyson out. Reasons come first, answers come second.

The same holds true for you. Why will you persist when you get knocked down? You already have powerful reasons to get back up; what are they? It is going to take everything you have got to become all you can be. From some final reservoir of courage and determination, you will summon all of your strength and triumph. You will persist and make it to the top.

The lessons in this book have provided you with the diet and success information, now it is time for action.

Persistence is the science of continuous movement. Action is the key to abundance. Action is what it takes. As long as we keep making efforts, even if we stumble, we are still moving, making progress and learning. Isaac Newton told us a body at rest tends to stay at rest, but a body in motion tends to stay in motion! Keep moving!

It is never too late to be who you "might" have been. Keep acting until you become who you want to become. It is never too late to get what you "might" have gotten. Keep looking until you have found what you are looking for.

The more you try, the more likely it is that you will find the right approach. You have to overcome the fear of failure by understanding that the more you fail, the more likely it is you will succeed at an exceptional level. Babe Ruth struck out almost twice as much as he hit home runs. Thomas Watson Sr., the founder of IBM (International Business Machines) said, "Do you want to succeed? Then, double your failure rate. Success lies on the far side of failure." Thomas Edison tried ten thousand types of filaments for the electric light bulb before he found the one that worked. Did he look at himself as a failure? No, he remained persistent. The only guaranteed way to fail is to not make the effort. I heard a success seminar speaker once say, "Successful people fail their way to the top." Taking action is always better than doing nothing, because if you fail, at least you know what doesn't work!

Courage Versus Conformity

People do not lack courage, they simply are overburdened by an abundance of conformity. Persistence requires courage, while quitting requires conformity.

It is better by far to live a vital life of commitment, rather than a shallow existence of compromise. After you commit to your goals, then you begin to move down a new trail, paths will open up to you that you never would have seen before. You will discover how you will become something more.

Keep in mind that the higher you rise, the greater and more clever is your opposition, and the greater will be the pressure to compromise. Always return to the basics when doubts arise. As I mentioned earlier, the greatest sports coaches the world has ever seen taught the basics over and over and over

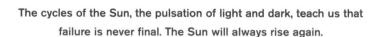

The cycles of the Sun, the pulsation of light and dark, teach us that failure is never final. The Sun will always rise again.

again. Practice the fundamentals daily. Conquer the critics by mastering fundamentals.

Have the raw courage to stand out. The great vice of the ages is conformity. Be strong and fear not, for all obstruction melts away before real strength of deed and sincerity of character. When you triumph, thrice blessed are you. Glory and honor be unto those who have the courage to win.

The time has come when every individual must rise from the slumber of indifference, from the orthodox complacency of the standard rules and regulations of society, and reach out, pioneering new fields of beautiful, ethical and spiritual progress. It is now time to experience the incredible majesty of living.

Instantaneous Change

At a certain point in our lives, after assiduously applying the principles of mind-mastery and circumstance creation, our lives are taken into the nourishing arms of destiny and we are catapulted forward to places beyond our wildest dreams. We enter hallowed halls of instantaneous change. Everything can change suddenly, without a single warning. In the **Bible** it says, "Behold, I show you a mystery; we shall not all sleep, but we shall all be changed, in a moment, in the twinkling of an eye..." (I Corinthians 15:51-52).

When real change happens in our lives, it happens instantaneously. The secret of "instant change" is to continue to persistently practice fundamentals until you hit what in non-linear mathematics is called a point of instability. In science and mathematics, it is known that a chain of events can have a point of crisis that can instantly magnify small changes. But chaos theory teaches us that such points are pervasive — they are everywhere. This means that no matter where your station in life, your work can be magnified instantly. You can arise out of obscurity to the very highest level of intensity in any field. But, to do so, you must practice fundamentals daily.

Go forth and win! Gather all you can of the Earth's good things. As you persist, remember: "That which you are seeking is also seeking you." Employ the trial and success method: learn from your mistakes and adjust your behavior accordingly.

It is for you to travel the path, no outside power can do it for you. It is as detrimental to have some outside force travel the path for you as it would be to tear open a cocoon before the butterfly has emerged. You have to free yourself through persistence, and in the struggle to obtain your freedom, you will have acquired the strength to fly.

Behold and understand that you are now standing upon the threshold of a splendid dawning Sun. With persistence, you hold the key to the future.

PERSISTENCE

1   Open your journal and review the top five yearly goals established in the Action Steps at the end of **Lesson 5: Goals**. Rewrite, next to each goal, exactly why you will faithfully persist until you achieve your top five yearly goals.

2   Consider the following aphorisms: "Do the thing you fear and the death of fear is certain," "Feel the fear and do it anyway," "Act in spite of your fear." Ask yourself: "How can I make conquering my fears fun?" Record the answer in your journal.

DON'T QUIT
(Author Unknown)

When things go wrong, as they sometimes will,
When the road you're trudging seems all uphill,
When the funds are low and the debts are high,
And you want to smile, but instead you sigh,
When care is pressing you down a bit,
Rest if you must, but don't you quit.

For life is strange with its twists and turns,
As everyone of us sometimes learns,
And many failures turn about,
When they might have won, had they stuck it out.

So don't give up though the pace seems slow,
You may succeed with another blow;
Success is failure turned inside out,
It's the silver tint of the clouds of doubt.

And you never can tell how close you are,
It may be near when it seems so far.
So stick to the fight when you're hardest hit,
It's when things seem worst that you must not quit.

THE FAR SIDE OF FAILURE

On the far side of failure,
Beyond the path of rejection
Far past the ghosts
Of doubt and dejection.

Just a bit farther
Than life's toughest question.
Over the stream running,
After each lost election.

Farther along
Than the extra mile.
Floating further
Than the lonely isle.

Beyond the sign:
"The buck stops here."
Over pools reflecting —
The faces of fear.

Over chasms deep
Where things seem worst,
Through hardened deserts,
Overcome by thirst.

Even surpassing
The road traveled less
Lies the hidden valley
Of massive success.

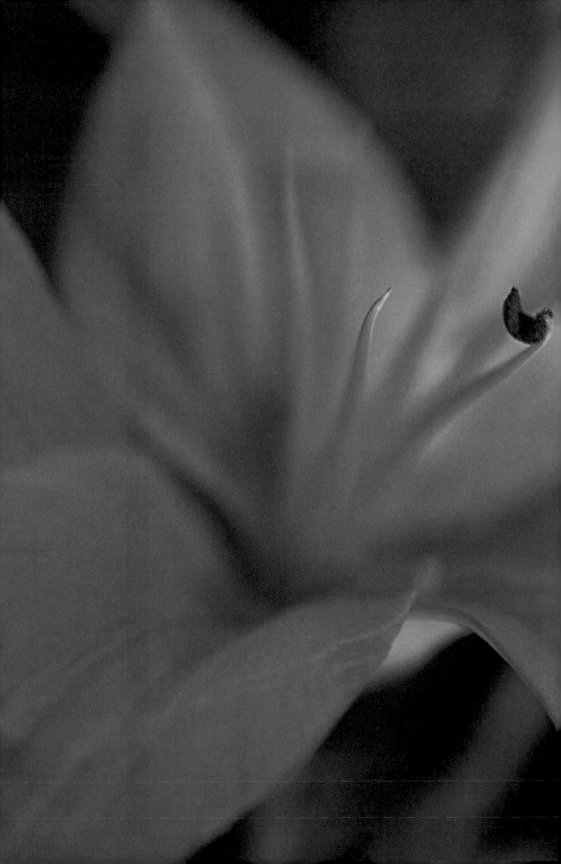

36

MY PERSONAL CHALLENGE TO YOU

"In the last analysis, great human achievement rests on perfect physical health." — *Emerson*

"It's a funny thing about life; if you refuse to accept anything but the best, you very often get it."
— *W. Somerset Maugham*

"What the caterpillar calls the end of the world, the master calls a butterfly." — *Richard Bach, Illusions*

"I challenge you to make your life a masterpiece.
I challenge you to join the ranks of those people who live what they teach, who walk their talk.
Live with passion!" — *Anthony Robbins*

"Champions aren't made in gyms. Champions are made from something they have deep inside them — a desire, a dream, a vision."
— *Muhammad Ali*

My challenge to you is to become the divine being you are capable of becoming. We are creators of circumstance, never creatures of circumstance. We can become anything we desire. We can fulfill every goal. We can achieve a state of total prosperity, perpetual health and youthfulness.

The cosmic laws are always in operation. The Laws of Nature are here, and they remain here. "As you think, so shall it be" is part of the code — it is written into everything. From the seeds of your thought spring all the events and material objects around you. From great thinking arises a great life.

You get out of life what you expect to get. If you expect massive abundance, you shall receive massive abundance. Your state of mind controls your state of results. You create your own reality. Cultivate within your garden-mind an abundant success consciousness.

Life is a self-fulfilling prophecy. Whatever you truly want will happen.

Dare to take possession of your own mind! Your thought habits are created by the mental food that your mind consistently dwells upon, just as your eating habits are created by the food you consistently eat. When you plant the seeds of prosperity in your garden-mind, they will always grow.

What you think dramatically affects the way you eat. What you eat dramatically affects the way you think. Food has a consciousness. One cannot remain positive long by ingesting a consciousness of fire, poison, pain and death. When one takes in positive, living food and positive, living thoughts, one also becomes positive and living! What an amazing truth this is! Dead food and negative thoughts lead to ruin.

Eat the divine food offered to us by the Sun-God Ra (Raw)! The Raw Law is unlimited. It does not end today or tomorrow. It persists for all time.

Increase your energy. Digestion is the number one energy zapper. To increase your energy, eat less and breathe more!

Make your body a supreme physical support system, so that it will carry you to distant goals and your most treasured dreams. Purify! Get there I say! From purity arises divinity.

Eden is here on Earth. It is right where you are at this moment. You are standing right now on your own "Acres of Diamonds." Paradise is a state of consciousness. All you have to do is purify yourself and you automatically arrive.

The Sunfood Diet Success System works — every time. Simplicity is the key. Use the 36 lessons in this book to help you lead a simple and beautiful life. As the philosopher Friedrich Nietzsche wrote: "To live simply and naturally is the highest and final goal."

The Sunfood Diet Success System places you in a magical world of continual renewal. When you stay this path long enough, many of the profound mysteries of the world will be opened to you. You will come to discover that for the complete reconstruction and rejuvenation of this planet and its inhabitants, there are tremendous projects afoot.

Life is an incredible adventure. You should spend every moment of your life fully alive, never bored. You should be growing, becoming better in every single way.

Surround yourself with those who can push you to your limits, who can challenge you to be everything you can be and more.

Transform all your trials and tribulations, your battles of mind and diet, your thirsting in the desert of knowledge, into flowing grace. Allow grace to embrace you.

Transform an ephemeral life into one of dynamic longevity. Allow age to ennoble you.

When your time is passed, let others say, "Now there was one who really lived life! There was one who chose the uncommon path, and achieved an uncommon destiny of health, happiness and success." The choice is yours: a long life of glory, or a short, uneventful life in obscurity. What will it be?

You are the heir to all the ages, in the foremost ranks of time. You are a genius, a masterpiece of Nature. Embrace the abundance life has to offer. Trust your judgment. Take action! (Nothing is more fulfilling than taking action). By your fruits you shall be known! As Emerson stated: "Your actions speak so loudly that no one can ever hear a word you are saying!"

What counts is action — acting instead of talking. When you decide to do something you must go all the way. You must know exactly why you are doing it. Then you must proceed with massive action without having doubts or remorse. Keep moving forward, until it is done.

Success is not a goal, but a process, a way of living, a series of habits. Successful people practice fundamentals every day. Successful people take daily consistent action towards their life's purpose.

Everything in life is cumulative. Everything counts. Stack the odds in your favor whenever possible. When you use any one of the lessons in this book today, you have made a positive choice for your future, your children's future, and the planet's future.

It is time to awaken, to think, to believe, to desire, to act in faith and fulfill. Within you are the seeds of greatness. Revel in the joy of your true Nature. Step into your mastery and climb the ladder of your destiny.

Fulfill your purpose! Walk your talk! Become more than you ever thought possible. Reach the highest state of perfection imaginable. Attract to yourself an abundance of spiritual, mental, emotional, physical and financial wealth! Cultivate a philosophy of perfect health consciousness. Enjoy every moment of life's adventure. Laugh your way to the top!

A great transformation in a single individual can alter the destiny of the human race.

What would your life be like if you were to do the impossible?

Take on heroic, sacred attributes. There is a mysterious, almost magical charm about the personality of true greatness. A magical being is a sight to behold.

Dare to be bold. Spiritual forces will come to your aid. The bolder you are, the more magnetic is your presence. Boldness has a mystical quality to it, it creates an invisible force-field around you that deflects all attacks and attracts every-thing you need.

Go after what you really want, that state which humankind has always aspired to, the manifestation of the divinity within, here and now. The spiritual power lies within you. It is the unlimited power which provides superhuman strength of body, mind and spirit. It is yours to use. Use it.

We sense there are two sides to our nature. You exist in this form as part animal, part deity; we are a spirit animated in a physical body. The glorious journey is to become as much of a deity as possible and ascend to our highest potential. To that end we desire a health which allows the full expression of our spirit through our physical body. You are a divine being who walks the Earth — start living like one.

Decide to be, and command forth, the youthful spirit. Become powerful, passionate, outstanding in your field. Accelerate the energy within you at any moment. Live your dreams. Succeeding is so much fun!

Best wishes on your journey. May the force be with you.

Keep facing the Sun and the shadows will fall behind.

The Master

A friend of the brave,
Gives strength to the weak.
Who loves the Beautiful,
And builds up the meek.

Who breathes in:
To win.
Who breathes out
All-doubt.

Who calls up high-daring,
And casts down despair.
To rule the Earth,
To run with the Fair.

The Solar Vibration
And wild charm,
Impeccable to live
Without causing harm.

The choice of word,
And dramatic timing.
Passion, deep meaning.
Eyes: clear and shining.

Light of foot,
Intuition,
Heavy wit, Grace,
Decision.

Glory,
Great Fortune,
The Effortless
In action.

The Grand Logic,
Magnetic.
Abundant
Symmetric.

The Cosmic Forge
A dance of the stars.
The Destiny,
The smooth sea —
Perfection.

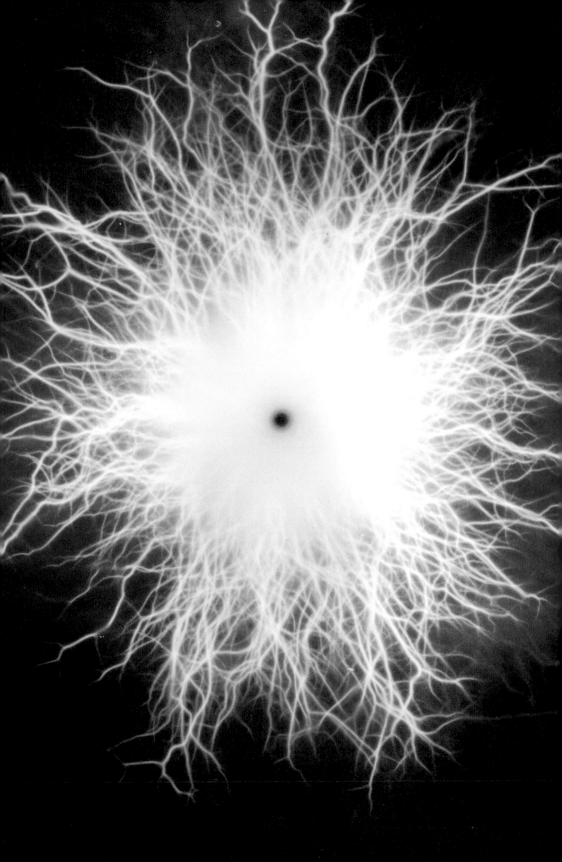

A MESSAGE TO ALL SUNFOODISTS

"And when much of the people were gathered together,
and were come to him out of every city, Jesus spake by a
parable: 'A sower went out to sow his seed: and as he
sowed, some fell by the way side; and it was trodden
down, and the fowls of the air devoured it. And some
fell upon a rock; and as soon as it was sprung up, it
withered away, because it lacked moisture. And some
fell among thorns; and the thorns sprang up with it, and
choked it. And others fell on good ground and sprang up,
and bore fruit a hundredfold.' And when he had said these
things, he cried, 'He that hath ears to hear, let him hear.'
And his disciples asked him, saying, 'What might this
parable be?' And he said, 'Unto you it is given to know
the mysteries of the Kingdom of God: but to others in
parables; that seeing they might not see, and hearing they
might not understand. Now the parable is this:
The seed is the word of God.'"— *Luke 8:4-11*

"There is nothing more powerful than
an idea whose time has come."— *Victor Hugo*

This book is the flower, you are the fruit. Go out and spread the seeds of good fortune. Let others devour your knowledge.

It is imperative for us as Sunfoodists to become attractive artists, wonderful parents, friendly farmers, great inventors, glorious statesmen, spiritual giants, magical millionaires, famous actresses and actors and mystical musicians. By our achievements we will attract attention to this lifestyle. We will spread this information by our inspiring example to the farthest corners of the world.

You are an incredible human being. I have tremendous respect for you being the type of person who took the time to read this book.

My message to you is to walk your talk; example is not the main thing influencing others, it is the only thing. Especially if you are teaching The Sunfood Diet Success System, first go to work on yourself, then set about the business of attracting new interest.

> The eye's an amazing student,
> And more telling than the ear,
> Fine words are important,
> But the example's always clear.

Unfortunately, in the past, there have been many promoters of raw plant-food diets who did not walk their talk. Therefore, their information was not accurate, and even though they carried the message forward transforming many lives, it did lead many people astray.

The Sunfood Diet is about massive abundance. The Sunfood Diet cannot be about restriction and denial. When you are teaching the raw plant-food diet, let people know that their choices are abundant. If they want to eat a lot or a little, it does not matter. If intuition is followed and the guidelines of this book are followed, the result of vibrant health and living in harmony with Nature will be achieved.

After many years of promoting a raw-food lifestyle, I have found that the best way to introduce The Sunfood Diet to other people is to be a shining example of health and vitality myself. This is always the best way to attract people to the Sunfood lifestyle.

Become the example. You are in a much better position to communicate with people when they approach you, rather than when you approach them. Have them ask you about your amazing state of health. I have had women approach me from out of the blue and ask to touch my skin or ask me what is my secret. When this occurs you are in a powerful position to forward this vital Sunfood information. When someone approaches you like this, when they see your vitality, your transformation, don't give away the farm. Make them work for the information. When they ask, "What's your secret?" Just smile and say, "It's a secret." That will arouse their curiosity and make it much more likely they will take action when you do eventually tell them about this information! It will also make the situation much more fun.

Aside from the charismatic power of your own example, I have found the top two approaches to help people discover the raw-food truth for themselves are as follows:

Approach 1. "Life is designed raw." Out of trillions of organisms that were alive at the beginning of time, are alive now and will be alive at the end of time, only one tampers with its food. You do not want to bet against those kinds of odds.

Approach 2. "You can't convince a child." Children naturally gravitate towards brightly-colored fruits. My friend Lenny Watson, a long-time raw-foodist and natural healer from Maui, tells us, "You don't start a child on macrobiotic food." Children intuitively know that their natural foods are raw fruits and vegetables.

As you communicate this information, people will say "no" to you. The best salespeople know how to do deal with doubters, pessimists, the disinterested and the apathetic. The best salespeople have overcome their fear of rejection. They just say, "Next." Move on to someone else. There are billions of people who need this information and millions who will listen and take action. Go forth, find them, leverage your mind to present this information to them in the most attractive way possible.

Some Do. Some Don't.

Some do.
Some don't.
Some will,
Some won't.
Some do now,
Some do later.
Some never do
And say : "See you later."

Some get it,
Some don't.
Some grasp it,
Some won't.
Some live,
Some die.
Some ask:
"Why?"
Why it is? Who knows.
It's just how it goes.

Some laugh,
Some cry.
Some are honest,
Some lie.
Some win,
And some tie.
Some say: "Just try."
Be curious.
Move on.
Some pro,
Some con.

Some fake it.
Some make it.
Work with it,
Not against it.
Some slip,
Some rise.
Some see
With clear eyes.

You can't
Change it,
Rearrange it.
It's the set up,
Just face it.
But you can
Change yourself.
To attract some —
Living wealth.

Your goal
You control.

Some believe,
Some achieve.
Some reach,
Some hold.
Some are shy,
Some are bold.
Some grow,
Some won't.
Some do.
Some don't.

Dynamic Communication

Start talking to people about raw foods. Become a dynamic communicator. The more precise our communication with ourselves and others, the more effective we are, because we humans are gregarious, social beings.

Communication is more than it seems. Discover how to communicate. First, tell your voice it is in harmony with the sounds of Nature. Then, tell your skin it glows with smooth perfection. Next, begin to talk health into every organ of your own or another's body. Tell yourself or another that their muscles are limber, shapely, and beautiful. Tell your mind, or another's mind, that it is functioning at peak efficiency. Master personal communication skills. Choose your body language, tone of voice, and words carefully.

Be aware of the 55:38:7 communication equation. 55% of your communication (as it is perceived by others) is non-verbal. This includes: physiology, body language, eye contact and gestures. 38% comes from the sound and tone of your voice. 7% of your communication is the based on the actual content of what you are saying.

Be there in the present moment with anyone you find before you throughout the day. Really listen to what they are telling you. Ask questions. Some of the most incredible stories I have ever heard came from seemingly boring people. I find something fascinating in every person I meet. When you are a good listener, you not only know what you know, but you also know what the other person knows.

Teaching is not about preaching, it is about asking questions. How can I know how I can help someone nutritionally if I do not know anything about them? By asking questions, I can discover everything I need to help!

Questions are answers. Just as you can focus your own brain's energy by asking yourself specific questions, you can also direct the focus of someone else's brain by asking her/him specific questions.

As individuals who live the Sunfood lifestyle, we should understand that the history of cooked food has caused more than raw food alone can cure. Other healing modalities, such as massage, yoga, meditation, walking, playing, and laughing all have their place. But the raw-food information is the key to the whole thing — it makes everything else work amazingly well. This information is absolutely vital to the future health and happiness of the planet. People can always use a boost, they need The Sunfood Diet Success System in their hands and hearts. Challenge yourself to push this message into the world. Speak up when you would have held your tongue.

Pass It On

If there is a blessing known,
If a better way is shown,
Pass it on.
Send it out on waves of thought.
Let it find one who has sought.
Pass it on.
Inspire it in each holy mind,
Let it produce after its kind.
Pass it on.
Let it travel down the years,
Let it dry another's tears,
Until in heaven the deed appears,
Please pass it on.

I want you to know that I feel tremendously fortunate to be a voice in the world for raw foods, superfoods, superherbs, living water, and the magical aspects of radical health transformation. I would like to thank you for your interest in becoming all that you can possibly be.

Together we must carry the Sunfood Diet message forward. Together we can turn this world into a paradise. You, who have glimpsed your true potential, will be among the leaders of a new dispensation on Earth.

"We, the new, the nameless, the hard-to-understand, we firstlings of a yet untried future — we require for a new end also a new means, namely, a new healthiness, stronger, sharper, tougher, bolder, and merrier than any healthiness hitherto. He whose soul longs to experience the whole range of hitherto recognized values and desirabilities, and to circumnavigate all the coasts of this ideal "Mediterranean Sea," who, from the adventures of his most personal experience, wants to know how it feels to be a conqueror and discoverer of the ideal — as likewise how it is with the artist, the saint, the legislator, the sage, the scholar, the devotee, the prophet, and the godly Nonconformist of the old style: — requires one thing above all for that purpose, great healthiness — such healthiness as one not only possesses, but also constantly acquires and must acquire, because one continually sacrifices it again, and must sacrifice it! — And now, after having been long on the way in this fashion, we Argonauts of the ideal, who are more courageous perhaps than prudent, and often enough shipwrecked and brought to grief, nevertheless, as said above, healthier than people would like to admit, dangerously healthy, always healthy again, — it would seem, as if in recompense for it all, that we have a still undiscovered country before us, the boundaries of which no one has yet seen, a beyond to all countries and corners of the ideal known hitherto, a world so over-rich in the beautiful, the strange, the questionable, the frightful, and the divine, that our curiosity as well as our thirst for the possession thereof, have got out of hand — alas! that nothing will any longer satisfy us!"

– Friedrich Nietzsche, Joyful Wisdom

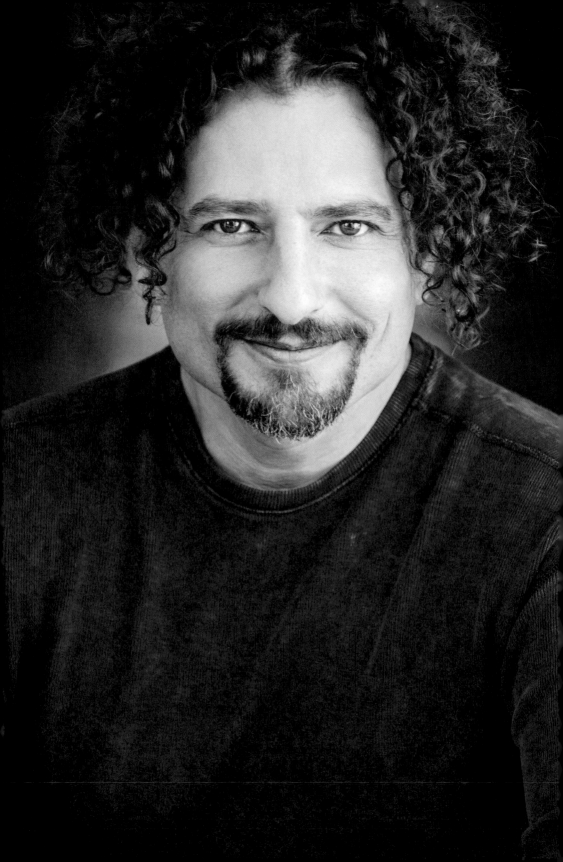

SELECTED POETRY

It was thought that ruled,
When Augustus fueled,
The ships of ancient Rome.
It was thought that led Columbus,
Over the Atlantic's foam.

It was thought that guided the astro-naughts,
To the Moon's Tranquillity Bay.
Thought is the power which rules the world:
This is the logic of today.

Thought alone is the building stone,
The total of which you're the sum,
The strangest secret of success in life is:
What you think about you become.

Behind the world's greatest minds,
Lies the primordial law,
Brilliant thoughts, radiant ideas,
To hold the world in awe.

The thinking mind creates the future,
All "luck" is a fraud.
Each mind is a creative force,
With the potential of a god.

Actualize your thoughts
Through deeds of splendor and renown.
Face your inner fears,
And they retreat without a sound.

Creative minds may free the Earth,
When action is taken thereon,
And Liberty to those who know:
What you think about — you become.

For thoughts command when people reach,
Outward towards the stars,
And it was thought which dropped the probe,
Onto the surface of Mars.

It was thought that ruled,
When the druids built
Astronomic Temples of stone and clay.
This is the testimony of the ancients:
And the logic of today.

And thoughts direct when empires sink,
In storms of steel and flame.
And it is by thought alone
That seeds are sown —
And it will always be the same.

The powerful thoughts
Of those who act,
Rush forth to fill the mass,
Of thoughtless minds
Who should invest their lives,
Growing gardens instead of grass.

Harmonize with the Earth and trees,
People and plant are one,
The greatest truth of all the world is:
What you think about you become.

Thought governs all organic life,
Inspires all right and wrong.
It's Nature's plan to give a helping hand,
To those whose thoughts are strong.

By thought you may ride to glory —
Let nothing bar your way,
And if you decide to rule your thoughts:
You've grasped the logic of today.

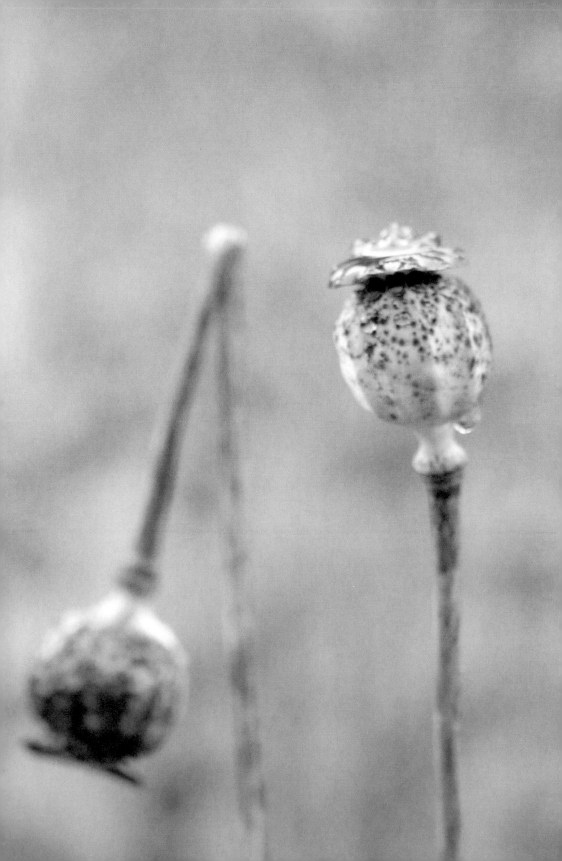

YE ARE GODS

"...Is it not written in your law, I said, Ye Are Gods?"

A fascinating abstraction.
The pranic interaction.

The Empyreal Living Sea.
Pantamorphic energy.

Galama. Air. Radiation.
You are a —
Perfect Creation.

Bubbling springs of sweet, clear blue.
Ye are Gods! I tell you!

Humans need little here.
The simple needs are few!
Some fruits to smell and herbs to feel,
Good thoughts for an evening meal,
The truths the immortals knew.

The secret trite
and simple rite:
"Air for dinner,
Makes a winner."

Bathed within
Oceans of gas
Billions of sparks unseen.
The purest fuel of immortal Life,
Burns so pure and clean.

No residue remaining.
No ash to remove.
Air alone sustaining.
Float instead of move.

The secret now revealed:
Grow in the open air,
Breathe and sleep with the earth,
Dream deeply of the fair.

To see the good in everybody,
Think what is only true,
Breathe in life above the strife,
And show what you can do.

Emanate the impeccably true,
Ye are Gods! I tell you!

Obey your own conviction,
Love. Wisdom. Perfection.

Touch what can't be touched,
See what can't be seen.
Let the drama unfold,
No need to intervene.

Float on intuition,
Go with what you feel,
Only what you sense is true,
Can ever become so real.

An energetic forcefield,
An energetic seeing,
Not eating for a living,
Is a new way of being.

Stop the world, right on cue.
Ye are Gods! I tell you!

Paradox is reality,
Life is Destiny.

"As above you so below".
See the living planet glow.

Rhythm and antiquity.
Deep unsolved history.

Stillness, solitude, open space.
The beauty of being in this place.

The Earth is bliss
Between the worlds.
At the dawn,
A mystery unfurls.

Clear view of Sun,
Sky, stars, clouds,
Moon, cliffrock, canyon.
Dance among the sounds.

Time enough to allow
Thought and feeling to range far.
From here to the end of the world and back.
Travel from star to star.

The more harmonious you become
To the beat of the vital heart,
The more you will attract to your being
The whole, instead of the part.

Surrender all your ideas,
Things are not what they seem.
Here, within all worlds,
We can only live our dream.

Action. Life. Manifestation.
You are a —
Perfect Creation.

Trust the spirit, desire it too.
Ye are Gods! I tell you!

Transmit the signal,
Harmonize the storm
The Ascended Masters
Are here in form.

Abundant love
You attract.
Abundant health,
No turning back;
Abundant life
It's a game, you see,
Abundant world
Fulfill your Destiny.

The Ascended Ones shower you;
Their vibration soon to strengthen you!
They seed your creative fire,
It's reality as you desire.

Be extremely quiet
Have no diet
And create,
Gather your spirit
Emanate:
The master work,
The philosopher's stone,
The elixir of life,
Few have known.

Materialized before you,
The mysterious, secret chain,
The Cosmic Circuit Board
Connecting every plane.

The white powder of gold
What Enoch left untold.

Ascended Master
Impeccable Faster
You are Creators upon this plane.

The NeFiLim
Are upon the Earth.
This is the moment
Of your rebirth.

As you ask you shall receive.
What you see is what you believe.
What you think in life you are.
Your breath alone will take you far.

With focus you surpass
All the expectations.
Manifestation is instant,
In this time of transmutations.

Float so high you find yourself
In constant states of joy and health!
Then you'll know with ease and grace.
The mystery of the secret face.

The divine force
In physical form.
Magic presence.
Beyond the norm.
Perfect potential.
Life abounds.
Slow the breath,
Hear cosmic sounds.

You're obsidian, volcanic
A pulsing ember, organic.
You're a limitless being, creating anew,
Ye are Gods! I tell you!

All is perfection,
All is divine.
Don't eat...listen
And soon you shall find.

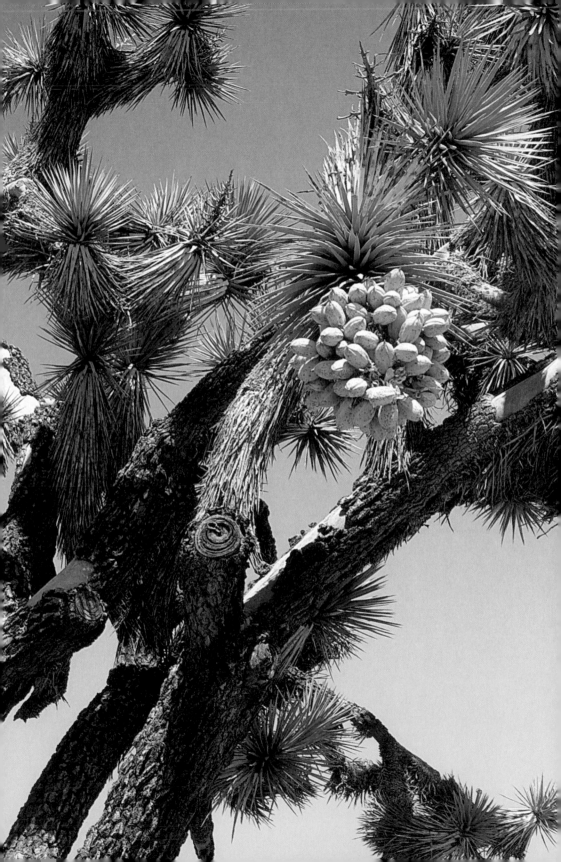

MAJESTY

Nature's test is:
The trial by fire.
To fall with the ash
Or rise ever higher.

You may become:
An elegant being.
A genetic titan
With entirely new meaning.

A spiritual giant.
Baroque, classic,
Masterful, effective,
Totally dynamic.
A great, bold spirit
With impeccable logic.
Embodied pure form
Majestic, high-gothic.

But a challenge awaits.
One truth you must face:

It stumbles the beggar,
It fells the queen,
A gift of the gods?
Or a curse cast unclean?

The eternal lie,
The primitive flame
Its sapping potential
The most dangerous game.

Its flaming wings:
Dispel the magic,
Bring paradise lost,
Give birth to the tragic.

Confusing the mind,
Emotions entwined,
Forging a path where
Life's not designed.

The flames are about
And nearing they seize:
Life, love, and laughter,
Even the trees.

The peril is high
The passion arising
The flames upon you
The urgency rising.

Choosing now
What to believe.
To trust in You.
Is not to deceive.

Summon the symbol,
A Courage long past.
The Sun-Fired crest,
Revive it at last.

It's a trial by fire.
None excepted
Who will pass?
Each is tested.

The cosmic law:
Of paradox shifting,
That which destroys
Is also uplifting.

The flaming wings of divine tragedy,
Can uplift you to a soaring majesty.

Must all the gods die?
Have you found out why?

Age ennobles
The legends untold
Thrust through the eons
The karmas unfold.

The Fates deciding
The zodiak throw,
The pantheon crumbles
Impending overthrow.

Obscuring the Sun,
The ominous clash,
Mind-states in ruin,
Consumers of ash.

Descending now
The savage curtain,
And for the noble
The test is certain.
It's the twilight of the gods,
The wolf-god's unleashed,
Will you choose beauty...
Or the beast?

The destruction, ecliptic,
Ruins, apocalyptic.

The queen stares
The cities in fire
But the phoenix flames
Are rising higher.

It's a trial by fire.
None excepted
Who will pass?
Each is tested.

The cosmic law:
Of paradox shifting,
That which destroys
Is also uplifting.

The flaming wings of divine tragedy,
Can uplift you to a soaring majesty.

The killing words,
The elegant whisper:
"You will become more than you were."

It's the cosmic law:
That opposition breeds
A fertile ash for
Transforming seeds.

The solar beat,
A rhythm drumming,
You are pure life
Pure becoming.

Gather your strength,
Arise from the ashes!
Grasp now
What intuition flashes!

The biological aim,
The inner direction,
The fulfillment of what
Was ordained at conception.

A new royal
Dynastic crown,
You may be reborn
Of the sky and ground.

It's a trial by fire.
None excepted
Who will pass?
Each is tested.

The cosmic law:
Of paradox shifting,
That which destroys
Is also uplifting.

The flaming wings of divine tragedy.
Can uplift you to a soaring Majesty.

Faustian life striving
For infinite space.
A rhythm alive
From Rome to Thrace.

The love of wild Nature,
The mysterious compassion,
The ineffable forsakeness
An intangible fashion.

Will-to-power,
The passionate striving,
Uncompromised truth,
Forever is driving.

The electric thrill
In overthrowing
Regressing life
Never growing.

Aristocrat features:
Wild-animal eyes.
Staring deeply,
See through the lies.

True conviction belongs to the wise,
There is no strength in compromise.

Surpass, overcome,
Overwhelm all denial,
In Nature there is
Only one trial.

It's a trial by fire.
None excepted
Who will pass?
Each is tested.

The cosmic law:
Of paradox shifting,
That which destroys
Is also uplifting.

The flaming wings of divine tragedy.
Can uplift you to a soaring Majesty.

The heavenly bodies,
Both hemispheres,
A celestial symphony,
The conjunction nears

The maximum moment
The cosmic flowing
The zodiak spinning
Inspiration growing.

The destiny appears,
The mind-world showing
The tarot spinning.
Vision overflowing.

Insight deep from
A simple deduction:
"Wrong thinking leads on to destruction."

Insight clear from
A cosmic instruction:
"All death is caused by internal obstruction."

Opposition leads
to transformation.
You are complete:
A perfect creation.

Draw in the knowledge
A meteor shower,
Tune in the body,
Embrace its power!

A feeling of flowing,
Wondrous grace,
To always be found
In the right place.

"You are the reflection of transcendent perfection."

Unstoppable volition.
Philosophic insight.
Mystic premonition.
This is your right.

Purify the body,
The cosmic receiver
Dismiss away doubt
The greatest deceiver.

It's a trial by fire.
None excepted
Who will pass?
Each is tested.

The cosmic law:
Of paradox shifting
That which destroys
Is also uplifting.

The flaming wings of divine tragedy.
Can uplift you to a soaring Majesty.

The planets in glory
The ocean in pearls
Throughout the ether
The nebulae swirls.

The desire for life,
A cosmic imperium
Begins a thought seeking:
Mind-world dominion.

You are the sculptor,
You build the worlds.
From the font of a thought
Your destiny unfurls.

The gehenna fire
The cosmic joke.
Disintegrate now
Its plume of smoke.

Extinguish the fire
In which life burns;
Release pain's liar
From whom one learns.

How many times
Will you rise from the ashes?
With each death,
The Phoenix flashes:
The perception brighter,
The mind more alive,
Sensitive, elastic,
A new call to thrive.

Dragon Mistress,
The ancient quest,
Put down the flame,
For massive success.

Abundant life of
Archaic Earth
Now undergoes
A Gothic rebirth.

Architect of archetypes
In the mind-world array.
Actualize your form
Tomorrow is today.

It's Twilight in Olympus.
A mystic rage for order
Magic-moment chaos:
The You World Order.

It's a trial by fire.
None excepted
Who will pass?
Each is tested.

The cosmic law:
Of paradox shifting,
That which destroys
Is also uplifting.

The flaming wings of divine tragedy.
Can uplift you to a soaring Majesty.

It's the ineffable truth,
The eternal test,
That fire captures
All but the best.

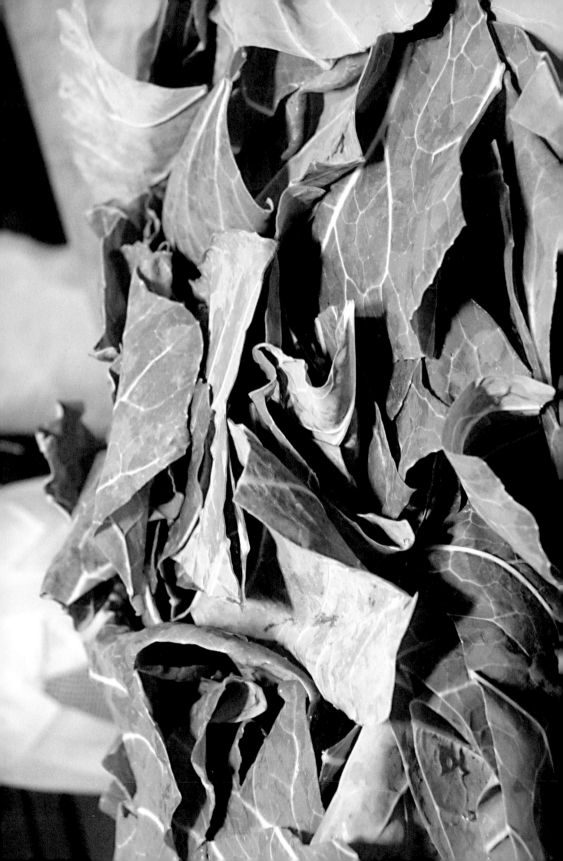

A P P E N D I X

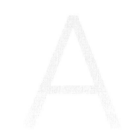

ANATOMY CHART

Is a human being a carnivore, herbivore or omnivore?

	CARNIVORE	HERBIVORE	HUMAN
1	Teeth are long, sharp and pointed. No flat molar teeth. Sharp canine teeth.	Front and canine teeth may be sharp or pointed. Back teeth are flattened for grinding.	All teeth are flattened, especially the back molars. Dullest canine teeth of all primates.
2	To facilitate tearing and biting, jaw can only move up and down (vertically).	To facilitate the grinding of vegetable foods, jaw can move both up and down (vertically) and side to side.	To facilitate the grinding of vegetable foods, jaw can move both up and down (vertically) and side to side (horizontally)
3	No lip or pouchy cheek structure.	Adaptable lip and pouchy cheek structure.	Refined lip and pouchy cheek structure.
4	Shape of the face allows the carnivore to dig into a carcass and rip out the entrails.	Shape of the face allows the animal to pull vegetation off of plants.	Shape of the face clearly indicates that humans have no ability to rip out entrails with their mouth.
5	Forward facing eyes; binocular vision.	Herbivores with predators: radial eyeset allowing for wide field of vision. Herbivores without predators: forward facing eyes; binocular vision.	Forward facing eyes; binocular vision. Humans have no natural predators.
6	Drinks water by lifting it into the throat with the tongue.	Drinks water by suction.	Drinks water by suction.
7	Tongue is rough and thin.	Tongue is smooth and thick to manipulate vegetable matter into the back molars for grinding.	Tongue is smooth and thick to manipulate vegetable matter into the back molars for grinding.
8	Zonary placenta.	Placenta non-deciduate.	Discoidal placenta.
9	Intestines are 3 times as long as the trunk of the body; their design facilitates rapid expulsion of fleshy matter.	Intestines are at least 8 to 12 times as long as the trunk of the body; they are designed for extracting all nutrients from plant fiber.	Intestines are at least 12 times as long as the trunk, and an integral part of the most sophisticated juice extractor in the world: the human digestive system.

	CARNIVORE	HERBIVORE	HUMAN
10	Liver contains uricase, an enzyme used to break down uric acid; it can break down 10 to 15 times as much uric acid as a herbivore.	Liver has a low tolerance for uric acid.	Liver has a low tolerance for uric acid.
11	Bowels are smooth and short for quick expulsion of waste matter.	Bowels are sulcified and complex for the reconstitution of waste matter.	Bowel walls are puckered, convoluted, and full of deep pouches for the reconstitution of waste matter.
12	Digestive system has the capacity to expel large amounts of foreign cholesterol.	Digestive system has no capacity to expel foreign cholesterol.	Digestive system has no capacity to expel foreign cholesterol.
13	Saliva is acidic.	Saliva is alkaline; it contains enzymes specifically designed to break down starchy carbohydrates.	Saliva is alkaline; it contains ptyalin, an enzyme specifically designed to break down starchy carbohydrates.
14	Blood is acidic.	Blood is alkaline.	Blood is alkaline.
15	Urine is acidic.	Urine is alkaline.	Urine is alkaline.
16	Cools itself primarily through action of the tongue and mouth (panting).	Cools itself primarily through perspiration.	Cools itself primarily through perspiration.
17	All four feet are clawed (to rip into flesh).	All four feet are hoofed (cloven) or hands and feet contain individual digits (fingers or toes) with nails.	Hands and feet contain individual digits with nails and opposable thumbs. Hands are perfectly designed to reach out, grab fruit and peel it.

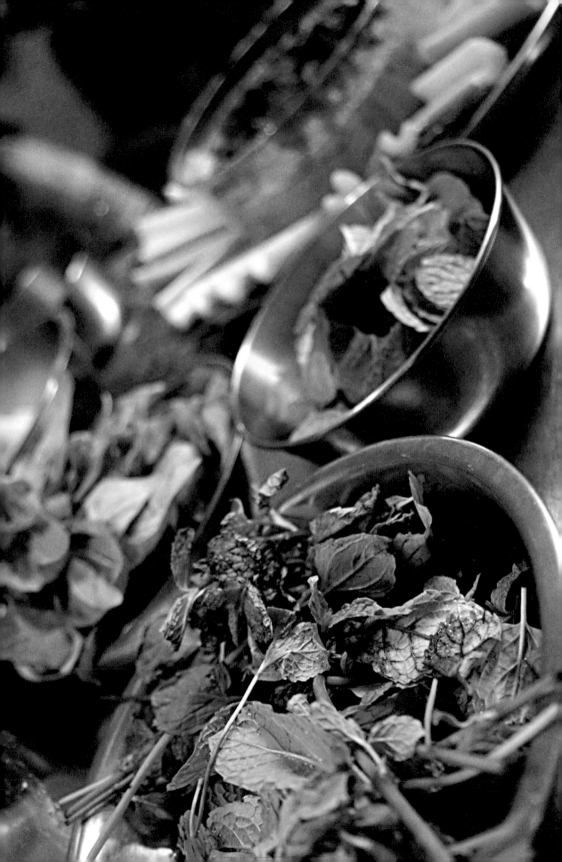

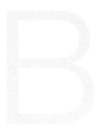

THE SUNFOOD DIET
Weekly Guideline and Menu Plan

Green-Leafy Vegetables, Fruits and Fats

A fruit is any natural food containing seeds (e.g. tomato is a fruit, cucumber is a fruit). Eat fruits with seeds (avoid seedless hybrid fruit).

All types of vegetables are great, however, preference should be given to green-leafed vegetables. Avoid juiced or cooked hybrid vegetables (i.e. carrots, beets, potatoes).

All types of raw plant foods that contain fats help transition over from cooked and processed foods to raw-plant-based nutrition. They satiate hunger. These include avocados, olives, coconuts, cacao beans, nuts, seeds, etc.

If one is sensitive to sugar, it is a good idea to add oils (flax, olive, hemp, etc.) or protein (spirulina, blue-green algae, maca powder) to smoothies or fruit salads. This will allow a slower time-release of sugar into the blood. If one is extremely sensitive to sweet fruits, replace sweet fruits in the morning with lemon water, cucumber, tomatoes, noni or other low-sugar fruits. Some sweet fruit, however, is necessary in the diet.

Eat nuts and seeds moderately. Quantities should be kept to less than 2.0-2.5 pounds (0.9-1.2 kg) of nuts per week. Eat nuts together with green-leafy vegetables for ideal digestion. If one is sensitive to nuts, then replace all nuts listed in the menu below with avocados, olives or seeds.

All daily menus should contain a healthy balance of green-leafed vegetables (i.e. chard, collards, lettuces, kale, spinach, etc.), sugary fruits (berries, melons, mangos, papayas, etc.) and fatty foods (i.e. avocados, olives, nuts, seeds, etc.). Chlorophyll foods build the structure of the body. Sweet fruits fuel the system with glucose. Fats lubricate and oil the tissues and joints.

Salad Dressings

For salad dressings, combine a raw plant fat with a sugar and a sour element. For example, we can blend half an avocado, a peeled orange and a skinned half of a lemon with a little water in the blender and pour that on our salad as dressing. If we look at most commercial salad dressings on the market, we can see they consist of three basic ingredients — a fat (oil, pasteurized dairy milk), a sugar (high fructose corn syrup) and vinegar. People love fats and sugars with greens because they complete The Sunfood Triangle! The sour element (vinegar, lemon juice) is a digestive aid to help break down fiber.

Water

The amount of water one drinks should be dictated by thirst. Raw fruits and vegetables contain so much high-quality water one may find that thirst markedly diminishes. If you do drink water, preferably drink primary source spring water or, in the alternative, drink a pure water charged with sea salt, Himalayan rock salt, MSM powder, a squeeze of lemon and/or a blade of grass. Drink at least 30 minutes before you eat a meal — drinking water after a meal dilutes the digestive juices and interferes with digestion. Pure water could include Trinity Springs Water or spring waters packaged in glass. Only use water delivered in glass if possible. Always charge distilled water to bring some life and structure into it. A clay egg water dispenser is the ideal water containment system.

Alcohol

One should preferentially choose wine over all other alcohols. Most wines have not been heat-processed. Seek out organic varieties with no sulfites added.

All beers are brewed (cooked). If one does choose to drink beer, one should preferentially choose dark beers with more minerals over refined commercial beers. Dark beers have a less dramatic effect on blood sugar levels.

Gradually letting go of alcohol will strengthen one's immune system, and decrease the risk of an early death in an accident. Remember, alcohol is the most dangerous drug of all.

Dairy Products

Any pasteurized dairy products have long-range destructive effects on health and the digestive system. The only reason pasteurized dairy products are found in stores is because they have a longer shelf life than raw dairy products, and thus they bring more money to the dairy industry.

If dairy products are included in the diet, they should be raw. Children who simply refuse to eat healthy portions of green-leafed vegetables may have raw dairy products in their diet for calcium, other alkaline minerals and DHA (long-chain omega 3 fatty acid). Raw goat's milk is superior to cow's milk because it is closer to human milk and easier to digest.

Raw almond or even processed rice milk are better options than soy (now genetically modified) and cooked cow's milk. Almond milk has a high-fat content, and may be used to "cut" tea or coffee.

Love and Prayer

Everything we eat could and should be saturated with love. Loving our food is the next massive health revolution.

Not only what we eat is important, but how we eat. Take a moment, before you eat a meal and bless the food. Say a prayer. Thank all the people, angels, animals, plants and insects who worked hard to provide you with abundant, beautiful food.

Below are two blessings I use at home and that we use at our raw-food retreats:

THE FAMILY PRAYER

Through this food
And this family
We give ourselves strength
To hold ourselves high
In the light that surrounds us
And is within us
For this is the water
Of the spring of life.

THANKS GIVING

Great spirit.
Thank you
For the all the beings
Who contributed to this meal
And for the vitality of this food.
We relish our bounty
And revere your creation.

Chewing

Be sure to fully chew every mouthful of food. The famous Dr. Fletcher recommended 50 chews per mouthful.

Try eating with chopsticks instead of kitchen utensils as they will help to slow the rate of your eating.

Sea Vegetables

With raw nutrition, sea vegetables have a balancing effect because they contain a dense amount of trace minerals and alkaline-mineral salts. Sea vegetables, however, grow in the sea, and are subject to intake the pollution found there. Reputable sources for these products are important.

Variety

Among wild primates, approximately 25 different raw plant foods are eaten each week. In a year, wild primates eat up to 115 different varieties of raw plant foods. This provides us with some great guidelines and goals for our own diet. Enjoy a wide variety of fruits, vegetables, nuts, seeds, seaweeds, sprouts, grasses, herbs, flowers and superfoods. Rotation is the natural way of eating — seasons help dictate our diet this way. Always err on the side of eating more variety and drinking more vegetable juices.

Transitional Strategy

Eat as high a percentage of raw-plant foods in your diet as possible. Feel free to eat large quantities of raw plant foods if you feel so inclined. Discover sources for raw organic foods either locally or through Internet mail order. Items that may be unfamiliar, such as hempseed oil, spirulina, maca or goji berries may be found at a natural-food store.

Any cooked foods should preferentially be eaten in the evening, and then only one type at a time. Always combine any cooked food with the evening's large salad and freshly-made vegetable juice.

Cooked starches should be those which are lower on the Glycemic Index Chart shown in **Lesson 11: The Secret Revealed**, such as yams or sweet potatoes.

Transitioning off of red meat initially, then pork, chicken, fish and finally cooked dairy products is an excellent way to let go of animal foods. For all the reasons I have outlined in this book, it is very important for our own health and success, as well as the health of the planet, to let go of these foods.

Remember the simple rule: Simplicity is bliss.

Three complete menu plans, corresponding to three stages of transition, are provided in the following pages: **The Basic Sunfood Diet, The 80/20 Sunfood Diet** and **The All-Raw Diet**. The concepts here are simple. These menus are provided to give you an idea as to what it is like to be a raw-foodist on a day-to-day basis.

You may choose to use raw-food recipe books to help create even more fantastic cuisine beyond the simple ideas I provide below. Discover a host of new ideas in this area of exciting cuisine. Learn to create dehydrated crackers at low temperatures, raw ice creams and many, many other culinary delights.

The menus are provided to give you an idea of where to start. They are not the "law." Be flexible. Be easy on yourself. Transition at your own pace.

Many different types of prepared raw-food treats are now available on the Internet and in healthfood stores. These are great for traveling and for snacking. Feel free to add those into your diet.

Unless otherwise stated, all menu items should be raw, plant-based and organic.

THE BASIC SUNFOOD DIET WEEKLY MENU

The Basic Sunfood Diet

At this level, the focus is to include significantly more raw plant foods and their juices into the diet. At this level, one should make the commitment to seek out organic foods.

This diet is about abundance, not denial. Therefore, on **Day 5: Friday** and **Day 6: Saturday** one may still eat their favorite meals in the evening but with a salad. Over time, as one eats more raw foods containing the three food classes along with a wide variety of superfoods and other raw plant foods, and less cooked foods, the taste buds will change and a dietary shift will happen automatically.

MONDAY BASIC

Breakfast

8 ounces (1/4 liter) of herbal tea. Squeeze in fresh lemon if desired. Use raw honey or maple syrup to sweeten.

One blended super smoothie containing: coconut water, berries (all types), maca powder (2 tablespoons) and coconut oil (2 tablespoons).

Or

1 shot (1 ounce) of wheatgrass juice.

2 persimmons.

2 slices of watermelon (not seedless).

Lunch

One small green-leafed vegetable salad. Squeeze lemon into the salad along with olive oil as dressing.

One sandwich made with toasted sprouted grain bread, avocado, clover sprouts, diced red bell pepper, red onion and diced cucumber.

Snacks

1 young coconut with inner flesh.

2 oranges.

1 handful of hempseeds.

Dehydrated flax crackers with guacamole.

Dinner

One large lettuce, cucumber, tomato, spinach, clover sprout and green onion salad with two avocados and a fresh-squeezed lemon and olive oil as dressing. Add raw sauerkraut or kim-chi to the salad as desired.

One meal of cooked starch (brown rice, baked yams and/or sweet potatoes are preferred over potatoes).

1/2 quart (1/2 liter) of freshly-made vegetable juice containing at least 60% green vegetables (i.e. celery, lettuce, broccoli, etc.), 40% other vegetables or fruits (i.e. apple, cucumber, etc.).

TUESDAY BASIC

Breakfast

8 ounces (1/4 liter) of herbal tea. Squeeze in fresh lemon if desired. Use raw honey or maple syrup to sweeten.

14 ounces (0.4 liters) of a blended berry smoothie containing: water, blueberries, blackberries, raspberries and strawberries. Add 2 tablespoons of hempseeds and/or 2 tablespoons of blue-green algae if desired.

Lunch

One small green-leafed vegetable salad with one avocado. Add fresh-blended lemon, basil, miso and avocado as a dressing.

One item of cooked starch (baked, no-salt corn chips would be preferred) eaten with one avocado. (All salted food products should be salted after cooking as the heat alters the salt making it harsh on the circulatory system and the kidneys).

Warm vegetable soup.

Snacks

2 oranges.

Two handfuls of pumpkin seeds.

Assorted green leaves (lettuce, spinach, endive).

Your favorite chocolate snack (made with raw cacao beans).

Dinner

Large salad containing 80% green-leafed vegetables (including spinach, sunflower greens, lettuce), 2-3 avocados, 1/2 cup of unhulled tahini and an orange squeezed as dressing. Add 10-20 Sun-ripened olives and raw dulse seaweed to the salad.

1 quart (1 liter) of freshly-made vegetable juice containing at least 60% green vegetables, 40% other vegetables or fruits (i.e. squash, peppers, cucumber, etc.).

Steamed vegetables (cauliflower or broccoli).

Hummus (preferably raw) with fresh vegetables and fruits: celery, broccoli, cauliflower, cucumbers and tomatoes.

Dehydrated or toasted wholegrain bread.

WEDNESDAY BASIC

Breakfast
8 ounces (1/4 liter) of herbal tea. Squeeze in fresh lemon if desired. Use raw honey or maple syrup to sweeten.
1 cantaloupe.

Or

Drink the water of 2 coconuts with a green, powdered, organic superfood formula in order to increase mineralization.

Lunch
1 shot (1 ounce) of fresh wheatgrass juice.
Greek salad containing: lettuce, tomato, cucumber, red onion, salt-cured black olives, 1-2 ounces (30-60 ml) of olive oil.
1 item of cooked starch (baked, no-salt corn chips would be preferred) eaten with one half an avocado.
1 sandwich made with toasted sprouted grain bread, avocado, clover sprouts, diced red bell pepper, diced tomatoes and diced cucumber).

Snacks
1 bowl of figs or cherries.
1 bowl of grapes.
1 handful of Brazil nuts.
Blended pudding containing: dates, avocado, cinnamon powder, Irish moss (a superfood from the sea) and distilled water.
One serving of cooked starch (wholemeal bread, wheat tortillas).

Dinner
Large salad containing 80% green-leafed vegetables, including kale or spinach, eaten with 20-30 raw walnuts or macadamia nuts and an orange squeezed as dressing.
One meal of cooked starch (brown rice or baked squash).
Warm vegetable soup.

THURSDAY BASIC

Breakfast

1/2 quart (1/2 liter) of freshly-blended peach and nectarine juice. Add 2 teaspoons of flax seed oil and/or 2 tablespoons of spirulina if desired.

Or

One blended super smoothie containing: apple, pear, berries (all types), bee pollen (2-3 tablespoons) and hempseed oil (2-3 tablespoons).

Lunch

2 bowls of berries (strawberries, blueberries, goji berries, Incan berries, etc.). One small lettuce salad with cucumber. Add 2-3 tablespoons of olive oil if desired.

One sandwich made with toasted sprouted grain bread, avocado, lettuce, clover sprouts, diced tomatoes, diced cucumber and cayenne powder.

One serving of cooked starch (brown rice or wholegrain bread).

Snacks

2 oranges or Asian pears.

One avocado eaten with sea salt.

1-2 handfuls of goji berries.

Your favorite prepared raw-food treat.

Dinner

Large salad containing 80% green-leafed vegetables, 30-40 almonds and an orange squeezed with hempseed oil as dressing. Add several servings of raw kelp seaweed to the salad. Add raw sauerkraut or kim-chi to the salad as desired.

Dehydrated or sprouted crackers or bread eaten with one-half an avocado.

Steamed vegetables (cauliflower or broccoli).

1/2 quart (1/2 liter) of freshly-made vegetable juice containing at least 60% green vegetables, 40% other vegetables or fruits (i.e. apple, cucumber, etc.).

FRIDAY BASIC

Breakfast

8 ounces (1/4 liter) of herbal tea. Squeeze in fresh lemon if desired. Use raw honey or maple syrup to sweeten.

1 honeydew melon or 1 whole or blended papaya with lime juice.

Or

Drink the water of 2 coconuts with a green, powdered, organic superfood formula in order to increase mineralization.

Lunch

1/2 quart (1/2 liter) of freshly-made vegetable juice containing green-leafed vegetables (i.e. spinach, collards, clover sprouts), apples and pears.

Cucumber, tomato, okra, zucchini mixed salad. Add organic, extra virgin, cold-pressed olive oil and a fresh-squeezed lemon as dressing.

One sandwich made with toasted sprouted grain bread, avocado, lettuce, oregano, sunflower greens, sliced tomato and diced cucumber.

Snacks

1 bowl of grapes (with seeds).

2 tangerines.

1-2 handfuls of goji berries.

Your favorite prepared raw-food treat.

Dinner

Large salad containing 80% green-leafed vegetables including parsley, 2 avocados, kelp and blended mango juice with stone-crushed, cold-pressed olive oil as the dressing.

Include your favorite meal here!

SATURDAY BASIC

Breakfast
Drink the water of 2 coconuts with a green, powdered, organic superfood formula in order to increase mineralization.

Or
1/2 quart (1/2 liter) of fresh-squeezed grapefruit juice.

Lunch
1 quart (1 liter) of freshly-made vegetable juice containing apples and celery. One sandwich made with toasted sprouted grain bread, avocado, clover sprouts, sliced tomato, diced zucchini and cayenne or garlic powder.

Snacks
One shot (1 ounce) of fresh wheatgrass juice.
2-3 apples or pears.
10-20 almonds or walnuts .
1 handful of Brazil nuts.
1 item of cooked starch (tortillas or baked, no-salt corn chips).

Dinner
Large salad containing 80% green-leafed vegetables including celery, kale, spinach and other greens, two avocados and organic, extra virgin, cold-pressed olive oil blended with lemon, a sprig of rosemary and raw apple cider vinegar as dressing. Add several servings of raw dulse seaweed and grated raw garlic to the salad.
Include your favorite meal here!

SUNDAY BASIC

Breakfast

14 ounces (0.4 liters) of herbal tea. Squeeze in fresh lemon if desired. Use raw honey or maple syrup to sweeten.

Or

Drink the water of 2 coconuts with a green, powdered, organic superfood formula in order to increase mineralization.

Lunch

1 bowl of strawberries and/or blueberries.
1 quart (1 liter) of freshly-made vegetable juice containing cucumber, lettuce, sunflower greens and yellow bell pepper.

Or

Seaweed salad containing: 2 cups dry dulse, 3-4 strips of sea lettuce, 6-8 shiitake mushrooms, 25 ground walnuts, 3 tablespoons of raw soy sauce (nama shoyu), 1 tablespoon of cayenne powder and the juice of one whole lemon.
One item of cooked protein (i.e. tofu).

Snacks

2-3 pears.
2 ribs of celery.
1 cucumber with 1/2 of an avocado sprinkled with powdered kelp.
Your favorite prepared raw-food treat.

Dinner

Large salad containing 80% green-leafed vegetables, 20-30 pecans, dulse seaweed and an orange squeezed with hempseed oil as dressing.
Include your favorite raw-food recipe here. Experiment!

THE 80/20 SUNFOOD DIET WEEKLY MENU

The 80/20 Sunfood Diet

At this level, the goal is to consistently eat 80% raw plant foods containing a balance of green-leafy vegetables, sweet fruits and raw plant fats along with superfoods. Once one has stabilized at eating 80% raw-foods, major improvements will be seen at the physical, mental, emotional and spiritual levels.

MONDAY 80/20

Breakfast

One blended super smoothie containing: apple, pear, berries (all types), spirulina or blue-green algae (2-3 tablespoons) and flax oil (2 tablespoons).

Or

Drink the water of 2 coconuts with a green, powdered, organic superfood formula in order to increase mineralization.

Lunch

1 shot (1 ounce) of wheatgrass juice.
One sandwich made with toasted sprouted grain bread, avocado, clover sprouts, sliced tomato, diced or shredded zucchini and red onion.

Snacks

5-6 ribs of celery and 1/2 cup of almond butter.
2 oranges.
Your favorite prepared raw-food treat.

Dinner

One large spinach salad containing cucumber, tomato and green onion salad with 2-3 avocados and fresh-squeezed lemon.
Popcorn made with cold-pressed coconut oil. (Even though the hard, waxy slivers from the kernels can be irritating to the intestines, popcorn with coconut oil is a healthier and tastier recommendation for those addicted to popcorn!).
Dehydrated or toasted wholegrain bread with one half a cup of raw, unhulled tahini.

TUESDAY 80/20

Breakfast

14 ounce (0.4 liters) of a blended berry smoothie containing: blueberries, blackberries, raspberries and strawberries. Add 2 tablespoons of cold-pressed hempseed oil and/or 2 tablespoons of spirulina or bee pollen if desired.

One medium or large papaya eaten whole or blended with fresh orange or lime juice.

Or

Drink the water of 2 coconuts with a green, powdered, organic superfood formula in order to increase mineralization.

Lunch

One small green-leafed vegetable salad containing soaked sunflower seeds, thyme, dulse seaweed and fresh-squeezed lemon.

One item of cooked protein (i.e. tofu).

2 oranges.

Snacks

1 small melon.

2 cherimoyas.

Assorted greens (lettuce, endive, bok choy).

15 water-soaked almonds.

Dinner

1 quart (1 liter) of freshly-made vegetable juice containing at least 60% green vegetables, 40% other vegetables or fruits (i.e. apple, cucumber, yam, etc.).

Large salad containing 80% green-leafy vegetables, 2 avocados and an orange squeezed with hempseed oil as dressing.

1 large bowl of Sequoia's Calcium Soup (see **Appendix C: Sunfood Recipes**).

Hummus (preferably JM's Almond Hummus see **Appendix C: Sunfood Recipes**).

Cooked quinoa eaten with unpasteurized soy sauce (nama shoyu). Baked squash may be included with this meal.

WEDNESDAY 80/20

Breakfast

2-3 apples.

10-20 pecans or macadamia nuts with lettuce.

1/2 quart (1/2 liter) of fruit juice containing: apples, celery and pears. Mix with 2 teaspoons of flax or hempseed oil if desired.

Or

One blended super smoothie containing: coconut water, berries (all types), cacao beans/nibs (2 tablespoons), maca powder (2 tablespoons) and coconut oil (2 tablespoons).

Lunch

Silicon Salad (see **Appendix C: Sunfood Recipes**). Add stone-crushed, cold-pressed, extra-virgin olive oil blended with orange juice as dressing.

10 pitted dates, 1 avocado and lettuce in a mixed salad. Squeeze an orange into the salad as dressing.

1 bowl of hummus (preferably raw) eaten with celery, tomatoes and cucumbers.

Snacks

2 mangos.

2 persimmons.

Assorted green leaves (lettuce, spinach, endive, dandelion, collards).

1-2 handfuls of goji berries.

Dinner

Large salad containing 80% green-leafed vegetables including kale or spinach eaten with 1 avocado and an orange squeezed as dressing. Add raw sauerkraut or kim-chi to the salad as desired.

Nori Rolls! Be creative. (see **Appendix C: Sunfood Recipes**).

Live Berry Pie! (see **Appendix C: Sunfood Recipes**).

THURSDAY 80/20

Breakfast
1/2 quart (1/2 liter) of freshly-blended peach and nectarine juice. Add 4 teaspoons of flax seed oil and/or 2 tablespoons of spirulina if desired. Almond milk: blend 40 soaked almonds with 8 pitted dates.

Lunch
2 bowls of berries (strawberries, blueberries, etc.).

Greek salad containing: lettuce, tomato, cucumber, red onion, salt-cured black olives and diced parsley. Add a dressing containing blended avocado, lemon and 1-2 ounces (30-60 ml) of olive oil.

Blended pudding containing: dates, avocado, cinnamon powder, Irish moss (a superfood from the sea) and distilled water.

One serving of cooked starch (brown rice, wholemeal bread, wheat tortillas).

Snacks
2 Asian pears.

1 handful of Brazil nuts.

1 handful of raw pumpkin seeds.

Dinner
Large salad containing 50% green-leafed vegetables along with tomatoes, cucumbers, parsley, cilantro, cayenne, 30-40 pecans and hemp oil as dressing. Add several servings of kelp seaweed to the salad. Add raw sauerkraut or kim-chi to the salad as desired.

1/2 quart (1/2 liter) of freshly-made vegetable juice containing at least 60% green vegetables (i.e. spinach, chard), 40% other vegetables or fruits (i.e. apple, cucumber, etc.).

One sandwich made with toasted sprouted grain bread, avocado, lettuce, clover sprouts, diced tomatoes, diced cucumber and cayenne powder.

Dehydrated or sprouted crackers eaten with guacamole.

FRIDAY 80/20

Breakfast

1 honeydew or sharlyn melon.

2 young coconuts, with coconut meat and water blended together in a cream. Add spirulina, hemp protein and 15 cacao beans. If young coconuts cannot be found, blend one avocado with mature coconut water.

Lunch

One smoothie containing: mango, orange and peach. Add 2-3 tablespoons of olive oil if desired.

One sandwich made with toasted sprouted grain bread, avocado, lettuce, sunflower greens, sliced tomato and diced cucumber.

Cucumber, okra, zucchini, onion mixed salad. Add organic, extra virgin, cold-pressed olive oil as dressing.

2 tangerines.

1 grapefruit.

Snacks

1 bowl of grapes (with seeds).

2 cherimoyas or white sapotes.

1-2 handfuls of goji berries.

Dinner

Large salad containing 80% green-leafed vegetables including parsley, 2 avocados and blended papaya seeds, mango juice, lemon juice, hempseed and vinegar as dressing.

1 quart (1 liter) of freshly-made vegetable juice containing at least 60% green vegetables (including 3 ribs of celery), 40% other vegetables or fruits (i.e. asparagus, apple, cucumber, etc.).

Include your favorite cooked-food meal here. (Notice how you feel in the morning)!

SATURDAY 80/20

Breakfast

1-2 cups of berries (strawberry, blueberry, etc.) blended with lemon. Add 1/2 avocado if desired.

One fruit smoothie containing freshly-blended papaya, oranges, hemp seeds, Incan berries and powdered grasses.

Or

Drink the water of 2 coconuts with a green, powdered, organic superfood formula in order to increase mineralization.

Lunch

1 cantaloupe.

1 quart (1 liter) of freshly-made vegetable juice containing apple, cucumber, ginger and kale.

One small green-leafy salad containing kale or spinach. Add one squeezed orange as a dressing.

20 raw macadamia nuts.

Snacks

2 mangos.

1/2 quart (1/2 liter) juice containing apple, cabbage, celery and parsley.

1-2 handfuls of goji berries.

Dinner

Sequoia's Calcium Soup (see **Appendix C: Sunfood Recipes**). (Make a thick, hearty raw soup and enjoy until satiated!)

Small salad containing 80% green-leafed vegetables (including kale or spinach), 2 avocados and organic, extra virgin, cold-pressed olive oil as dressing.

One large serving of spaghetti-sliced zucchini bathed in raw sauce (containing blended soaked pine nuts, basil, garlic and lemon).

SUNDAY 80/20

Breakfast

No breakfast.

Lunch

One smoothie containing: a mango, an orange, a peach, water and 20 cacao beans.

1/2 quart (1/2 liter) of freshly blended fruits containing apples, pears and berries. If desired add one cup of raw sunflower seeds (soaked for 6 hours) with 1 teaspoon of cinnamon powder and blend them in with the mixture.

Snacks

10-15 almonds.

2 apples.

2 ribs of celery.

Assorted greens (spinach, baby bok choy, endive).

1 zucchini.

Dinner

Large salad containing 80% green-leafed vegetables, 1 avocado, dulse and kelp seaweed and an orange blended with 1/2 cup of raw, unhulled tahini as dressing. Add raw sauerkraut or kim-chi to the salad as desired.

Include your favorite raw-food recipe meal here!

THE ALL-RAW DIET WEEKLY MENU

The All-Raw Diet

The All-Raw Diet is real magic. One must take up The All-Raw Diet when ready — we want to avoid the "yo-yo" effect (too much too fast before one is ready and capable of the daily health disciplines). Remember, the all-raw diet may not be appropriate for everyone, especially those with an extreme vata dosha (excessive thinness), a preponderance of air and water in their constitution or those who do not have the physical and emotional grounding for it.

Calories

If we think of food as body fuel, then we can understand that the energy provided by food is measured in calories. According to the current standards, a male adult requires about 18 calories per day, per pound (40 calorics pcr kg) of body weight. Women require about 16 calories per pound (35.5 calories per kg) of body weight. Growing children and teenagers require about 20 calories per day, per pound (44.4 calories per kg) of body weight. An increase in caloric needs is also determined by physical exercise. For example, a 165-pound (74.3 kg) male may need 2,970 calories for a normal day's routine. However, if the same man engages in vigorous activity throughout the day, caloric needs may double, up to 5,940 calories.

As an example, a caloric sample of the foods from the diet plans is provided. I have outlined this below to demonstrate that enough calories are easily available on The Sunfood Diet:

Menu Item:	Calories
Two young coconuts (spoon-meat & water)	800
Eight oranges	1000
Three avocados	1350
One large bowl of spinach	150
Four cucumbers	100
Four tomatoes	150
Four green onions	25
One lemon	75
TOTAL CALORIES	3,650

Quantities On The All-Raw Diet

Feel free to eat large quantities of raw fruits and vegetables if you desire. Most of you will eat less than I recommend here in these menu plans, however, I want you to feel free to enjoy abundant natural foods. Over time you can refine your diet, increase your assimilation, enjoy a liquid diet more often and eat less and less. Follow the guidelines laid out in The Sunfood Triangle. Natural raw nutrition coupled with daily exercise is the foundation of perfect health. The All-Raw Menu is designed for an active 145-175 pound (66-80 kg) individual. Those of a lighter weight and/or who are less active can adjust the quantities down accordingly.

Women, suggested daily maximum intake:
6 pounds (2.7 kg) of fruit
2.5 pounds (1.1 kg) of vegetables (one-third in salad, two-thirds in juice)
0.25 pounds (0.11 kg) of nuts or seeds

Men, suggested daily maximum intake:
7.5 pounds (3.6 kg) of fruit
3 pounds (1.4 kg) of vegetables daily (one-third in salad, two-thirds in juice)
0.33 pounds (0.15 kg) of nuts or seeds

MONDAY ALL-RAW

Breakfast

One blended super smoothie containing: apple, pear, berries (all types), cherries, spirulina, chlorella or blue-green algae (2-3 tablespoons) and coconut oil (2-3 tablespoons).

Or

Drink the water of 2 coconuts with a green, powdered, organic superfood formula in order to increase mineralization.

Lunch

1 shot (1 ounce) of wheatgrass juice.
One sandwich made with dehydrated flax crackers, avocado, clover sprouts, sliced tomato, diced zucchini and red onion.
2 oranges.
3 sticks of celery.

Snacks

2 mangos or oranges.
1 avocado with powdered cayenne and kelp.
Your favorite prepared raw-food treat.

Dinner

One large lettuce, cucumber, tomato, clover sprout and green onion salad with one handful of raw sunflower seeds, two avocados and a fresh-squeezed lemon.
Fats Guacamole. (see **Appendix C: Sunfood Recipes**).

TUESDAY ALL-RAW

Breakfast
One large honeydew melon or papaya eaten whole or blended with orange or lime juice and 20 cacao beans.

Or
One blended super smoothie containing: coconut water, berries (all types), maca powder (2 tablespoons) and coconut oil (2 tablespoons).

Lunch
One small green-leafed vegetable salad (containing kale, spinach and celery) with 10-20 walnuts and fresh-squeezed lemon.
4 oranges.

Snacks
1-2 handfuls of goji berries.
1 handful of Brazil nuts.
2 bowls of cherries.

Dinner
Large salad containing 60% green-leafed vegetables (i.e. romaine lettuce, endive, parsley, malva, collards, kale), 2 avocados, diced radishes, cayenne pepper and a lemon squeezed as dressing. Add raw sauerkraut or kim-chi to the salad as desired.
1 quart (1 liter) of freshly-made vegetable juice containing at least 60% green vegetables (i.e. chard, celery, parsley, lettuce), 40% other vegetables or fruits (i.e. apple, cucumber, yam, pumpkin, etc.).

WEDNESDAY ALL-RAW

Breakfast

1 quart (1 liter) of freshly-made orange juice mixed with 1/2 avocado and/or 3 teaspoons of flax seed or hempseed oil. (Mixing a fat with a sugar for breakfast will time-release the sugar for more endurance energy).
2 apples.
10-20 pecans or macadamia nuts with lettuce.

Or

Drink the water of 2 coconuts with a green, powdered, organic superfood formula in order to increase mineralization.

Lunch

Cucumber, parsley, tomato, 10 olives, 5 pitted prunes, 5 pitted dates in a mixed salad. Squeeze an orange into the salad as dressing.

Snacks

2 apples.
2 persimmons.
Assorted greens (spinach, green cabbage, lettuce, endive).

Dinner

Large salad containing 60% green-leafed vegetables eaten with 1/2 cup of raw nuts and an orange blended with thyme, sage, raw apple cider vinegar and hempseed oil as dressing. Add several servings of raw dulse seaweed to the salad. Add 30-40 Sun-ripened olives (if available).

THURSDAY ALL-RAW

Breakfast

1/2 quart (1/2 liter) of freshly-made grapefruit juice.

2 large pomegranates and 3 oranges cut and juiced on a citrus juicer. Blend with 2-3 tablespoons of flax or hempseed oil if desired.

Lunch

Silicon Salad. (see **Appendix C: Sunfood Recipes**).

2 bowls of berries (strawberries, blueberries, etc.).

8 dried prunes.

Snacks

2 mangos.

2 Asian pears.

Assorted greens (kale, spinach, baby bok choy, tak soy).

Dinner

Large salad containing 80% green-leafed vegetables, 20-30 almonds, onions and an orange squeezed as dressing. Add several servings of raw dulse seaweed to the salad.

Nori Rolls! Be creative. (see **Appendix C: Sunfood Recipes**).

FRIDAY ALL-RAW

Breakfast
3-4 oranges, tangelos or tangerines (eat the white pith too!).
10-20 macadamia nuts with lettuce.

Or
Drink the water of 2 coconuts with a green, powdered, organic superfood formula in order to increase mineralization.

Lunch
Cucumber, tomato, okra, diced radishes, zucchini mixed salad. Add organic, extra virgin, cold-pressed olive oil as dressing.

Snacks
2 oranges, tangelos or tangerines.
Assorted greens (spinach, baby bok choy, endive).
1-2 handfuls of goji berries or Incan berries.

Dinner
Cucumber, okra, zucchini, avocado and onion mixed salad. Add organic, extra virgin, cold-pressed olive oil as dressing.
1 quart (1 liter) of freshly-made vegetable juice containing at least 60% green vegetables (including 3 ribs of celery), 40% other vegetables or fruits (i.e. pear, zucchini, asparagus, radish, etc.).

SATURDAY ALL-RAW

Breakfast
30-40 berries (strawberry, blueberry, etc.) mixed with lettuce or mixed with 1 avocado.
1 Papaya mixed with lettuce or mixed with one half an avocado.

Or
Drink the water of 2 coconuts with a green, powdered, organic superfood formula in order to increase mineralization.

Lunch
1 cantaloupe.
1 cup (0.25 liters) of wheatgrass juice blended or juiced with 3-4 apples or 1 quart (1 liter) of freshly-made vegetable juice containing at least 50% celery, 50% apples or pears.

Snacks
2 apples.
15 water-soaked almonds.
1 handful of pumpkin seeds.

Dinner
Large salad containing 80% green-leafed vegetables (including kale, spinach, celery, clover sprouts), 2 avocados and organic, extra virgin, cold-pressed olive oil blended with basil as dressing. Add several servings of raw dulse seaweed, sea lettuce and grated raw garlic to the salad. Add raw sauerkraut or kim-chi to the salad as desired.

SUNDAY ALL-RAW

Breakfast
No breakfast.

Lunch
The water of 1 coconut.
1 quart (1 liter) of freshly-made vegetable juice containing at least 60% green vegetables (i.e. nettles, dandelion, collards), 40% other vegetables or fruits (i.e. Asian pear, broccoli, cauliflower, radish, etc.).

Snacks
2 apples or pears
2 ribs of celery.
1-2 handfuls of goji berries or Incan berries.
Your favorite prepared raw-food treat.

Dinner
Large salad containing 80% green-leafed vegetables, 1 avocado, sea lettuce, kelp seaweed and an orange and lime blended with unhulled black tahini and raw apple cider vinegar as dressing. Add 8 pitted dates to the salad for added zest.
Cosmic Pepperman's Raw Chocolate Chip Mint Ice Cream. (see **Appendix C: Sunfood Recipes**).

There are so many options for designing beautiful meals with raw plant foods. Bring in two or more raw-food recipe books to enhance your kitchen. These recipe books contain a wide variety of recipe ideas and combinations, which reiterate and expand on the ideas in this book.

I do have a wonderful secret to share with all prospective live-food chefs. It would seem that the most ideal foods for human consumption would contain all three food classes simultaneously (review **Lesson 11: The Secret Revealed**). Since this does not occur, the secret to making totally satisfying live-food recipes is to combine all three categories of food (sugar, fat and chlorophyll) into one meal.

One of the most famous raw-food recipes is Dr. Ann Wigmore's "Energy Soup." Her soup contains avocado, apple and wheatgrass juice among other items. The three main ingredients are a fat, a sugar and a chlorophyll food. Dr. Ann would feed this balanced recipe to some of her patients as their sole nutrition for three months and they were often completely healed. Doctor Ann's entire "Energy Soup" recipe may be found in her last book, **The Blending Book**.

I have developed some excellent healing combinations based on the Sunfood Triangle. Below I have included my favorite recipes, juices and blends. All the ingredients in the following combinations should be 100% raw and organic.

Many of these combinations require a juicer or blender; I recommend the Green Star Juicer, the Commercial Champion Juicer, the Miracle Wheatgrass Juicer, the Excalibur Dehydrator, the Cuisinart Food Processor and any of the Nutri-Bullet/Magic-Bullet line of Blenders. I personally own and use them all. These are essential household appliances to create a healthy future for you and your family.

RECIPES

Avocado Burritos
8 leaves of romaine lettuce
2 avocados
2 jalapeno peppers
4 tomatoes
1 orange

Mix and mash the avocados, peppers and tomatoes. Squeeze on the orange for sweetness. Place avocado mix into a lettuce leaf and roll up. Remove the jalapeno peppers if serving this dish to young children.

Cosmic Pepperman's Raw Chocolate Chip Mint Ice Cream
Water from 3 young coconuts
Pulp from 5 young coconuts
1 cup pistachios
1/2 cup hemp seeds
1 cup macadamia nuts
1/2 cup NoniLand honey
1 tablespoon spirulina
1 medium-sized ripe avocado
3 tablespoons chopped fresh mint (chocolate mint if available)
2 tablespoons coconut oil/butter
1/2 cup of crushed cacao beans (raw chocolate)

Blend coconut pulp and coconut water in a strong blender. Strain coconut pulp through a fine mesh strainer or nut milk bag. Pour the coconut blend back into the blender. Add all ingredients except the cacao beans. Blend on high until creamy. Sprinkle cacao into the cream. For best results chill the cream in a freezer for several hours then pour into an ice cream maker. Follow ice cream maker directions, then serve!

Ecuador
1 cherimoya
4 kale leaves
1 avocado

Pick the seeds out of the cherimoya. Dice the kale. Cut, dice and mash avocado together with the other ingredients. The very center "stamen-like" growth in the heart of the cherimoya is excellent for replenishing male sexual fluids. This is a balanced meal.

Fats Avocado Salad

4-5 handfuls of wild greens (dandelion, lamb's quarters, malva, mustard, etc.)
2 avocados
40 olives
2 tbsp of organic, extra-virgin, stone-pressed olive oil or hempseed oil
1 pinch of sea salt or pink Himalayan salt

Mix in a salad. Combining olives with avocados is a powerful mixture. This is a trace mineralizer (wild greens and natural salts are loaded with trace minerals) and a bone builder (as fats help with the assimilation of calcium). I feel I am on top of the world when I eat this!

Fats Guacamole

3 avocados
3 ripe jalapeno peppers
1 habanero pepper
3 tomatoes
1 bunch of cilantro
1 ripe yellow lime

Mix and mash. Squeeze lime into the mixture. The lime juice acts as an antioxidant allowing the mixture to keep longer and taste better. Keeping the avocado pits in the mix will also help the guacamole to last longer.

JM's Almond Hummus

2 cups of water-soaked almonds

(strained after 8 hours of soaking)
6 sun-dried tomatoes
1 peeled clove of garlic
2-3 tablespoons of tahini (preferably black, unhulled tahini)
3-4 tablespoons of olive oil
1 sprig of basil
1 sprig of thyme
1 sprig of oregano
1 pinch of sea salt
Juice of four lemons

Start the almonds early. Allow to soak in pure water for 8 hours. Pour off the water and start the recipe with these almonds. Squeeze the juice from four lemons. Add all ingredients in a blender or food processor. Blend and serve.

Live Berry Pie

Pie crust:
2 cups of soaked almonds
1 cup of shredded coconut
1/2 cup of monukka raisins
The juice of one lemon
1 teaspoon of cinnamon
1/2 teaspoon of nutmeg

Mix all crust ingredients together in a food processor and press into a pie shell.
Binder: 2 cups of berries (blueberry, blackberry, raspberry and strawberry)
1 cup of peaches

Blend well in a food processor or blender. Stir the binder into the crust shell. Manicure the top of the pie with berries. Refrigerate for two hours before serving. This is a great recipe for children.

Nori Rolls

6-8 sheets of raw, sun-dried (not toasted) nori seaweed
2-3 avocados
1 bunch of clover sprouts
1 bunch of cilantro
1 cucumber

Dice all ingredients. Mix avocados, clover, cilantro and cucumber into a flat spread on the nori sheets. Roll each sheet tightly with a sushi mat. Cut into bite-sized portions. Add raw soy sauce (nama shoyu) if desired. Like all seaweeds, nori is an excellent source of trace minerals.

Raw Candy

10 dates
10 almonds
An assortment of superfood samples

Pit the dates. Insert an almond into the pit hole of each date. Pure decadence! Dip these treats into cacao nibs (broken cacao beans), nutmeg, allspice, bee pollen, spirulina, powdered blue-green algae or other favorite additives.

Raw Chocolate

2 young coconuts
20 cacao beans (preferably peeled)
10 raw cashews
3-5 tablespoons of maca (powdered root from Peru. Amazing high-protein superfood aphrodisiac, strengthener and fertility enhancer.)
3-5 tablespoons of NoniLand honey.
3 tablespoons of hempseed oil
2 tablespoons of coconut oil/butter
2-3 pinches of sea salt (preferably celtic sea salt or Himalayan pink rock salt)
2-3 sprinkles of cinnamon

Open up the two young coconuts and pour the water into the blender. Spoon the inner soft flesh out of the coconut and put that also in the blender. Add all ingredients and blend! This is guaranteed to satisfy any chocoholic. If you are a chocolate lover, please review my book **Naked Chocolate** for more ideas!

Sea Salad

10 strips of dulse seaweed
1 avocado
1 head of lettuce
4 tomatoes

Mix in a salad. Squeeze the lemon into the salad. Dulse is an excellent source of sodium and trace minerals and is a wild food.

Silicon Salad

1 head of romaine lettuce
4 cucumbers
4 tomatoes

6 okra
2 nopales
2 red bell peppers
3 tablespoons of horsetail herb
1 avocado or 1 ounce (30 ml) of organic, stone-crushed, extra-virgin olive oil

Cut, dice, mix in a salad. Add avocado or olive oil for dressing. Excellent for silicon, which the liver can biologically transmutate into calcium. Silicon creates beautiful, elastic skin; remedies brittle fingernails; and keeps the hair from turning prematurely grey. Silicon also relieves the pain of tendonitis and related tendon and ligament inflammation.

Winter Solstice
10 dates
10 dinosaur kale leaves (also known as black or lacinto kale).
1 avocado

Cut the avocado into ten pieces. Pit the dates. Place a date with an avocado slice inside a kale leaf like a burrito. I lived on this food mixture for nearly the entire winter of 1997-1998.

Juices & Blends

Almond Milk
40 soaked almonds
8 pitted dates
2 tablespoons of cinnamon powder

1 tablespoon of nutmeg

Mix and blend with distilled water. Almond milk is best when almonds and dates are mixed in an 8:1 ratio. An excellent warming drink for the winter. This drink replaces any egg nog!

Aloe & O.J.
2 aloe vera leaves
10 oranges
1 papaya
2 noni fruits

Juice the oranges on a citrus juicer. Fillet the aloe leaves until the green skin is removed. Blend aloe "gel" with orange juice. Aloe vera heals the skin and mucous membranes. Aloe vera juice is excellent for ulcers and hemorrhoids. Organic, non-GMO papaya is a great addition to this drink. Another great additive is fresh noni. To add noni, wait until the fruits are soft and have a strong odor. Blend the whole fruit including seeds with a little water until you are left with a liquid mush. Strain this mush. Add the remaining liquid to the aloe, orange juice and papaya drink above. Noni is rich in monoatomic elements and activates dormant superpowers.

Athlete
2 cucumbers
5 ribs of celery
10 kale leaves

1 lemon

Juice. I recommend this drink to all athletes. Alkalinity, juvenile water, sodium and calcium...everything is there.

Captain's Powerhouse
Two handfuls of greens (preferably wild)
2 spoon meat coconuts with water
2 avocados

Blend. We used to drink this in my office daily.

Cherimoya Cream
1 avocado
2 cherimoyas

Remove pit, seeds and skins from the avocado and the cherimoyas. Put the fruits in a blender. Blend. This is a splendid combination which one must taste to believe.

Estrogen Booster
2 yams

Juice. This drink is for young women looking for a boost, menopausal women, or anyone looking to taste something great.

Feijoa & O.J.
10 feijoas (pineapple guavas)
10 oranges

Cut all fruits in half. Juice on a citrus juicer. The smooth feijoa balances the acids in the oranges. This is my favorite sweet winter juice.

Iron Boost
10 strawberries
10 raspberries
1 slice of watermelon
1 handful of parsley

Mix, blend and serve! Red fruits, especially berries, contain high amounts of iron. Red watermelon has the highest iron content of any fruit. Parsley has the highest iron content of any green-leafy vegetable. This is an excellent drink for women just before, and following, menstruation.

Medicine
1 ripe red jalapeno or orange habanero pepper
5 ribs of bok choy
10 kale leaves
Juice. This drink helps detoxify the lymphatic system and boost the immune system. This drink relieves swollen glands in the throat. This is true medicine.

Molotov Cocktail
4 apples
1 clove of garlic

1 quarter slice of an onion root
1 red jalapeno pepper
1 slice fresh ginger root

Two cups of this drink a day: one for Breakfast, one with Dinner. In conjunction with The Sunfood Diet plan I have outlined in this book, this drink is likely to burn out all digestive parasites within 30 days.

Performance

1 glass of coconut water
1 heaping tablespoon of spirulina

Spirulina is the highest protein food on planet Earth. Coconut water is the highest source of electrolytes found in nature. Both spirulina and coconut water are alkaline. Together, they can drive any athlete to superior performance in all areas. This is one of my secret drinks I recommend for athletes.

Pièce De Résistance

5 apples
1 lemon

Shave off the outer skin of the lemon, leaving the white pith. Juice. I was originally introduced to this recipe years ago by Jay Kordich's book **The Juiceman's Power Of Juicing**. It is one of the all time best. I have been to Jay's beautiful home and we actually juiced this combination together — what a treat!

Potion Of Invincibility

2 heads of red-leafed lettuce
1 head green cabbage

Juice. A creamy drink. A powerful mineral boost. This is great to drink following a workout. My colleague Caleb "Kale" named this potion.

Raw Courage's Eyesight Enhancer

4 oranges
4 lemons
4 limes
2 grapefruits
2 tangerines
10 feijoas (pineapple guavas)

Juice on a citrus juicer. Mix well and serve. These alkaline citrus fruits are internal cleansers and help to alleviate internal debris, even in the fine capillaries of the eye. This is an excellent drink to use on a juice fast.

Rejuvenator

1 bunch of kale
4-6 ribs of celery
1 cucumber
1 burdock root
1 lemon
1-2 apples (optional)

Burdock root is a blood purifier and an excellent base to help the body create hormones. Burdock contains one of the highest amounts of organic iron in any food. Kale provides a dense source of alkaline minerals. Cucumber and celery soften the taste. The lemon should be shaved down to the white pith. Apples may be added to sweeten (although better results occur without them). This is, all-around, perhaps the most effective vegetable juice combination I have found. This is a great juice to drink every day.

Remineralizer
8 ribs of celery
12 kale leaves

Juice. Loads the body with sodium and calcium. This is an important drink for those who have been taking mineral-depleting chemical medicines, antibiotics or insulin as it restores heavy minerals to the body.

Sequoia's Calcium Soup
10 kale leaves (preferably dinosaur kale)
1 handful of parsley
2 cloves of garlic
1/3 of a red onion
2 lemons
1 avocado
1 tomato
2 yellow bell peppers
1 handful of dulse strips
1/2 teaspoon celtic sea salt
1 tablespoon of unpasteurized miso
3 tablespoons of flax oil
20 pumpkin seeds

Shave off the outer skin of the lemons, leaving the white pith intact. While blending all ingredients, add spring water to reach a thick, soupy consistency. This is a great raw soup for kids! And an excellent way to introduce important heavy minerals and calcium into a child's diet.

Super Smoothie
1 apple
1 pear
1 small bowl of blueberries, blackberries, raspberries and strawberries.
2-3 tablespoons spirulina
2-3 tablespoons of flax seed oil

Place all contents in a blender. Add distilled water and mix until the desired consistency is reached. This is an excellent breakfast drink in the winter. The pectin in the apples and pears stimulates a bowel movement. The berries are blood builders. The spirulina adds trace minerals. The flax oil allows a slower time-release of fructose into the blood.

REMEDIES

My recommendation is to begin any disease or injury treatment program by first undergoing a series of colon irrigations. Unless the colon is clean and functioning properly, the body will be bathing in its own waste and will be less than able to heal or assimilate foods to optimal efficiency.

Burns

In my experience, fresh, raw aloe vera gel helps heal burns faster than any other substance — raw manuka honey is a close second. Raw, fresh aloe vera gel (or in the alternative, raw honey) should be topically applied one to two times a day (first degree burns), three to four times a day (second degree burns) and five to six times a day (third degree burns). Accelerated healing will be noticed immediately.

MSM (methyl-sulfonyl-methane) lotion may be applied directly onto burns as long as the wounds are closed, the skin is not raw and the blisters are not oozing.

Eating aloe vera gel, avocados, olives, olive oil with parsley and spirulina will help accelerate the healing of burns. Adding MSM powder to one's drinking water (2 tablespoons per liter) is also valuable to rejuvenate the skin. Avoid all dietary cooked oils when healing from burns.

Common Cold

Once your body is significantly detoxified by eating a balanced Sunfood Diet you will experience fewer and fewer flus and colds. An old saying goes: "You don't catch a cold; you eat a cold." Cooked foods and animal foods can depress the immune system making one susceptible to illnesses. Raw plant foods strengthen the immune system. Consider the ramifications of this startling fact in terms of saved time, energy and expense!

Typically, cold symptoms make their appearance when the seasons change. This is when the body becomes more sensitive and detoxifies toxins more rapidly. Paul Bragg, the life-extension specialist, recommended in his books to fast four times a year (for seven days) during each change of seasons. As you purify your diet, take note of the seasonal appearance of colds, it will provide you with some interesting insights.

I know not everyone is ready right now to make a radical improvement in their diet, so I have provided my "Cantaloupe Cold Cure." I have prescribed this to many people over the years. I often hear their thanks days, weeks, even months later. If you or a loved one has a cold that just seems to hang on, try the following:

Cantaloupe Cold Cure

If sick with flu or cold symptoms, go to bed early. Upon awakening do not eat anything until 12 noon. After 12 noon eat an entire ripe cantaloupe. Do not eat anything else for the next 4 hours.

This will "break" a cold or the flu.

For the more disciplined individual, fasting (not eating) whenever sick works best. Energy is channeled away from digestion into strengthening the immune system and cleaning out toxins.

Eating only juicy alkaline fruits or their juices (figs, papayas, oranges, tangerines, grapefruits, berries, etc.) while sick also accelerates the recovery. Try the "Alkaline-Fruit Blend" described in **Lesson 7: The Sunfood Diet**, under the Recommendations For Rapid Results section.

If flu symptoms persist, daily drink 0.5 quart (0.5 liter) daily of the "Medicine" drink described in **Appendix C: Sunfood Recipes**.

Eczema

Eczema is a detoxification (often of drugs or medications) through the skin or a fungal condition that erupts from the skin, yet is actually located in the underlying joint or on the bones. Because it can be worsened by eating cooked eggs and cooked fat, especially pasteurized milk and cheese, these foods should be abandoned.

To help alleviate symptoms of this condition, after bathing, rub fresh aloe vera gel, fresh noni fruit, MSM lotion, coconut oil, avocado and/or papaya into the eczema every day.

To root out eczema from the joints and bones, please study and review my **LongevityNOW Program**, which contains detailed strategies on how to approach intractable conditions such as eczema.

If you have eczema (dry skin and eruptions) also consider at least 6 colonics initially to allow the body to detoxify through the colon, rather than through the skin. If colon hydrotherapy is not available, daily warm-water enemas while fasting on non-sweet vegetable juice (e.g. celery, cucumber) will be helpful.

A raw herbal cleanse can work wonders for those with eczema, as I have seen first hand several times.

Eyesight

From years of observation and study, I am convinced that the primary cause of poor eyesight is the habit of reading in the dark or with dim lighting. To maintain excellent eyesight for a lifetime, please be sure to read under bright full-spectrum lighting or outdoors whenever possible.

Eating a diet rich in raw plant foods typically immediately halts a continuous degeneration in eyesight. Eating raw foods can gradually restore poor eyesight, but this can take years. The raw foods most associated with improving eyesight are all berries (especially goji berries and blueberries), grapes, lychees, cold-pressed algae oil (DHA) and all plants containing rich pigments (such as turmeric, spirulina and dark green vegetables).

To heal the eyes, stop eating cooked fats — especially animal fats. Large molecules of cooked fat, devoid of their lipase enzyme, can lodge in the fine capillaries of the eyes creating blockages and weakening the eye's fine-tuned motor muscles. A 1995 study of 2,000 people, cited in the book **Surgery Electives**, linked the consumption of (cooked) saturated fat to blindness.

Also, to help improve poor vision, only drink pure water or fresh juices for liquids. Inorganic minerals from tap water can enter the body, filter through the system and damage the fine capillaries in the eyes.

Avoid all caffeine (coffee, tea, soft drinks) as it damages the fine nerve tissues in the eyes.

Table salt should be avoided as it tends to raise the blood pressure. This puts excessive pressure on the tiny capillaries in the eyes.

Several books describe specific programs including eye exercises you can do to restore eye strength and vision. **Relearning To See**, by Thomas R. Quackenbush, may be beneficial for you to study.

Hair Loss

Hair loss is a progressive decrease in hair growth typically resulting in baldness in men. It usually occurs due to poor oxygenation, acidification of the body due to a poor diet, a dietary deficiency of zinc and/or copper and a lack of Sunlight. Genetic predispositions also play a factor.

Rubbing the oil of a slice of crushed hot pepper directly into the hair loss area with your fingers will help dissolve waxy deposits that may have sealed off hair follicles. This oil will also cause blood flow to that area of the scalp oxygenating and enlivening the dormant follicles. Be cautious, pepper oil is very strong and can burn the skin — only 1/4 of a small pepper is required. Apply stone-crushed, cold-pressed, extra virgin olive oil or hempseed oil two to five minutes after the pepper oil as this will tone down the pepper heat and soothe the skin. Follow this procedure every day in the morning or evening for three weeks.

Dietary choices to restore hair loss should include significantly more organic alkaline fruits (papayas, figs, oranges); for vitamin C, a wide variety of organic green-leafed vegetables to reverse any acid-condition in the body; poppy and pumpkin seeds for zinc and occasional dulse or nori seaweed for trace minerals.

For excellent scalp care, use only organic, plant-based shampoos on the hair. Sometimes I simply use a dilute solution of lemon or orange juice as shampoo; I also occasionally use jojoba or sweet almond oil to maintain scalp and hair moisture and to avoid hair knots. Commercial shampoos and conditioners contain highly toxic chemicals and damage the scalp over time.

Mucous Congestion

Mucous congestion is a detoxification of the lungs and sinuses associated with sinusitis, nasal discharges, headaches, earaches, eye pain and fatigue. Mucus acts to both protect the system, by acting as a buffer for the sensitive internal organs, and as a transporter of toxins out of the body — typically through the lungs, mouth and sinuses.

Anyone with a mucous problem should avoid raw or cooked dairy products of all types. Dairy products are notorious mucus-formers. Simply avoiding all dairy products is often found to eliminate sinusitis.

Direct Sunlight on the chest and face will accelerate healing this condition. Sunlight helps dry out mucus and recharge the sinus chambers.

Eating plenty of hot peppers (cayenne, jalapeno, habanero) will thin and flush sinus mucus.

Mucus and wax may have combined to form a hard ball in the inner ear. If you suffer persistent earaches, consider having your physician or naturopathic doctor flush your ears with warm water.

Muscle Soreness

Sore muscles are the result of too much lactic acid and uric acid having accumulated in the muscle tissue.

To counteract acids in the muscle tissue, drink at least half a quart (0.5 liter) of green-vegetable juice. The "Potion Of Invincibility" described in **Appendix C: Sunfood Recipes** works extremely well. The alkaline minerals in green juices neutralize acids.

Spirulina, hempseed products, MSM powder and supplemental enzymes work wonders in easing muscle-soreness.

Restorative yoga followed by long, hot epsom-salt baths or hot springs soaking may also help relieve muscle soreness.

Nail Biting

Nail biting is caused by an alkaline mineral deficiency and/or a parasitic infection. People typically bite their nails when nervous or stressed. This is an instinctive action to recycle the alkaline minerals (calcium) found in the nails into the body to neutralize the acids formed by stress.

Consuming plenty of calcium-rich, green-leafed vegetables, such as parsley or kale along with plenty of other alkaline plant foods, will help restore a mineral balance in the body. Plenty of garlic in the diet tends to flush out parasites.

My cousin, a life-time chronic nail biter, completely reversed this condition by eating raw plant foods. He noticed a major shift after drinking a glass of parsley juice each day for two weeks. Results were also excellent after eating a bulb of elephant garlic every day for two months with his salads.

PMS (Pre-Menstrual Syndrome)

The body can use menstruation as a channel for detoxification. As toxicity is channeled out of the lymph for elimination during the monthly cycle, old substances will enter the blood. Because we crave what is in our bloodstream, cravings for toxic foods may surface during the cycle. These cravings appear just before or following a menstrual period — be aware and prepared for this. To get past cravings, eat cacao beans (raw chocolate nuts) and avocados. Cacao beans supply magnesium and other nutrients that ease PMS (this is the natural way to meet the PMS chocolate craving). Avocados are excellent foods to help regulate the female cycle.

PMS is essentially a detoxification episode that always has physical, mental and emotional components. Severe PMS is the result of a toxic, cooked, animal-food diet (especially now with all the hormones fed to farm animals). The cleaner your body is by eating raw plant foods, the less PMS you will experience. After several months to a year of eating raw plant foods, nearly all PMS symptoms will disappear.

If candy, cooked chocolates or cooked carbohydrates are eaten this can lead to an overproduction of insulin, which exacerbates PMS symptoms. Eat fruit to keep the blood sugar regulated throughout a PMS episode. On the day before, and on the day after, your menstrual cycle, drink at least one quart (one liter) of the "Iron Boost" drink described in **Appendix C: Sunfood Recipes**. When the body is totally purified, menstrual flow will be minimal. This is not a cause for alarm as it is the natural way of all mammals. When eating a diet of raw foods, avoiding nuts and seeds will greatly diminish menstrual losses.

Psoriasis

The quality of the skin (its glow, shine, radiance) reflects the state of the internal organs. The skin is specifically representative of the condition of the liver. Acne, rashes, spots, and other skin conditions are all indicative of challenges in the liver as well as issues involving anger and/or stress. In a purely physical sense, the skin disease psoriasis is connected with liver dysfunction and enzyme deficiencies — especially a lipase deficiency.

To heal psoriasis, one needs to daily select an appropriate type of fat (one which digests well). Fats that are easier on digestion include: fresh young coconut flesh, coconut oil, hempseed oil, flaxseed oil. One must ease into heavier dosages of fat in the diet as a weak liver (typical in those who have psoriasis) can be challenged by an excessive fat intake — even if raw.

To overcome psoriasis, all cooked fats, especially egg and milk products (cheese, milk, butter, dairy ice cream) should be completely avoided.

For those with psoriasis, six to ten colon irrigations should be undertaken.

After two months of this treatment, one should fast on water for three days, then conduct a gall bladder flush (drink eight ounces of stone-crushed, cold-pressed, extra virgin olive oil followed by 8 ounces of freshly-squeezed lemon juice) (see **Lesson 10: Detoxification**). This will help flush the liver and gall bladder.

Rub avocado, extra-virgin, cold-pressed olive oil, sweet almond oil, or fresh aloe vera directly into the affected skin. Get the Sun shining directly on to the affected area. Sunlight will accelerate the healing process.

Regularly ingesting green-vegetable juices, anti-fungal, liver cleansing herbal teas, mineral-rich sea vegetables, organic, cold-pressed oils and nutrient-rich, whole-food, superfood, green powders. Avoiding the excessive intake of fruit and other sugars will also be beneficial.

Skin

For beautiful, healthy, glowing skin, eat plenty of foods rich in silicon (cucumbers, horsetail herb, nettles, lettuce, nopales, okra, radishes, etc.). Regularly eat the Silicon Salad described in **Appendix C: Sunfood Recipes**. Silicon-residue foods help to restore the elastic skin of youth.

For vibrant skin, sulfur-residue foods should also be eaten. Sulfur, "the beauty mineral," provides smoothness and shine to the skin. Sulfur is found in aloe vera, wild grasses, cruciferous vegetables (broccoli, cauliflower), ripe bell peppers, ripe hot peppers, onions, garlic, rain water, some egg-smelling spring waters and MSM powder.

For an excellent skin complexion, rub one or more of the following items against the skin two to four times a week: papaya pulp, avocado, cucumber, spirulina, fresh noni fruit and/or aloe vera.

For dry skin, rub hempseed oil, jojoba oil and MSM lotion directly into the skin. This will alleviate dryness quickly. Or use avocado on the skin directly. Avocado oil is similar to our skin's oil.

To help dissipate scars, try applying the following formula directly to the skin every other day for several weeks: two tablespoons raw aloe vera gel, one tablespoon of parsley juice and one tablespoon of spirulina. MSM lotion used alternately with a topical vitamin C cream also works wonderfully.

Thyroid Imbalance

The thyroid is a large endocrine gland situated at the base of the neck. The thyroid controls the basal metabolic rate. An underactive thyroid slows the metabolic rate and increases the possibility of obesity. An overactive thyroid speeds up the metabolism often leaving one excessively thin with bulging eyes.

For any type of thyroid imbalance, I recommend removing canola oil, safflower oil, corn oil, soybean oil and margarine, along with inorganic salt (table salt), as well as all conventionally-grown pesticide-sprayed food from the diet. Seed oils slow thyroid function. Excess inorganic sodium is positively charged, and is attracted to the negatively-charged thyroid gland and leads to dysfunctions. Pesticides and heavy metals are also attracted to the thyroid and cause endocrine imbalances.

Adding significantly more organic foods, raw foods, green vegetables (not cruciferous/brassica family), green herbs, spirulina, blue-green algae, and goji berries to the diet will help thyroid imbalances. The calming effect of the alkaline minerals, raw enzymes and the restorative effect of the B-vitamins found in green vegetables, green herbs, spirulina, blue-green algae and goji berries act to balance the thyroid and other endocrine glands.

Liberal amounts of iodine from kelp seaweed often corrects a hypothyroid situation (two to four tablespoons of raw kelp seaweed flakes taken daily). Additionally, adding maca root powder (two to four tablespoons daily) and/or raw coconut oil butter (two to four tablespoons daily) will increase thyroid function. Maca (even though it is a cruciferous vegetable) has a balancing effect on the endocrine system and directly supports the thyroid. Coconut oil butter raises metabolism and helps reverse thyroid stagnation.

Additionally, Sunlight on the skin has been shown to stimulate the thyroid to increase hormone production. Edible clays (bentonite and others) as well as enzyme supplements are often helpful as well.

Hyperthyroidism (overactivity of the thyroid) is a more difficult situation and has many causes that are all related to internal toxicity and an excessive amount of acid-forming minerals in the body. An individual with this condition should have their iodine levels checked by a naturopathic doctor or physician. (If iodine is absent, two tablespoons of raw kelp seaweed should be daily added to the diet). If levels are excessive, no sea vegetables or iodized salt of any kind should be included in the diet. Additionally, adding raw polyunsaturated seed oils (flax, hemp, etc.) as the major fat source in the diet can slow thyroid function. Also, one with this condition should take 30 deep breaths daily in the ratio of 1:4:2 as described in the Action Steps found in **Lesson 22: Breathing (Pranayama)**. This will help calm an overactive system.

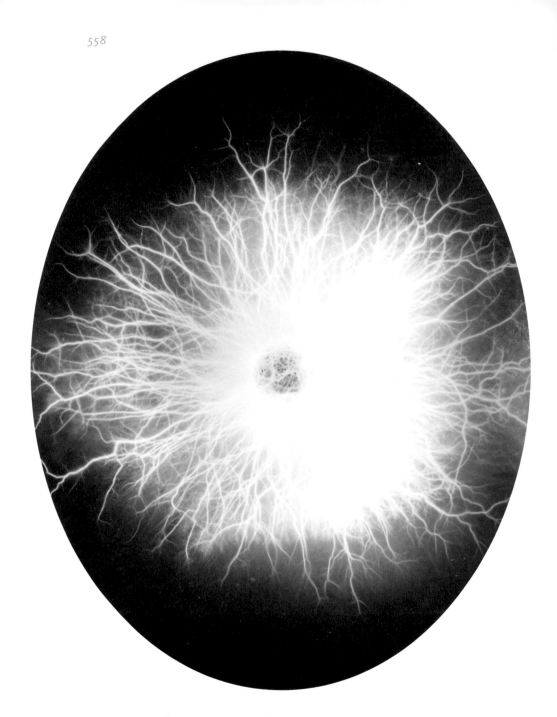

A magnificent Kirlian photograph
of raw organic Mangosteen powder.
This product is one of the greatest immune boosting and
anti-inflammatory substances ever.

PERMISSIONS

The author and publisher wish to express thanks and appreciation to those listed below who granted permission to use the following material:

Avery Publishing Group for permission to quote from **Enzyme Nutrition** by Edward Howell, (c) 1985; published by Avery Publishing Group, Inc., Garden City Park, New York; (800) 548-5757.

Campbell Thomson & McLaughlin Ltd. for permission outside of the United States and Canada to quote from **Shattering The Myths Of Darwinism** by Richard Milton.

Chelsea Green Publishing Company for permission to quote from **Whole Foods Companion** by Diane Onstad.

Dell Books for permission to quote from **Illusions** by Richard Bach.

Essence Of Health for permission to quote from **Fruit The Food And Medicine For Man** and **Diet, Health and Living on Air**.

Health Research for permission to quote from **Man's Higher Consciousness** by Professor Hilton Hotema.

Inner Traditions International for permission in the United States and Canada to quote from **Shattering The Myths Of Darwinism** by Richard Milton.

The University Of Chicago Press for permission in the United States and Canada to quote from **Year Of The Gorilla** by Dr. George Schaller.

The author and publisher made all reasonable efforts to contact all other literature sources quoted in the text.

PHOTOGRAPHY

Photography by
AARONA PICHINSON, AMY GAYHEART, DANIELLE CARNEY AND
DAVID WOLFE

AARONA PICHINSON PHOTOGRAPHY
www.aaronapichinson.com

DANIELLE CARNEY PHOTOGRAPHY

AMY GAYHEART PHOTOGRAPHY
www.amygayheart.com
(Amy is quite possibly the best graphic artist ever!)

KIRLIAN IMAGES
(Christopher Wodtke, www.kirlian.com)

ALOE VERA

ASPARAGUS

AVOCADO

BROCCOLI

CACAO BEAN

CACAO BUTTER

CACAO POWDER

DAISY

DURIAN

FIG

GOJI BERRY

JUJUBE

MALVA

NETTLE

RADISH

STAR FRUIT

INDEX

D

Q

R

universal karmic law, 53
Unlimited Power, 20, 59, 360
uranium, 143, 280
uranium dating system, 143
uranium-lead methods, 143
uric acid, 205, 239, 507, 552
urine, 159, 183, 188, 259, 291
utilitarianism, 126

V

vata, 253, 531
vegan, 12, 112, 119, 135, 162, 184, 234, 254, 304, 309, 319, 436, 551
vegetables (hybrid), 189, 291, 509
vegetables (non-starchy), 194, 195, 231, 264
vegetables (root), 188
vegetables (sea), 222, 233, 241, 243, 255, 263, 273, 293, 298, 303, 305, 310, 312, 329, 410, 412, 512, 513, 517, 519, 520, 521, 522, 525, 527, 530, 533, 535, 536, 538, 539, 543, 547, 552, 555, 556, 557
vegetarianism, 40, 108, 109, 112, 119, 134, 135, 147, 162, 194, 226, 234, 239, 254, 255, 302, 304, 584
villi (intestinal), 432
Visionary (poem), 64, 67
vitamin A, 98
vitamin B-12, 104, 301, 302, 303, 304, 305, 327
vitamin B-12 analogues, 303, 305
vitamin B-12 supplement, 305
vitamin C, 98, 101, 167, 197, 215, 223, 241, 242, 264, 324, 327, 552, 556
vitamin D, 253, 343
vitamin E, 327
vitamin K2, 305
vitarian diet, 274
vivisection (animal experimentation), 117, 119
volcanic material, 143

W

wadging, 337
wakame, 285
Walden, 387
Walker, Dr. Norman, 165, 172, 257, 386
walnuts, 165, 196, 199, 518, 521, 522, 534
wandlung, 130
warming foods, 202, 270

warmth (eating for), 202, 270
water, 56, 75, 76, 78, 88, 93, 98, 99, 102, 117, 125, 147, 159, 163, 164, 165, 166, 167, 170, 179, 180, 181, 184, 189, 193, 195, 200, 203, 204, 209, 210, 211, 222, 227, 228, 236, 239, 240, 241, 242, 243, 250, 255, 258, 265, 266, 268, 269, 270, 272, 274, 297, 310, 312, 313, 327, 332, 338, 341, 416, 431, 434, 435, 436, 437, 438, 506, 509, 510, 512, 516, 517, 518, 518, 521, 522, 524, 525, 526, 528, 529, 530, 531, 533, 534, 535, 537, 538, 539, 541, 542, 543, 544, 545, 546, 547, 548, 551, 552, 555, 581
water (distilled), 313, 437, 510, 518, 527, 544, 546
water content of fruits, vegetables and nuts, 180, 181
waterfalls, 279, 434
watermelon, 229, 233, 266, 390, 412, 516, 545
watermelon seed (as aphrodisiac), 412
watermelon seedless, 188, 290
Watson Sr., Thomas, 453
Watson, Lenny, 471
Weaver, Don, 331
weight gain (eating for), 248, 252, 253
weight loss, 159, 169, 202, 235, 249, 250, 436
well water, 281
West, Dr. C. Samuel, 158, 205, 266
whale, 131, 349
wheat, 211, 223, 259, 291, 292, 518, 527
wheat (sprouted), 186
wheat bread, 259
wheatberries, 201, 241
wheatgrass, 186, 216, 255, 335, 516, 518, 521, 524, 533, 538, 540
wheatgrass juice, 216, 516, 518, 521, 524, 533, 538, 540
Whitehead, Alfred Lord, 55
Whiting, Lillian, 35
Whole Body Dentistry, 339
Whole Foods Companion, 415, 559
Wigmore, Dr. Ann, 95, 261, 303, 540
wild food, 228, 242, 245, 291, 292, 293, 297, 298, 299, 300, 301, 303, 305, 327, 337, 543
wine, 242, 427, 510
wolfberry, 40, 222, 227, 252, 257, 268
wooden floors, 280
World Health Organization, 203
World War II, 344
wounds (open), 344
www.davidwolfe.com, 6, 105, 199, 238, 587, 588
www.fruittreefoundation.org, 119, 580, 582, 587, 588

X

Y

Z

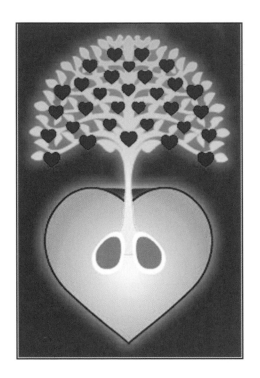

The Fruit Tree Planting Foundation

www.ftpf.org

"NOTHING IN THE WORLD GIVES ME MORE SATISFACTION THAN PLANTING FRUIT TREES. AS I HAVE ALWAYS CHOSEN TO CHANNEL MY ENERGY AND FINANCES INTO ENVIRONMENTALLY-FRIENDLY, SUSTAINABLE AND HEALTHY DIRECTIONS, I FOUNDED THE NON–PROFIT FRUIT TREE PLANTING FOUNDATION AS A PLACE WHERE WE COULD ALL VOTE WITH OUR MONEY FOR A BETTER, HAPPIER, MORE ABUNDANT, FORESTED FUTURE ON EARTH. PLEASE READ OUR MISSION STATEMENT AND DECIDE THAT YOU WANT TO DONATE TO THIS WORTHY CAUSE." — *David Wolfe, JD*

Mission Statement

The Fruit Tree Planting Foundation's primary mission is to plant 18 billion heirloom varieties of edible fruitful trees on the planet Earth and encourage their growth under organic standards (no pesticides, sprays or fertilizers). Trees create shade, calling forth water from the Earth. This living water creates health abundance and attracts more vegetation and animals. Living water and forests restore a positive equilibrium to the hydrological cycle of the planet thus normalizing weather patterns.

We believe in thinking big and that if you set a goal, you get a goal. Planting 18 billion fruit trees is possible and can spring out of the inspiration, drive and soul of just one human being.

Our Specific Goals:
• To spearhead a variety of planting programs. These programs are aimed at enriching the environment, providing nutritious food sources for wild and rescued animals and improving human health by bringing shade and producing delicious, fresh, locally-grown raw fruits.
• To secure planting lands and then organizing the placement of fruit trees and other trees that benefit the surrounding air, water and soil resources and provide food sources for people and animals. We aim to reestablish native plant ecosystems wherever possible.
• To make available an abundance of delicious, fresh, locally-grown, raw fruits and undergrowth vegetables of the highest quality to all the peoples — especially the homeless.
• To encourage each person on this planet to plant at least 3 fruitful trees.
• To provides support, resources and guidance for those interested in planting fruit trees.

We have come together through a love of trees, nature and a desire to foster harmony between the human race and mother earth, her plants and creatures, thus restoring this planet through each of our actions. It has been estimated that the planting of 18 billion trees (that is three planted by each person on this globe) would reverse the atmospheric pollution damage.

We choose trees that yield edible fruit, nutritious leaves or roots or are fruitfully useful in some other manner. Thus through our plantings we are creating rich, ecological, life-sustaining, organic diversity all over America and, eventually, the world. As we replant we bring not only vibrant health to humanity through fostering the accessibility of delicious fresh local fruits and vegetables but we also restore the plants that sustained the lives of the first peoples of this Earth, all the while following the contours of the land creating natural waterways that increase the reproductive strength of each fruit forest and designing our plantings in ways that alleviate erosion.

Please unite with us in the care of mother earth and in the reforestation of her once rich forest cover. Begin now to plant and care for trees wherever you are and send us photographs of your tree adventures and plant friends. We delight in donations of your time, money or barter.

To donate to The Fruit Tree Planting Foundation, please visit www.ftpf.org and follow the instructions to donate online or you may send check or money order made payable to:

THE FRUIT TREE PLANTING FOUNDATION
WWW.FTPF.ORG
PO Box 900113
San Diego, CA 92190
USA

Donations of any amount are accepted. Consider donating anywhere from $5 to $5,000. Please visit our website: www.ftpf.org

For your tax records, our registered non−profit organization will send you a confirmation that we received your tax−deductible donation.

"IN SPITE OF EVERYTHING, HUMANITY IS ADMIRABLE."
— Jean Giono, author of The Man Who Planted Trees

"WHEN YOU EAT A FRUIT, THANK THE PERSON WHO PLANTED THE TREE."
— VIETNAMESE PROVERB.

David Wolfe's Peak Performance Archives available at this new website:

www.thebestdayever.com

(**Warning!** The contents of this website may cause you to have The Best Day Ever!)

A special message from David Wolfe

I have so many tapes of my past lectures, so many notes I have taken over the years, so many great health and success secrets, so many incredible bits of information that my office and I are overloaded. I literally spent a couple years wondering what to do with all this great stuff! Should I put it into more books? More DVDs? More audio recordings? This stuff is not doing the planet any good sitting here in my office! Then I met a man who recommended that we start a subscription website. We did! We took my material and combined it with information and seminars by the leading women and men in the nutrition and peak performance field. Now all this material is online at thebestdayever.com and I am so excited!

On this one website you will have access to a literally priceless amount of the most valuable, peak-performance nutritional seminars, documents, interviews, product reviews and videos ever assembled in one place, at one time!

www.thebestdayever.com demonstrates how to:
- Shed those stubborn, unwanted pounds.
- Experience up-to-date information from America's foremost raw lifestyle authorities (both women and men).
- Leap ahead of the curve in the health and peak performance field.
- Achieve an extraordinary level of energy.
- Radically rejuvenate yourself physically, emotionally and spiritually.
- Achieve a remarkable level of sensuality, charisma and sex appeal.
- Enjoy every second of life and really experience The Best Day Ever!
- Explode your creativity.
- Sleep 2–4 fewer hours each night and wake up feeling better than ever!
- Add years (if not decades) to your lifespan.
- Take immediate advantage of secret, yet crucial diet information.

This incredible website gives you complete ACCESS to my text, audio and video library containing dozens of lectures and CONFIDENTIAL files on nutrition, health, minerals, rejuvenation programs and exotic information. Including information on how to heal some of the most stubborn conditions known to humanity.

Also, the website includes professional nutrition coaching forums where you can get up-to-the-moment answers to your questions. You will also hear live interviews with me on a monthly basis, where I answer your questions and bring you up to date on the latest and greatest. Also, if you are interested, you can tap into my monthly diary blog.

I am a BIG believer in saturating oneself with positive, empowering information. www.thebestdayever.com has been designed to literally bombard you with inspirational text, audio and video. Much of the material on the site you can download directly onto your computer or iPod and use whenever you want!

www.thebestdayever.com is essentially my uncensored online magazine that allows you to instantly access the latest, most fascinating information in the field. No more waiting by the mailbox. All I do, all day, every day is pursue and live the cutting edge of health, beauty, nutrition, peak performance, vegetarian diets and especially raw-food diets. This information allows you to leap miles ahead of the curve and create astounding rejuvenation and healing now without having to make the same mistakes tens of thousands of others have made.

Why am I doing this? Because the information that is in my brain and computer is expanding far faster than I can publish it in books. I have been perplexed as to what to do with it all. Eventually, the answer appeared: create an online magazine for you! This site was created to give you immediate access to leading edge information to help you instantly enhance the quality of your life.

This is the first time in the history of my career as a peak-performance consultant that I've packaged together so many compelling, life-changing programs into one jam-packed website. Nothing like this website is available on the Internet. This is truly a one-of-a-kind phenomenon. The future is now!

www.thebestdayever.com is constantly updated. This is an ever-growing resource for you and your whole family to enjoy.

If you are inspired to achieve an exceptional state of health, success, beauty, fitness, awareness, joy, sensuality, accomplishment, peak performance and most important fun then these Peak–Performance Archives are for you!

Check it out and HAVE THE BEST DAY EVER!!!

www.thebestdayever.com

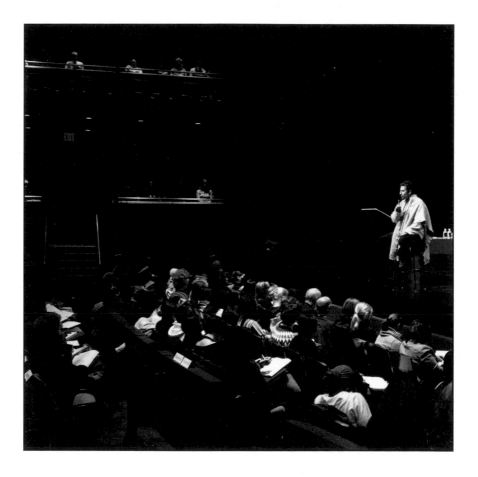

Bring the latest health and nutrition seminars into your home (without ever leaving home) by joining thebestdayever.com!

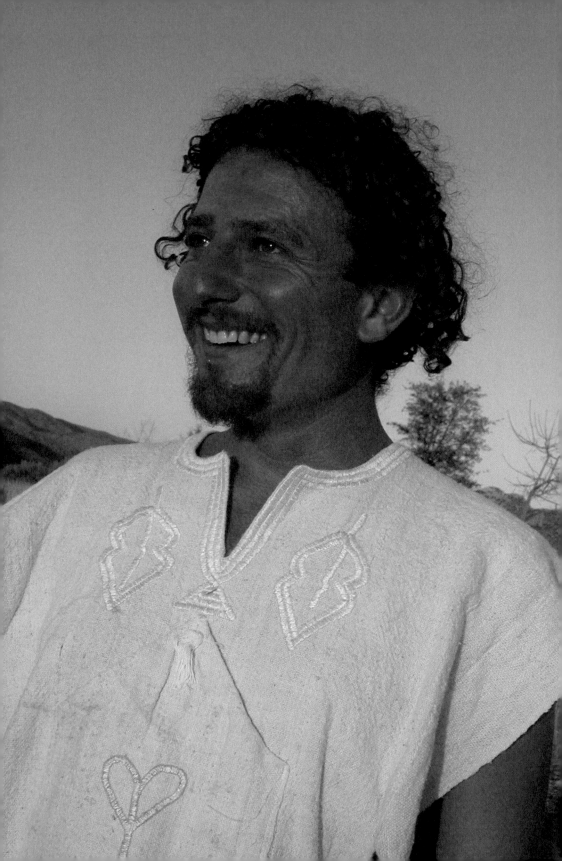

ABOUT THE AUTHOR

DAVID "AVOCADO" WOLFE

David "Avocado" Wolfe is considered by peers to be one of the world's leading authorities on nutrition. David develops and distributes some of the world's most wonderful and exotic organic food items. David was the first to bring raw and organic cacao beans/nibs (raw chocolate), goji berries, Incan berries, cacao butter, cacao powder, powdered encapsulated mangosteen, maca extract, cold-pressed coconut oil, and Sacred Chocolate™ into general distribution in North America. Known for extraordinary quality control and ethical production, these products, and many others developed by David, lead the field.

The son of two medical doctors, David brings a unique perspective on health and nutrition to the world of superfoods. He holds degrees in mechanical and environmental engineering, political science, a Juris doctor in law degree, and a master's degree in living-food nutrition. He has studied at many institutions, including Oxford University.

Since 1995, David has given well over 2,500 health lectures and seminars in the United States, Canada, Europe, the South Pacific, Central America, and South America. As part of his action-packed schedule, David also coaches and feeds Hollywood producers and celebrities as well as some of the world's leading business people and entrepreneurs.

The author of **The Sunfood Diet Success System**, **Naked Chocolate**, **Eating for Beauty**, **Chaga: King of the Medicinal Mushrooms**, **The LongevityNOW Program** and **Amazing Grace**, he hosts several health, fitness, and adventure retreats each year at various retreat centers across the world. You may view his current schedule at www.davidwolfe.com. David is the founder of and leading contributor to the Internet's leading peak performance and nutrition magazine: www.thebestdayever.com. He is also founder of the nonprofit Fruit Tree Planting Foundation (www.ftpf.org) whose goal is to plant eighteen billion fruit trees on planet Earth.

Other than his passion for nutrition, David's favorite hobbies include drumming, gardening, hiking, yoga, literature, writing, alchemy, chemistry, wild adventures, hot springs soaking, planting fruit trees, spending time with loved ones, and having The Best Day Ever!

David Wolfe's Websites:
www.davidwolfe.com

Shops:
www.longevitywarehouse.com
www.sacredchocolate.com

Education:
www.thelongevitynowconference.com
www.thebestdayever.com
www.rawnutritioncertification.com

Charity:
www.ftpf.org

Social Media:
www.facebook.com/DavidAvocadoWolfe
www.twitter.com/DavidWolfe
www.youtube.com/DavidAvocadoWolfe

RESOURCES

Bulk Organic Raw Foods, Raw Superfoods, Superherbs, Exotic Foods, Longevity Recipe Books, Health and Longevity Books, Grounding/Earthing Technologies, Zappers, David Wolfe's Products, Special Supplements and much more!

WWW.LONGEVITYWAREHOUSE.COM

Telephone: 805-870-5756
International: +001-805-870-5756
support@longevitywarehouse.com

www.longevitywarehouse.com

David Wolfe's on-line magazine:

www.thebestdayever.com

Found a family,

Plant a forest,

Rule your mind,

And laugh with the gods.